Tomographic Methods in Nuclear Medicine: Physical Principles, Instruments, and Clinical Applications

Editor

Bhagwat D. Ahluwalia, Ph.D.

Associate Professor
Department of Radiological Sciences
University of Oklahoma Health Sciences Center
Oklahoma City, Oklahoma

CRC Press, Inc.
Boca Raton, Florida

Library of Congress Cataloging-in-Publication Data

Tomographic methods in nuclear medicine.

Includes bibliographies and index.

1. Tomography. I. Ahluwalia, Bhagwat D. [DNLM:
1. Tomography, Emission Computed. WN 160 T661]
RC78.7.T6T65 1989 616.07'57 88-35200
ISBN-0-8493-6198-2

This book represents information obtained from authentic and highly regarded sources. Reprinted material is quoted with permission, and sources are indicated. A wide variety of references are listed. Every reasonable effort has been made to give reliable data and information, but the author and the publisher cannot assume responsibility for the validity of all materials or for the consequences of their use.

Direct all inquires to CRC Press, Inc., 2000 Corporate Blvd., N.W., Boca Raton, Florida, 33431.

International Standard Book Number 0-8493-6198-2

Library of Congress Card Number 88-35200
Printed in the United States

FOREWORD

The introduction of computed tomography in the early 1970s had a profound influence on nuclear medicine. First, it drove "nukes" from static imaging of organs into dynamic studies of physiology, especially in the heart. Second, it gave credence to the computer as an integral part of imaging systems, so much in fact that a revolution in all approaches to diagnostic imaging has occurred over the last 15 years. These two influences combined initially to stimulate the evolution of cardiovascular nuclear medicine, and subsequently the development of tomographic techniques for nuclear imaging. Computed tomography was the first successful application of reconstruction mathematics to tomographic imaging. Perhaps its most significant influence was that computed tomography captured the imagination of several bright and ingenious young physicians, physicists, and engineers, whose contributions over the past few years have yielded such clinical breakthroughs as magnetic resonance imaging, digital angiography, digital radiography, real-time ultrasound, and single photon and positron emission tomography.

It has been an exciting 15 years. Yet many challenges remain, including several which may be particularly amenable to tomographic nuclear imaging. Most of these challenging applications are discussed in this text, and I shall mention only one in this Foreword. This single application has such potential that its realization could help millions of people and save billions of dollars in health care costs. In addition, it could open a multitude of promising avenues of research. The 1990s have been described by several savants as the "Era of the Neurosciences" and "Decade of the Brain". Advances in understanding of fundamental biochemical and neurophysical mechanisms in the brain promise ultimately to yield new ways for diagnosis of mental diseases and conditions, and novel approaches for their treatment. Early intervention in these problems, and perhaps even prevention in some cases, may evolve from knowledge gained in basic science laboratories and applied in clinical settings where the appropriate diagnostic tools are available. Tomographic techniques in nuclear medicine promise to be among the pivotal tools needed to realize these advances.

No one entering or working in diagnostic imaging today can afford to remain ignorant of the techniques of nuclear tomographic imaging, or of the scientific and technical base from which they evolve. These techniques are at the leading edge of some of the most exciting research arenas in medical and biomedical research, and their importance to clinical medicine will undoubtedly be even greater in the future than they are today. Consequently, I am very pleased that Dr. Ahluwalia has compiled this text which offers a breadth of coverage of nuclear tomography that is unavailable in other texts on nuclear imaging.

William R. Hendee, Ph.D.
November 7, 1988
Chicago

PREFACE

The attention to the subject of tomographic methods in nuclear medicine is fairly new. Tomographic methods and instrumentation have undergone quite rapid development in the last decade. The first tomographic organ imaging performed with radionuclides was initiated by Kuhl in 1964. In 1971, the basic concepts were applied by Hounsfield in the development of X-ray transmission computerized tomography. However, the tomographic methods in nuclear medicine have not yet achieved the level of recognition gained by CT in diagnostic radiology.

Methods available to nuclear medicine for tomographic viewing include positron emission, single photon emission, and planar tomography. Nuclear methods provide pathophysiological as well as morphological information on both the regional and the localized level. Likewise, there is a variety of instruments for usage. There is no volume in print which deals with all these methods and which provides system details and other aspects of these topics.

This book deals with each topic in a comprehensive fashion to provide a ready reference of the work done on the subject. The book is a compendium of physical principles, system descriptions, instrument quality assurance, and clinical applications of tomographic methods in nuclear medicine. Each chapter is written by the individuals who have directly contributed to the pertinent field. The editor and authors have worked cohesively in presenting topics in a comprehensive manner. The objective is to provide a resource volume of general applicability for nuclear medicine physicians, medical physics students, nuclear medicine scientists, and researchers in organ imaging and image processing techniques.

B. Ahluwalia, Ph.D.

THE EDITOR

Bhagwat "Wally" Ahluwalia obtained B.Sc.(Honours) and M.Sc.(Honours) degrees in physics from Panjab University, Chandigarh, India, and a Ph.D. in physics (nuclear radiation) from Boston University in 1972.

After receiving his doctoral degree, Dr. Ahluwalia began his career in medical physics as a clinical instructor andFellow inMedical Physics at the University of Colorado Medical Center, Denver. His primary involvement was nuclear imaging and radiation therapy. In 1973, he started a National Institutes of Health fellowship in medical physics at the Department of Radiology, Massachusetts General Hospital, Harvard University, Boston. After that he served as Assistant Physicist at MGH and Associate at Harvard University Medical School until 1977. At MGH, Dr. Ahluwalia was actively engaged in imaging with positron emitters, tumor localization, and therapy. In the fall of 1977, he joined the University of Oklahoma.

His active interests are teaching, research, and clinical medical physics related to nuclear medicine imaging, radiation therapy, and radiation safety. Dr. Ahluwalia has authored and coauthored a number of articles.

ACKNOWLEDGMENTS

Numerous individuals have assisted me and other authors in preparation of this book. Support from the staff of the University of Oklahoma Health Sciences Center, Department of Radiological Sciences deserves a special mention. For typing assistance related to Chapters 1 and 4, and overall correspondence to authors, thanks are due to Mrs. Dorothy Bell. I am grateful to Ms. Carolyn R. Martel, medical artist, for the illustrations in Chapter 2. I am greatly indebted to Ms. Glenda Sims for providing me general technical assistance for the entire manuscript and valuable suggestions. Special thanks are due to Dr. Sang Yiel Baik, who was helpful in collecting reference material on various topics and has provided other computer assistance. I thank Dr. Sidney P. Traub, Professor and Chairman, Department of Radiological Sciences, for continued encouragement and support.

Special contributions of my wife, Ekta, and my children Ana, Atul, and Sumit, and Grandma for their understanding and support are acknowledged.

Finally, I appreciate the support and patience of the staff of CRC Press, and in particular, the assistance of Ms. Anita Hetzler, the senior coordinating editor.

Dedicated to my teachers
William R. Hendee
and
Gordon L. Brownell

CONTRIBUTORS

Bhagwat D. Ahluwalia, Ph.D.
Department of Radiological Sciences
University of Oklahoma Health Sciences Center
Oklahoma City, Oklahoma

Amjad Ali, M.D.
Department of Diagnostic Radiology and Nuclear Medicine
Rush-Presbyterian-St. Luke's Medical Center
Chicago, Illinois

Ralph Blumhardt, M.D.
Department of Radiology
The University of Texas Health Sciences Center
San Antonio, Texas

Wei Chang, Ph.D.
Department of Radiology
University of Iowa
Iowa City, Iowa

William D. Erwin
Department of Radiology and Nuclear Medicine
Rush-Presbyterian-St. Luke's Medical Center
Chicago, Illinois

Ernest W. Fordham, M.D.
Rush-Presbyterian-St. Luke's Medical Center
Chicago, Illinois

Mark W. Groch, M.S.
Department of Radiology and Nuclear Medicine
Rush-Presbyterian-St. Luke's Medical Center
Chicago, Illinois

Bruce H. Hasegawa, Ph.D.
Department of Radiology and Bioengineering Graduate Group
University of California
San Francisco, California

William R. Hendee, Ph.D.
American Medical Association
Chicago, Illinois

R. Edward Hendrick, Ph.D.
Department of Radiology
University of Colorado Health Sciences Center
Denver, Colorado

Michael A. King, Ph.D.
Department of Nuclear Medicine
University of Massachusetts Medical School
Worchester, Massachusetts

Dennis L. Kirch, M.S.E.E.
Cardiology Associates
Valley View Hospital
Denver, Colorado

J. A. Lancaster
Department of Radiology
The University of Texas Health Sciences Center
San Antonio, Texas

John C. Lasher, M.D.
Department of Radiology
University of Colorado Health Sciences Center
Denver, Colorado

Ulrich Raff, Ph.D.
Department of Radiology
University of Colorado Health Sciences Center
Denver, Colorado

Andrew Todd-Pokropek, M.Phil.
Department of Medical Physics and Bio Engineering
University College London
London, England

TABLE OF CONTENTS

Chapter 1

PROMISING IMAGING MODALITIES

B. Ahluwalia

For a nuclear medicine imaging modality, the major requirements are to provide three-dimensional information, minimize the effect of overlying and underlying activity and structure, good resolution, and regional quantitation. Until about 10 years ago, the nuclear medicine imaging modality was limited to planar imaging. Cross-sectional imaging of the brain was undertaken by Kuhl and Edwards in 1963.[1] Progress in transverse section imaging has been quite slow due to the developments in instrumentation, radiopharmaceuticals, and computer systems. In the early 1970s, the positron imaging modality was utilized to provide transverse sections of organs with biological radionuclides. Nuclear medicine imaging equipment, radiopharmaceuticals, and computer systems have since undergone developments. Imaging modalities such as single-photon emission computed tomography (SPECT) and positron emission tomography (PET) offer great promise in the future. PET developments have displayed various frontiers for development of SPECT.

In this chapter, the future of imaging modalities is reviewed. Pertinent instrumentation and clinical applications of SPECT and PET are discussed in individual chapters in the book. For brain imaging, biological requirements for a radiopharmaceutical are ability to cross blood-brain-barrier (BBB) and to distribute in the brain, proportional to the blood flow. Once in the brain, the tracer should stay fixed for a time sufficient for SPECT data acquisition. To cross the BBB the complex has to be lipophilic, the molecules small in size, and possessing no charge. Iodine-123-labeled *p*-iodo-*N*-isopropylamphetamine (^{123}I-IMP) has been widely used for brain imaging and regional blood flow. ^{123}I-IMP has been shown to be quite promising for SPECT imaging.[3]

The growth and utility of SPECT for central nervous system disease has centered around the use of iodinated amphetamines and amphetamine derivatives. The accumulation of ^{123}I-IMP is proportional to blood flow. These amphetamine compounds cross the BBB and are retained, to a large extent, by the cerebral cells. The exact mechanism of uptake is not clear.[3,4] The IMP compounds are cleared from circulation in the first few minutes. This compound is useful for the study of cerebral infarctions, transient ischemia, and epilepsy. Other problems which will control the success of this imaging agent are availability and cost.

Routine myocardial perfusion imaging is performed with ^{201}Tl for noninvasive evaluation of coronary artery disease. Due to the low energy of radiation, ^{201}Tl is not a suitable agent. Furthermore, ^{201}Tl has a long half-life and serial imaging cannot be performed. A new technetium-labeled radiopharmaceutical, ^{99m}Tc-carbomethoxyisopropyl isonitrile (^{99m}Tc-CPI), has favorable characteristics. It accumulates in the myocardium and rapidly clears from lung and liver.[5] ^{99m}Tc-CPI can be prepared on site and can be applied for evaluation of acute myocardial infarction. This agent has great promise for SPECT imaging in evaluation of global and regional ventricular function. It does not redistribute into zones of ischemia, at least for several hours.

It is anticipated that new receptor-based radiopharmaceuticals will play an important role in the study of pathophysiology and organ imaging. Advanced SPECT imaging systems, radiolabeled amines, and radiolabeled isonitrile have opened new avenues for cerebral and myocardial imaging. For brain imaging, some investigators claim that the lesion size, location, and correlation of the areas with a clinical picture is superior to X-ray transmission. It is yet to be seen how the information obtained with these imaging agents correlates with magnetic resonance imaging (MRI).

SPECT imaging will still be affected by modifications in attenuation corrections. Most methods assume uniform attenuation in the thorax region, however, the attenuation is non-uniform in this region. This attenuation correction plays an important role as far as net image quantitation is concerned. The major target of the imaging modalities is to provide quantitative information from the transverse sectional images. SPECT imaging needs modification for quantitation.

Attenuation correction is more complex in SPECT than in PET. Due to the higher energies of annihilated gamma, the scatter contribution is less than the 140 keV gamma from ^{99m}Tc. Similarly, the attenuation correction factor is much higher for technetium imaging than PET. The attenuation correction for PET depends upon the total distance along the line of flight. Attenuation corrections are simple in PET. Although most of the workers for SPECT assume a uniform attenuation factor, a true attenuation factor must be measured for each pixel for adequate correction in SPECT. In PET, sequential transmission and emission data are accumulated which is only possible when working with short-lived radionuclides. Furthermore, the quantitation will always be limited to the organ size in both PET and SPECT.

One of the major limitations of SPECT imaging is that studies can be performed only at equilibrium and rapid time sequential studies cannot be performed. This is due to limitations of the equipment and the time involved in imaging. This drawback can be overcome by adopting multi-ring cameras or multi-planar cameras for sequential imaging. The cost of such equipment will be comparable with the cost of PET imaging devices.

It is evident that three important modalities, PET, SPECT, and MRI, are the imaging modalities of the future. PET imaging has undergone great advances in technology and radiopharmaceuticals, however, due to the complexities and instrumentation, it will be limited to the larger diagnostic centers. Advances of PET are being translated into SPECT with the availability of ^{123}I and ^{99m}Tc radiopharmaceuticals. The growth utilization of SPECT is slow but forthcoming, and true organ quantitation is yet to be seen. Developments in instrumentation are also expected to improve the sensitivity of the SPECT system.

Chapters 2, 3, and 4 deal with the reconstruction theory and instrumentation of SPECT imaging. Chapter 5 covers the clinical applications of SPECT. Chapter 6 provides a brief review of PET instrumentation and organ imaging applications. Chapters 7, 8, 9, 10, and 11 deal with some of the other section imaging techniques used in nuclear medicine.

To summarize, PET and SPECT both have important roles to play in the future of nuclear medicine imaging. PET imaging offers more than SPECT, as a host of biological tracer-labeled radiopharmaceuticals are available and their pertinent kinetics are well understood. It is anticipated that studies of organ pathophysiology performed with positron emitters will provide guiding pathways for development of SPECT receptor radiopharmaceutical and organ imaging applications.

REFERENCES

1. **Kuhl, D. E. and Edwards, R. Q.,** Image separation radioisotope scanning, *Radiology,* 80, 653, 1963.
2. **Kuhl, D. E. and Edwards, R. Q.,** Cylindrical section radioisotope scanning of the liver and brain, *Radiology,* 83, 926, 1964.
3. **Lee, R. G., Hill, T. C., Holman, B. L., et al.,** N-Isopropyl-I-123-p-iodoamphetamine brain scans with single photon emission tomography. Discordance with transmission computed tomography, *Radiology,* 145, 795, 1982.
4. **Holman, B. L., Lee, R. G. L., Hill, T. C., et al.,** A comparison of two cerebral perfusion tracers, N-isopropyl-I-123-p-iodoamphetamine and I123-HIPDM in human, *J. Nucl. Med.,* 25, 25, 1984.
5. **Holman, B. L., Sporn, V., Jones, A. G., et al.,** Myocardial imaging with Tc-99m-CPI. Initial experience in human, *J. Nucl. Med.,* 28, 13, 1987.

Chapter 2

THEORY OF TOMOGRAPHIC RECONSTRUCTION

A. Todd-Pokropek

TABLE OF CONTENTS

I. INTRODUCTION

Tomographic reconstruction techniques have been employed in a variety of medical applications. Some of the original references are in X-ray CT (computed tomography) scanning,[1-3] MRI (magnetic resonance imaging) (NMR),[4,5] impedance imaging,[6] ultrasound,[7] and nuclear medicine for both single photon emission computed tomography (SPECT)[8-11] and positron emission tomography (PET).[12,13] An even greater range of applications has been found in nonmedical areas ranging from astronomy[14] to (and in particular) molecular biology.[15-17] The basic mathematical methods of reconstruction techniques have tended to be rediscovered over and over again by workers in rather specific areas, unaware of the work of others in different areas. Three useful general review papers in the area of radiology/nuclear medicine are References 18 to 20 which provide a short survey of some of these techniques. An attempt at a general approach to tomographic reconstruction is presented here, followed by a brief discussion of some of the special problems in nuclear medicine, specifically attenuation and scatter correction.

Tomography is one example of an inverse problem. We have a set of observations, **g**, for example, numbers of photons detected, related in some way to a set of values, **f**, for example, the radiological density of a whole set of positions within the patient. In general, we may be able to state that **g** and **f** are related, for example as a set of simultaneous equations

$$\begin{aligned} g(1,1) &= a(1,1,1,1)\, f(1,1) + a(1,1,1,2)\, f(1,2) \\ &\qquad \cdots\, a(1,1,N,N)\, f(N,N) \\ g(1,2) &= a(1,2,1,1)\, f(1,1) + a(1,2,1,2)\, f(1,2) \\ &\qquad \cdots\, a(1,2,N,N)\, f(N,N) \\ \\ g(N,N) &= a(N,N,1,1)\, f(1,1) + a(N,N,1,2)\, f(1,2) \\ &\qquad a(N,N,N,N)\, f(N,N) \end{aligned} \tag{1}$$

may be represented in matrix notation as

$$g = A\, f \tag{2}$$

where **A** is the matrix of coefficients a(i,j,i′,j′) as given in the set of simultaneous equations above. We must solve the above equations to find the unknown set of values **f** from the known values **g**, which may be expressed as finding **f** from

$$f = A^{-1}\, g \tag{3}$$

where $\mathbf{A}^{-1}$ is the matrix inverse of **A**. However, although we can state the problem in such simple terms, this does not imply that it is able to be done. The inverse $\mathbf{A}^{-1}$ may not exist, i.e., a solution to the set of simultaneous equations may not exist. Even if it does exist it may not be possible to compute.

Tomography is a specific type of inverse problem where the set of values **f** represents the values of some parameter (radioactivity, etc.) at every point either in a slice (see Figure 1) or in true 3-D volume (see Figure 2), and **g** are the external observations. The relationship **g = A f** is called the Radon transform. What is desired is some usable method for solving this equation. This problem will be considered essentially in 2-D, that is, trying to solve for values in a single transaxial slice.

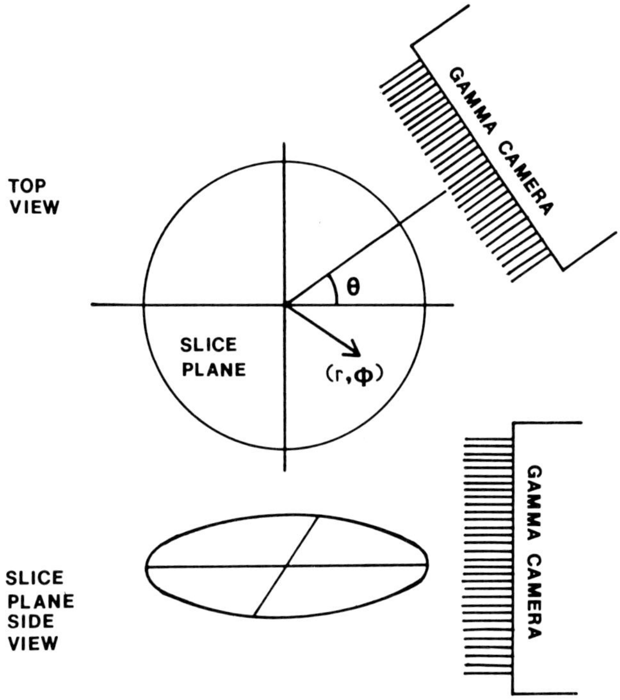

FIGURE 1. Diagram of a transaxial slice in a SPECT tomographic system. The camera rotates about the axis of rotation viewing the slice place at some angle θ.

The special problems associated with tomography are that the matrix **A** is very large, very sparse, e.g., many of the coefficients A(i,j,i′,j′) are equal to zero, and finding its inverse can be very unstable; small errors in the observed data can lead to large errors in the solution. Some good general references are References 15 to 18.

II. MATHEMATICAL OVERVIEW

The most powerful method for looking at the tomographic reconstruction problem is that of Functional Analysis.[21,22] In summary, this approach considers that space of functions, all of which are possible solutions, and then reduces the number of possible solutions, leaving what may be termed the "desirable" solutions. Such methods provide a powerful insight into the reconstruction problem and will be referred to in passing in certain sections of this chapter. The following section, however, assumes only a knowledge of simple matrix algebra and some familiarity with the Fourier transform.

A. The Radon Transform (How the Data Are Sampled)

As illustrated in Figure 1, it is assumed that when an observation is made it is along some path which is normally termed a ray. In tomography, it is convenient to call this set of observations projections and to use the symbol **p** to represent them. Thus, one given observation $p(\xi,\theta)$ corresponds to some function of the values $f(x,y)$ along the corresponding ray. The ray is categorized by a pair of values, θ its angle, and ξ its perpendicular distance from a line drawn through the center of rotation. (In 3-D the ray is categorized by three values, ξ, θ, and Φ, as was shown in Figure 2.) Normally, it is assumed that $p(\xi,\theta)$, or in 3-D $p(\xi,\theta,\Phi)$, is the line integral, i.e., the sum of the values found along the ray. Thus

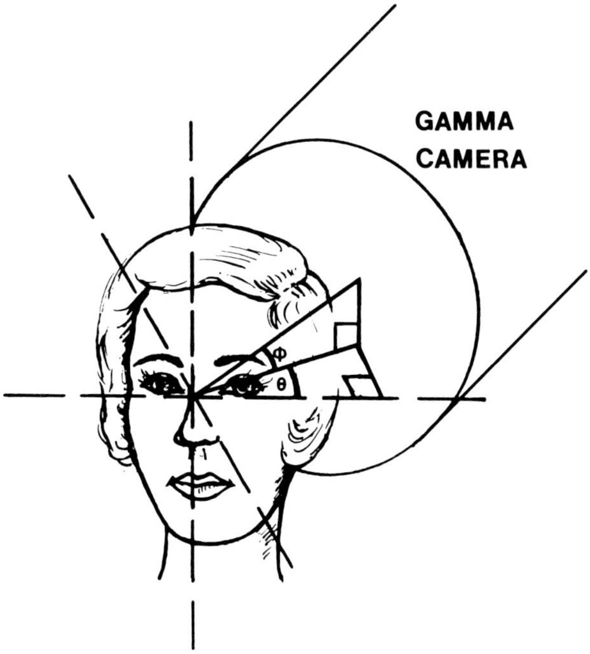

FIGURE 2. The geometry of SPECT system considered here in 3-D. The camera is pointing at a patient, for example, using a converging (cone beam) collimator, and the angle of view is defined by a pair of angles θ and I.

$$p(\xi,\theta) = \int_s f(x,y)ds \qquad (4)$$

where s is a variable directed along the ray. Thus, one projection line is the set of values of p(ξ,θ) for all values of ξ for a specific value of θ, as illustrated in Figure 3. Note the distinction between a projection line and a ray line. The Radon transform[23-25] therefore converts the set of values f(x,y) into a set of projection values p(ξ,θ). Angle θ is defined in Figure 3.

The first relationship which needs to be defined is that relating the coordinates x,y to ξ,θ. As shown in Figure 3, it may easily be demonstrated that the equation of the ray line is

$$\xi = x\cos(\theta) + y\sin(\theta) \qquad (5)$$

and thus the line integral may be re-expressed as

$$p(\xi,\theta) = \int_R f(x,y)\ \delta(\xi - x\cos(\theta) - y\sin(\theta))dxdy \qquad (6)$$

where δ[ξ − x cos (θ)] is a δ function which is zero for all values other than δ (0), that is, for all points not lying along the line ξ − x cos(θ) = 0, in the domain R. Thus (for all values of ξ and θ), the Radon transformation generates a set of observed projection values from a set of "true" values within the patient. The 3-D form of this operation is normally called the X-ray transform,[23] and the term "Radon transform" is restricted to the 2-D case given above.

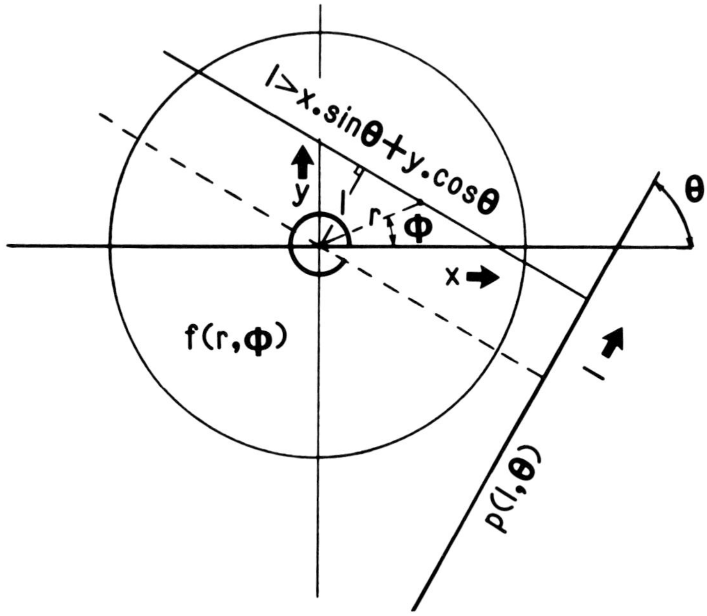

FIGURE 3. The geometry of tomographic reconstruction, relating the projection ray at some offset 1, the projection line at some angle θ, and a point in the reconstruction slice with cartesian coordinates (x,y) and polar coordinates (r,I).

B. Tools: Forward- and Backprojection

Two useful tools need to be defined, forward- and backprojection. Forward-projection is essentially the same as the Radon transform itself, that is, the operation of obtaining line integrals along rays to give projections from some set of values. Unfortunately, as will be stressed in the next section, the Radon transform is defined only for continuous distributions, that is, where f(x,y) exists for **every possible** value of x and y, and therefore p(ξ,θ) can be obtained for every possible value of ξ and θ. Let us imagine, however, that we have a set of discrete values f(x,y), that is, f(x,y) is known only at a certain number of sample points spaced Δx and Δy apart. It is still possible to define the operation of forward-projection as

$$p(\xi,\theta) = \sum_i \sum_j f(i,j)\ \delta(\xi - i\Delta x \cos(\theta) - j\Delta y \sin(\theta)) \tag{7}$$

or in matrix notation

$$p = Ff \tag{8}$$

where i and j are the discrete coordinates within f, **F** is a matrix of coefficients, and the δ function has not been properly defined as yet. This (discrete) operation in NOT identical to the Radon transform.

Similarly, we may define an operation called backprojection. In forward-projection, we sum all the values of f(i,j) that lie along some ray ξ,θ to give a projection value p(ξ,θ). It is possible to imagine the opposite process. Take a projection value p(ξ,θ), and add it to every pixel f(i,j) that lies along the corresponding ray ξ,θ to generate the result, f′(i,j) such that

$$f'(i,j) = f(i,j) + \sum_\xi \sum_\theta p(\xi,\theta)\ w(i,j,\xi,\theta) \tag{9}$$

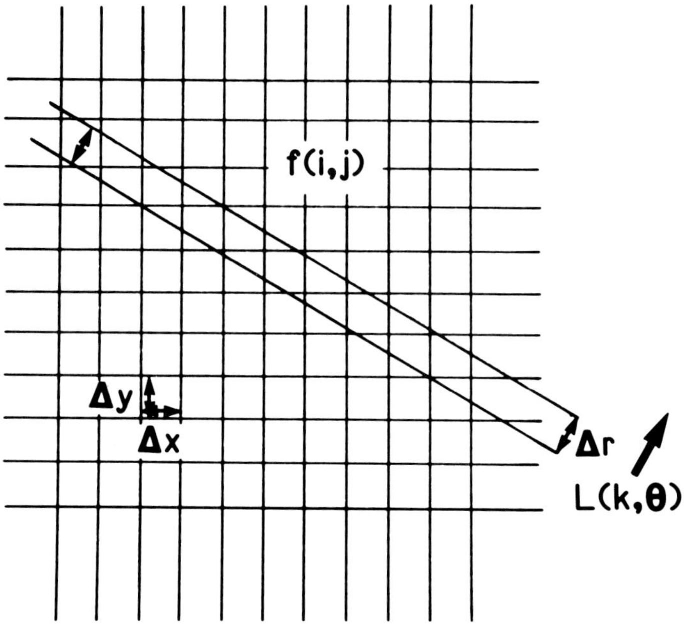

FIGURE 4. Diagram showing how a thick projection ray passes through the reconstruction array, where the intersection between the thick ray, and the finite pixels gives rise to a series of polygons of different shape and area.

where w is an appropriate weight, as is explained later. This operation needs to be repeated for every value of ξ and θ. It can be performed both for discrete data and in principle for continuous data. It is convenient to express this operation as **B** such that

$$f_b = B\ p \tag{10}$$

Thus, the operation of backprojection (i.e., applying the backprojection operator **B**) creates a set of values $\mathbf{f_b}$ from the complete set of projections **p**. The backprojection operation takes every point $p(\xi,\theta)$ for all angles θ and positions ξ and backprojects its value into the array of data $\mathbf{f_b}$. It is assumed that the initial values of $\mathbf{f_b}$ are zero. In certain cases only the backprojection of a single projection line will be considered, that is, the operation $\mathbf{f_b} = \mathbf{B_\theta}\ p(\theta)$, for a given value of θ.

The question of the weights (w) to be used has been glossed over. Normally[26] when a given projection value is "added" to a point i,j in $\mathbf{f_b}$ it is weighted such that the sum of all such values when added together along the ray line is equal to the original value $p(\xi,\theta)$. If $\mathbf{f_b}$ is continuous, then the value $p(\xi,\theta)$ is weighted by $\Delta\xi/L$ where L is the total length of the ray of width $\Delta\xi$. If $\mathbf{f_b}$ is discrete, as shown in Figure 4, the weight is chosen as being $\Delta\xi(i,j)/L$ where $\xi(i,j)$ is the area of that part of the ray that passes though the pixel i,j divided as before by the total area of the ray L. A similar trick may be used for forward projection of discrete data. A weight may be determined corresponding to the area of the ray line as it passes though a pixel. Note that a ray, in such a discrete domain may be imagined as having an area. The determinations of these weighting factors are approximations, and many different techniques have actually been used in the algorithms in practice, primarily in order to achieve greater speed.[26,27]

C. The Inverse Radon Transform

At first sight, the tomographic inverse problem seems very straightforward. The Austrian mathematician Radon published a proof finding a solution to the inverse transform in 1917.[28]

His proof may not have been the first and was certainly not the last. He stated that the unknown

$$f(r,\Phi) = \frac{1}{2\pi^2}\int_0^{\pi}\int_{-\infty}^{+\infty}\frac{\partial/\partial\xi[p(\xi,\theta)]}{\cos(\theta - \Phi) - \xi}\,d\xi d\theta \tag{11}$$

although many alternative forms can and have been determined (see, for example, Barrett[23]). This solution is exact, but $f(r,\Phi)$ in polar coordinates or $f(x,y)$ in Cartesian coordinates can be found only when $p(\xi,\theta)$ has been determined for all values of ξ and θ and also where $p(\xi,\theta)$ can always be differentiated, or in other words, there are no discontinuities. Thus, we can solve the tomographic problem, in principle, provided we have an infinite number of observations. Therefore, this transform does not appear immediately to be of any practical use; however, using the tools of forward- and backprojection, methods can be developed for its solution and shown later.

D. General Matrix Inverse

Another approach is to handle the problem directly in the discrete domain and forget about the continuous domain. Let us therefore imagine that a finite set of readings $p(k,t)$ has been found corresponding to a set of desired (unknown) values $f(i,j)$. It is possible normally to express the relationship between the two as a set of simultaneous equations between the observed projections values p and the unknown image values f:

$$\begin{aligned}
g(1,1) &= a(1,1,1,1)\, f(1,1) + a(1,1,1,2)\, f(1,2) \\
&\qquad \ldots\, a(1,1,N,N)\, f(N,N) \\
g(1,2) &= a(1,2,1,1)\, f(1,1) + a(1,2,1,2)\, f(1,2) \\
&\qquad \ldots\, a(1,2,N,N)\, f(N,N) \\
&\vdots \\
g(N,N) &= a(N,N,1,1)\, f(1,1) + a(N,N,1,2)\, f(1,2) \\
&\qquad \ldots\, a(N,N,N,N)\, f(N,N)
\end{aligned} \tag{12}$$

which is simply just the familiar matrix equation with respect to projections **p** and the true image **f**

$$p = A\,f \tag{13}$$

as given in Equations 1 and 2. Since we may assume that **A** can be determined for the given system, we may use standard methods for solving the set of simultaneous equations. All that is required is finding the set of inverse coefficients $\mathbf{A}^{-1}$, after which one merely (matrix) multiplies that matrix by the set of observations **p**. The requirement for infinite sampling has apparently been circumnavigated.

Several important observations may be made. Let us suppose that we must find $f(i,j)$ for some set of values $0 < i < N - 1$, $0 < j < N - 1$; then there are N^2 unknowns. For example, if we wish to find $f(i,j)$ for a 256×256 matrix of points, then there are 65536 unknowns and therefore, there must be at least 65536 simultaneous equations. Thus, the size of the matrix **A** is at least 65536×65536 and has 4.3×10^9 elements, although many of them are either zero or nearly zero. It is computationally not very easy to find $\mathbf{A}^{-1}$, neither is it very efficient. Thus this technique, which may be called direct matrix inversion, is not really appropriate, although it has been attempted.[26,29]

E. Solutions to Ill-Posed Problems

As stated in the Introduction, even if it were possible to compute a solution by direct matrix inversion, an important additional problem has been ignored. There is no guarantee that such a set of simultaneous equations has any solution at all. Even when the number of equations is increased by increasing the number of observations, there is no guarantee that a **unique** solution exists. This situation is particularly aggravated in that none of the observations that can be made are necessarily exact; themy may be noisy. Thus, we require a method to solve this set of equations which will give a reasonable answer, even when the data (observations) are noisy. Unfortunately, the reason that the direct application of the inverse Radon transform was inappropriate is the same reason that the matrix inverse method may give unacceptable solutions: the basic reconstruction problem itself is "ill-posed".[30,31] In simple terms this means that, for a given set of observations, there may be **many** possible solutions, all of which are consistent with the data. There is no single "correct" solution but a multiplicity of possible solutions. Some method needs to be used to select the most "reasonable" solution from the set of possible solutions. Several techniques may be employed: windowing, maximum entropy, regularization, etc., which are discussed later.

III. ITERATIVE ALGORITHMS

Although we know that difficulties exist in trying to find a good solution, we still can continue to ignore them and can try another (brute force) approach to solving such a system of equations. It seems appropriate to try an iterative approach.[13,32] Let us take as a basic premise that if a set of values $\hat{\mathbf{f}}$ can be found such that when forward-projected the set of values

$$p' = F\,\hat{f} \tag{14}$$

is such that $\mathbf{p}'$ is the same as (tends to) the observed values $\mathbf{p}$, then $\hat{\mathbf{f}}$ is the desired solution. Unfortunately, as suggested previously, $\hat{\mathbf{f}}$ may not be the unique solution, wherein lies the basic limitation of the method; however, it may be a solution which, with respect to some criterion, is acceptable.

The following approach seems reasonable. Let $\mathbf{f}^n$ be the nth guess at $\hat{\mathbf{f}}$. Therefore, if $\mathbf{p}^n$ is the result of forward-projecting $\mathbf{f}^n$, we can define an error term $\mathbf{e}^n$ such that

$$\begin{aligned} e^n &= p - p^n \\ &= p - F\,f^n \end{aligned} \tag{15}$$

or

$$e^n(\xi,\theta) = p(\xi,\theta) - \{\text{forward-projection}\}\ f^n(i,j) \text{ at } \xi,\ \theta \tag{16}$$

Thus, one can imagine that as the set of error values **e** tends to zero, so the estimated solution $\mathbf{f}^n$ tends to the true solution. The backprojection operation can be used to achieve this. The error terms can be backprojected and subtracted from the current estimate $\mathbf{f}^n$ such that

$$f^{n+1} = f^n - B\,e^n \tag{17}$$

or

$$f^{n+1}(i,j) = f^n(i,j) - \sum_{\xi,\theta}\sum e^n(\xi,\theta)\, w(i,j,\xi,\theta) \tag{18}$$

where $w(i,j,\xi,\theta)$ is an appropriate set of weights. An iterative process of this type in tomography is generally known as the algebraic reconstruction technique (ART).[32] The question of convergence is far from simple.[22] A rather superficial approach is given both in the next section and with respect to maximum entropy and conjugate gradient algorithms.

A. ART

The basic ART algorithm is essentially as described above.

A first estimate of the set of values $\mathbf{f}^0$ is made. One such starting point is for each $f(i,j)$ to be made equal to $p(\xi,\theta)/N^2$ where $\mathbf{f}$ is a matrix of size $N \times N$. That is, all values of $f(i,j)$ are equal and their sum is equal to the sum of the observed values. It should be noted that there is usually an implicit assumption in such techniques, which is that sum (θ), the sum of the values for each projection at each angle θ, where

$$\mathrm{sum}(\theta) = \sum_{\xi} p(\xi,\theta) \tag{19}$$

should always give the same value for all value of θ.

The first guess at the solution $\mathbf{f}^0$ is then forward-projected, subtracted from the observed values, and error terms $\mathbf{e}^0$ generated. These are backprojected, subtracted from $\mathbf{f}^0$ to give $\mathbf{f}^1$, and the iteration continued until the observed values $\mathbf{f}^n$ do not change, or until the sum of the error terms $e(\xi,\theta)$ is less than some threshold (or some other criterion). This process is carried out projection line by projection line, that is, each set of values for the error for some angle θ_1 is backprojected before the next computation of the error is estimated for some other angle θ_2.

Various selections of the order of the angles, when forward- and backprojection is performed angle by angle, have been tried. The simplest method is to take the angles in successive order. The two most common variations are to take angles in random order, or in orthogonal pairs, 0°s followed by 90°s followed by 45°s followed by 135°s, etc. maximizing the angular difference between successive operations.

There are many variations on these basic techniques, however. Very commonly, the method is damped. Instead of subtracting the whole of the error term from the current estimate of the solution, some constant λ times the error may be subtracted such that

$$f^{n+1} = f^n - \mu \, B \, e^n \tag{20}$$

where λ is typically $0 < \lambda < 1$, but λ may also vary as a function of iteration number, etc.[27] Using a fixed λ, as illustrated in Figure 5, the iteration will reach the desired solution (will converge) more slowly, but it will not tend to overshoot and swing backward and forward (or at least that is the hope). Various methods attempting to optimize the choice of the coefficient λ have been tried, but they are beyond the scope of this chapter.[22,32]

As described by Gordon, Bender, and Herman,[15] an additional constraint is normally imposed in that $\mathbf{f}^{n+1}$ is never allowed to become negative and is actually chosen as the maximum of zero and ($\mathbf{f}^n$ plus the backprojected error term).

Many variants of basic ART exist. An interesting modification has been called multiplicative ART.[33] Here, instead of adding the correction term $\mathbf{e}^n$ obtained by subtraction of the estimated $\mathbf{p}^n$ and observed projections $\mathbf{p}$, an error term $e^n{}_m(\xi,\theta)$ is derived from the ratio of $p^n(\xi,\theta)$ and $p(\xi,\theta)$. Thus, each element of $\mathbf{e}^n{}_\mathbf{m}$ gives a value which is the current over- or underestimation of the projection value, for each value of ξ,θ. This error term is backprojected and used to multiply each corresponding element in $\mathbf{f}^n$. Multiplicative ART, when the initial estimate is positive, ensures that the final estimate will also be positive. It should be noted that, in many cases, it is known that the desired solution cannot contain negative values.

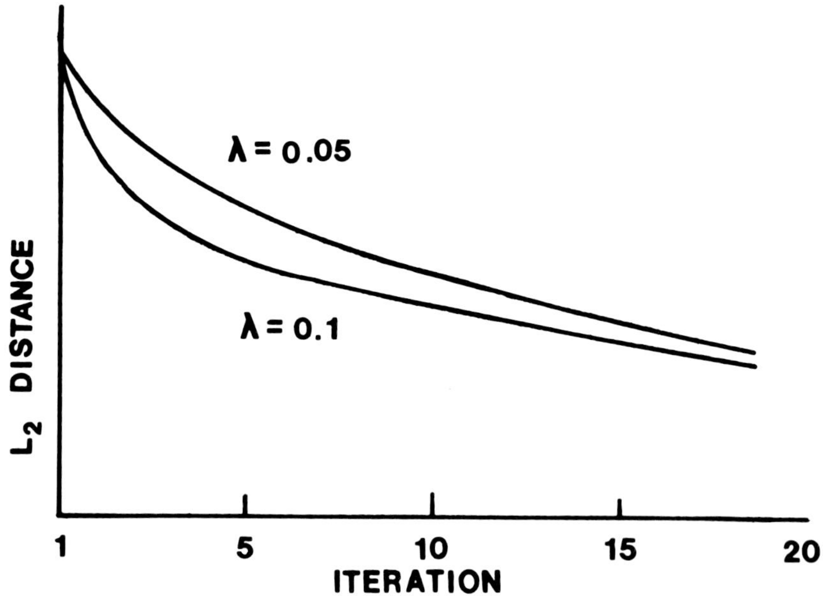

FIGURE 5. A plot of the least squares (L2) difference between a reconstruction and the true object, as a function of iteration number, for two different relaxation coefficients lambda.

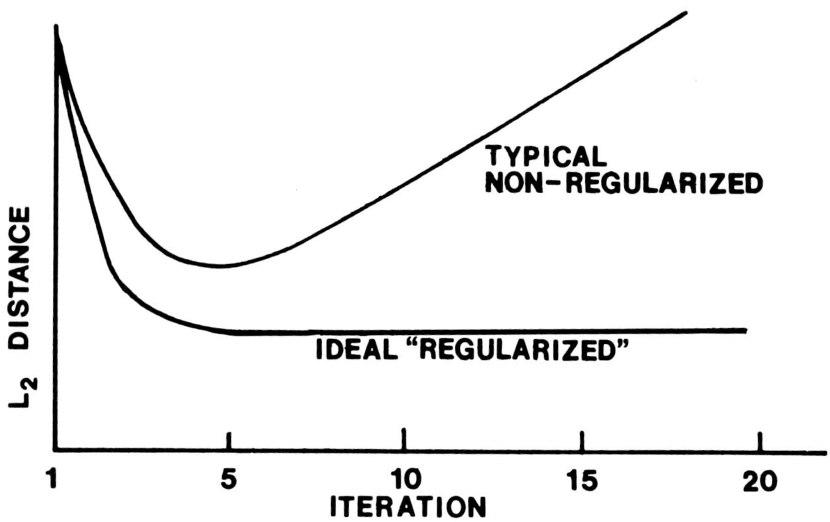

FIGURE 6. The behavior (in diagrammatic form) of two different reconstruction procedures, called "regularized" and "nonregularized", in terms of the least squares (L2) distance as a function of iteration number. The nonregularized algorithm is seen to diverge after a certain number of iterations.

It may be observed (see Figure 6) that with increasing iteration number many ART algorithms appear to converge initially and then diverge afterward. No completely satisfactory measure of convergence exists. A convergence criterion needs to be defined.[32] Some which have been used are

1. The root-mean-squared difference (RMSD) between observed and estimated projections

$$\mathrm{RMSD} = \{\Sigma[(p(\xi,\theta) - p^n(\xi,\theta)]^2\}^{1/2} \tag{21}$$

2. The variance (VAR), the difference between the nth estimate of **f** and its mean value

$$VAR = \Sigma[f^n(i,j) - f_{mean})^2] \tag{22}$$

where f_{mean} is the mean value of f.

3. The entropy(H) of the image defined as

$$H = -k\,\Sigma[fn\,\ln(fn)] \tag{23}$$

where

$$f^n = f^n(i,j)/f_{mean} \tag{24}$$

As a further alternative, a χ^2 statistic has sometimes been used[34] as a convergence criterion such that

$$\chi^2(f) = \sum_{\xi,\theta}\sum \frac{[F(i,j,\xi,\theta)\ f(i,j) - p(\xi,\theta)]^2}{VAR(\xi,\theta)^2} \tag{25}$$

where VAR $(\xi,\theta)^2$ is the uncertainty or variance in the estimated projection data at a point ξ,θ and F (i,j,ξ,θ) is an element of the forward-projection operator as previously. This may be shown to be equal to

$$\chi^2 = (\mathbf{f\ M\ f}) - 2(\mathbf{v\ f}) + c \tag{26}$$

where

$$M_{ij} = \sum_k F_{ik}\ F_{jk}/VAR_k \tag{27}$$

$$v_i = \sum_k F_{ij}\ p_k/VAR_k \tag{28}$$

$$c = \sum_k p_k^2/VAR_k \tag{29}$$

where k represents the pair of variables ξ,θ. This χ^2 value is another measure of the distance between the current estimate of the solution and the observed projection data. Such norms must be defined carefully when considering the convergence of reconstruction and other iterative processes.[35]

B. ART2 and ART3

Other important modifications to the basic ART algorithm have been made and normally entail special handling of the iteration when negative values are observed in the current estimates of the solution $\mathbf{f^n}$. The basic ART2 algorithm as is follows.[32] Let

$$f'^{n+1}(i,j) = f'(i,j) + e^n(\xi,\theta)\ w(i,j,\xi,\theta) \tag{30}$$

where f′ is an intermediate result and used such that

$$f^{n+1}(i,j) = \max[0, f'^{n+1}(i,j)] \tag{31}$$

This permits intermediate negative results to exist but still forces the final result to be positive. Such algorithms are by definition nonlinear. Convergence is often difficult to establish, but has been stated to be the minimum variance solution when fully consistent.

ART3[32] is slightly more complex. As before, an error term e^n (i,j) is calculated

$$e^n(i,j) = \begin{cases} p_e & \text{if} \quad abs(p_e) > 2\epsilon \\ 2p_e - \epsilon & \text{if} \quad \epsilon < p_e < 2\epsilon \quad \text{or} \quad \text{if } -\epsilon > p_e > -2\epsilon \\ 0 & \text{if} \quad abs(p_e) < \epsilon \end{cases} \tag{32}$$

where

$$p_e = p(\xi,\theta) - p^n(\xi,\theta) \tag{33}$$

and ϵ is an error tolerance which may be fixed or variable. This has the effect of limiting the correction term such that, if less than some given ϵ, no change is made. This is supposed to reduce oscillation in the solution.

C. Simultaneous Iterative Reconstruction Technique (SIRT)

SIRT[36] is very closely related to ART. In conventional ART the forward- and backprojection of error terms is normally performed angle by angle. Alternatively, the error term can be cumulated for the complete set of angles for a given point i,j and then applied once. This latter method is generally called SIRT.

This method has potential advantages in computation time has and has possible merit in terms of the signal-to-noise ratio in the reconstructed image. In practice, however, results are almost equivalent to conventional ART.

IV. 2-D FOURIER RECONSTRUCTION

As a complete alternative to such iterative techniques, a number of so-called analytical reconstruction methods have been proposed. These obtain the (or rather a) solution in one single operation. The most common class of analytical methods uses the Fourier transform to obtain a solution, making use of the central slice theorem. This may be stated as follows:

The Fourier transform F{ } of a function p(x) is defined as

$$\begin{aligned} F\{p(x)\} &= p(u) \\ &= \int_{-\infty}^{+\infty} p(x) \cdot \exp(-i\ 2\pi ux)dx \end{aligned} \tag{34}$$

where i is the square root of -1.

In two dimensions for a function p(x,y)

$$F\{p(x,y)\} = p(u,v) = \int_{-\infty}^{+\infty}\int_{-\infty}^{+\infty} p(x,y) \cdot \exp(-i\ 2\pi(ux + vy))dx\ dy \tag{35}$$

The central slice theorem states that, for a projection $p(\xi,\theta)$, then its Fourier transform $F\{p(\xi,\theta)\}$ is identical to a profile through the 2-D Fourier transform of $f(r,\theta)$, the object, at that same angle θ. The Fourier transform of the projection is given by

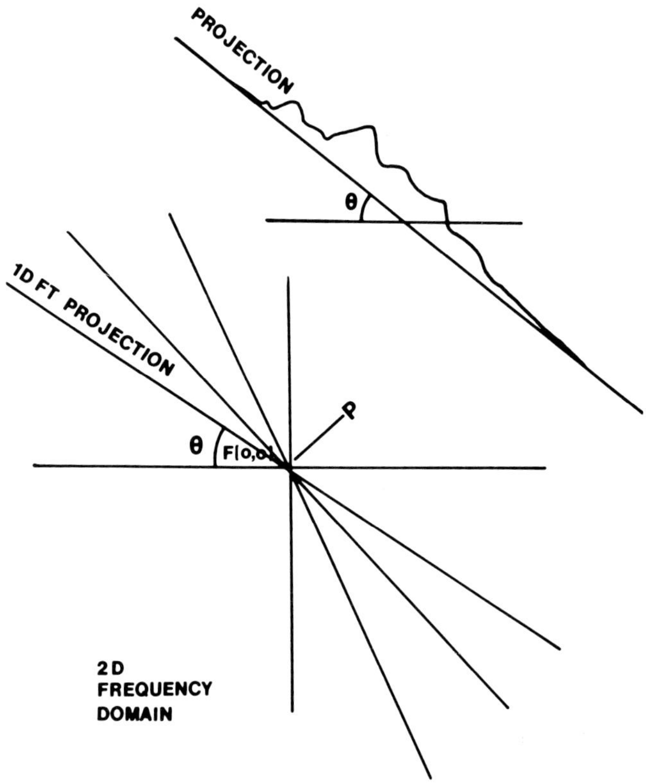

FIGURE 7. A diagram of the central slice theorem, showing a projection line at a certain angle θ, whose Fourier transform corresponds to a slice through the 2-D Fourier transform of the object at that same angle.

$$\int p(\xi,\theta) \cdot \exp(-i\omega\xi)d\xi = \iiint f(x,y)\ \delta(\xi - x\sin\theta - y\cos\theta)dx\,dy\,\exp(-i\omega\xi)d\xi \quad (36)$$

where ω is the spatial frequency along the projection line.

After reordering and eliminating ξ, this becomes

$$= \iint f(x,y)\ \exp[-i(f_x x + f_y y)]dx\,dy\ \delta(-x\sin\theta - y\cos\theta) \quad (37)$$

where f_x, f_y are the spatial frequencies in the image plane. Thus, a central slice through the 2-D Fourier transform of the function f is equal to the Fourier transform of the projection at the corresponding angle itself. To reconstruct f(x,y) from the set of projections, however, we need first to reconstruct $F(f_x,f_y)$ from the set of slices through it, as illustrated in Figure 7. This may be performed directly by interpolation between the slices. This unfortunately is not a simple operation.[17] In particular, it should be noted that the sampling is much finer at the center of the Fourier transform of f and decreases linearly with increasing frequency.

A. Filtered Backprojection

This section is slightly more mathematically difficult and should be skipped if the reader has difficulty.

The inverse Radon transform as given in Equation 11 may be restated after slight modification such that

$$f(r,\Phi) = \frac{1}{2\pi^2} \int_0^{\pi} \int_{-\infty}^{+\infty} \frac{\partial/\partial\xi[p(\xi,\theta)]}{\xi' - \xi} \, d\xi \, d\theta \quad (38)$$

where

$$\xi' = x \cos(\theta) + y \sin(\theta)$$

As stated previously, the object to be reconstructed f(x,y) is supposed to be continuous, bounded (e.g., equal to zero outside some region), and the partial derivative of the observed projections $p(\xi,\theta)$ must be continuous. Note that this assumption is violated if the projection contains any sharp steps! The inner integral in the above equation contains a singularity when $\xi = x \cos(\theta) + y \sin(\theta)$ and it therefore normally is evaluated in the Cauchy principal value sense, i.e., as the limit of the process

$$\lim_{R->\infty} \int_{-R}^{+R} f(x)dx \quad (39)$$

This is again a manifestation of the fact that the reconstruction is weakly singular, and its solution can be considered as ill-posed such that small changes in the input data, the observed projections, can lead to large changes in the reconstructed values. Thus, while many possible methods of reconstructing an image from its projections exist, what we would like to find is one which is as stable as possible in the presence of noise.

One method of proceeding is as follows (based on that developed by Horn;[37] see also Reference 38 for an alternative derivation). First, separate the inner integral into two parts, from $\xi < -\infty$ to $\xi < -\epsilon$, and $\xi < +\epsilon$ to $\xi < +\infty$. Thus, the inner integral is simply the sum of these two parts for the limit of $\epsilon = 0$. Integrating by parts gives:

$$f(x,y) = \lim_{\epsilon->0} 1/\epsilon \; p(\xi'-\xi,\theta) + 1/\epsilon \; p(\xi'+\epsilon,\theta) + \int_{|t|\geq\epsilon} (-1/t^2) \; p(\xi,\theta)dt \quad (40)$$

which may be rewritten as

$$\lim_{\epsilon->0} \int_{-\infty}^{+\infty} F(t) \; p(\xi,\theta)d\xi$$

where

$$F(t) = 1/\epsilon^2 \quad \text{for} \quad |t| < \epsilon$$
$$= 1/-t^2 \quad \text{for} \quad |t| \geq \epsilon \quad (41)$$

such that:

$$f(r,\Phi) = 1/2\pi^2 \int_0^{2\pi} \lim_{\epsilon->0} \int_{-\infty}^{+\infty} F(t) \; p(\xi,\theta)d\xi \; d\theta \quad (42)$$

The above may then be separated into two processes:

$$f(r,\Phi) = 1/2\pi^2 \int_0^{2\pi} g(\xi',\theta)d\theta \quad (43)$$

which is actually the familiar backprojection operation, and

$$g(\xi',\theta) = \lim_{\epsilon -> 0} \int_{-\infty}^{+\infty} F(\xi' - \xi)\, p(\xi,\theta) d\xi \tag{44}$$

which is a convolution with some sort of filter.

It should be noted that in order to compute the above integrals they must be replaced by summations, which is not necessarily a trivial task. A useful insight into the reconstruction process is given by the observation that for a given point in the reconstruction, the integral is determined the sum of both by the rays passing effectively through the point, and all the remaining rays. The weights of rays not passing through the point decrease as an inverse function of the distance squared. The sum of the weights of the rays passing through the point itself is equal to zero.

B. A Basic Reconstruction Using Filtered Backprojection

Consider the backprojection operator, generating $f(r,\theta)$, here given in polar coordinates as opposed to the usual Cartesian coordinates, from the integral of $p(r,\theta)$ with respect to θ. It may be proved[39] that

$$F\{f(r,\theta)\} = \rho\, F\{p(r,\theta)\} \tag{45}$$

where ρ is the radial spatial frequency and also:

$$1/\rho = F\,\{1/r\} \tag{46}$$

The above suggests the following simple and well-known reconstruction procedure. First, backproject the projections, then filter the result with a ρ function. The order of these two operations may be reversed. Thus, we end up with the process of filtering the projections with ρ, that is, by a ramp in the frequency domain (i.e., a filter which simply increases linearly with increasing frequency), and then backprojecting. This approach suggests that to obtain the same results as the inverse Radon transform, the weighting function to be used $F(t)$ is actually $F^{-1}\{p\}$, where $F^{-1}\{\ \}$ is the inverse Fourier transform.

Thus, it has been found (in two ways) that before backprojection it is necessary to perform a filtering operation such that the modified projection $p'(\xi,\theta)$ is given by, in discrete notation

$$p'(\xi,\theta) = \sum_{\xi'} F(\xi - \xi')\, p(\xi',\theta)\Delta\xi \tag{47}$$

where $\Delta\xi$ is the uniform interval between rays. A suitable form[40] for F is

$$F(k) = -w_k/(k\,\Delta\xi)^2 \qquad \text{for} \qquad k \neq 0 \tag{48}$$

otherwise

$$F(0) = -2 \sum_{k=1}^{N} F(k) \tag{49}$$

where w_k are weights associated with the kth value, and are chosen so as to "stabilize" the result. N is the size of the filter array. Values have been chosen by Ramachandran and Lakshminarayanan[41] as $w_k = 2$ for k odd and zero for k even. Shepp and Logan (1974) chose w_k as $4 \cdot k^2/(4 \cdot k^2 - 1)$. Many other choices are possible. As Horn[37] stated, the choice of filter function is "usually discussed in a somewhat *ad hoc* fashion in terms of the need to low-pass the projection data in order to avoid aliasing or undersampling. Clearly this is wrong since in order to avoid the effects of undersampling, low-pass filtering has to be performed before sampling. The derivation of these weights as an exercise in numerical quadrature seems more insightful."

V. PRACTICAL CONSIDERATIONS

There are a number of practical considerations which need to be developed in order to make the previously discussed methods useful, for example, the use of filters to improve the signal-to-noise ratio.

A. Filters

In tomographic reconstruction, it is important to limit the high frequency components before the reconstruction (ramp) filter is applied. For this reason, various smoothing window functions normally are used. For a discussion of window functions in general, see Hamming[43] and in SPECT, see Budinger.[18] These are smoothing functions which are multiplied by the basic ramp to create the final effective filter (in the frequency domain). Some examples of windows commonly used in tomography are

1. The Shepp and Logan window

$$w(f) = \mathrm{sinc}(f/2f_m) \tag{50}$$

where

$$\mathrm{sinc}(x) = \sin(\pi x)/(\pi x) \tag{51}$$

2. The modified Shepp Logan filter

$$w'(f) = w(f)\,(0.4 - 0.6\cos(\pi\, f/f_m)) \tag{52}$$

3. The Hann window

$$\begin{aligned} w(f) &= 0.5 + 0.5\cos(\pi\, f/f_m) && \text{if } f \leqslant f_m \\ &= 0 && \text{if if} > f_m \end{aligned} \tag{53}$$

4. The Hamming window

$$\begin{aligned} w(f) &= 0.54 + 0.46\cos(\pi\, f/f_m) && \text{if } f \leqslant f_m \\ &= 0 && \text{if if} > f_m \end{aligned} \tag{54}$$

5. The Butterworth filter

$$w(f) = [1/(1 + f/f_m)^{2n}]^{1/2} \tag{55}$$

where n is an arbitrary constant

6. The Parzen window:

$$w(f) = 1 - 6(f/f_m)^2 (1 - f/f_m) \quad \text{if} \quad f \leq f_m/2$$
$$= 2(1 - f/f_m)^3 \quad \text{if} \quad f_m/2 < f \leq f_m$$
$$= 0 \quad \text{if} \quad f > f_m \qquad (56)$$

There are certainly many others. There seems little to choose between these filters from theoretical consideration and they must be judged in practice, that is, by considering their effects on the final sharpness and signal-to-noise ratio of the resulting image. Note that these 1-D filters could have also been used as 2-D filters on the reconstructed image, although computationally 2-D filters are likely to be more costly to implement.

Note also that there is no need to restrict such filters to smoothing filters; some refocusing or sharpening of the image may be performed and is indeed performed by some manufacturers, as illustrated in Figure 8.

B. Noise

The two basic equations defining the characteristics of noise in tomography define the frequency spectrum of the noise and the signal-to-noise ratio in the reconstructed image. The frequency spectrum of the noise is essentially filter function shaped[43] such that

$$N(f) = \text{FILT}(f)^2/f \qquad (57)$$

where N(f) is the nose Wiener or power spectrum, FILT(f) is the filter used in filtered backprojection in the frequency spectrum, and f is the spatial frequency. Thus, if no window function is used, FILT(f) = f, and the noise spectrum is ramp shaped. The power spectrum of a function f(x) is defined as $[F\{f(x)\}]^2$.

The signal-to-noise ratio as a first approximation is given by[44]

$$\text{FSD} = k\, N_p^{3/4}/N_c^{1/2} \qquad (58)$$

where N_p is the number of pixels in the reconstruction containing data, N_c is the number of counts (events detected), FSD is the fractional standard deviation (coefficient of variation), and k is a constant. This equation commonly is named after Budinger.[45]

These equations serve as a good starting point; however, they do not specify what the pixel size is, they exclude attenuation and the shape and size of a region, they make the assumption that the noise on a projection is constant, and in any case they are only appropriate at the center of an object. Many of these points have been addressed by Alpert et al.,[45] who suggest the following modification to obtain the variance at a point x,y

$$\text{VAR}(x,y) = k \iint p(\xi,\theta)\, A(\xi,\theta)^2\, h^2(\xi' - \xi)^2\, d\xi\, d\theta \qquad (59)$$

where $p(\xi,\theta)$ are the projection values, $A(\xi,\theta)$ is the attenuation correction, h is the reconstruction filter, and k is a constant.

It is important to remember that the signal-to-noise ratio in tomography is considerably worse than conventional imaging (with Poisson-distributed values) for the same number of counts, as illustrated in Figure 9, and is not white but filter shaped, as illustrated in Figure 10. Thus, the tomographic process is a high frequency noise amplifier.

An approximate rule of thumb is that to obtain the same statistical accuracy (signal-to-noise ratio) in tomography, about five times as many counts need to be collected as for a conventional image. In fact, considering that further degradation of the signal to noise ratio will occur as a result of attenuation correction, etc., probably even more counts need to be collected. SPECT in particular is very photon-limited.

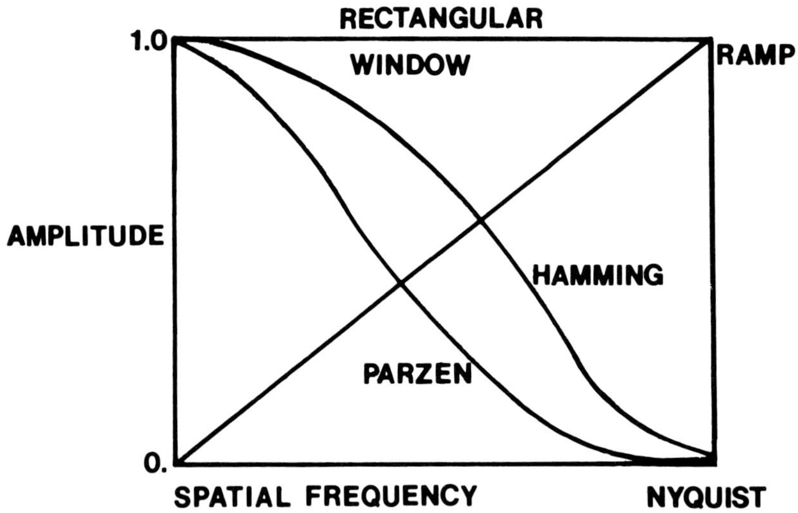

FIGURE 8. Plots of different window functions showing amplitude as a function of spatial frequency from zero up to the Nyquist frequency.

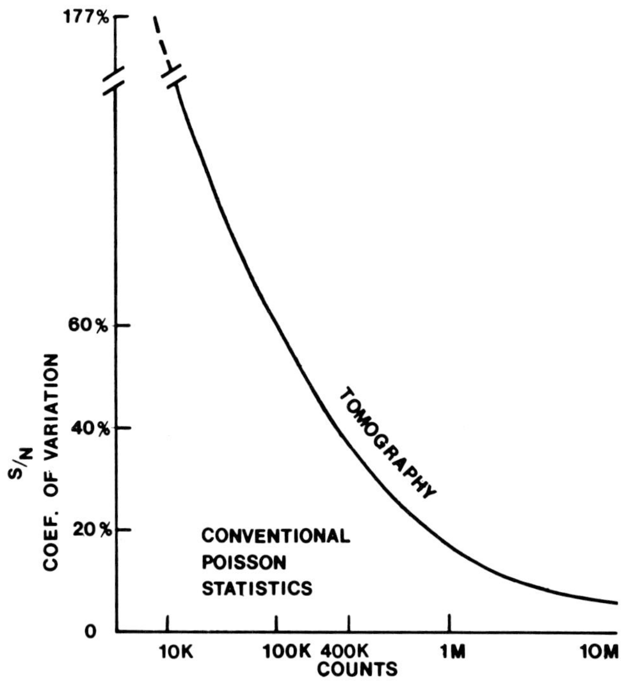

FIGURE 9. A graph of signal-to-noise ratio, expressed as the coefficient of variation in percent as a function of the number of counts collected in a slice for an object occupying 1000 pixels. The equivalent value for a conventional planar image is also plotted.

An alternative approach which can improve the signal-to-noise ratio considerably in certain applications is, instead of reconstructing the data and then estimating sums of pixels within certain regions of interest, to estimate the value of the integral of the image within the region of interest directly from the projections without reconstruction.[46] The effect of this is to manipulate the ''noise color''.

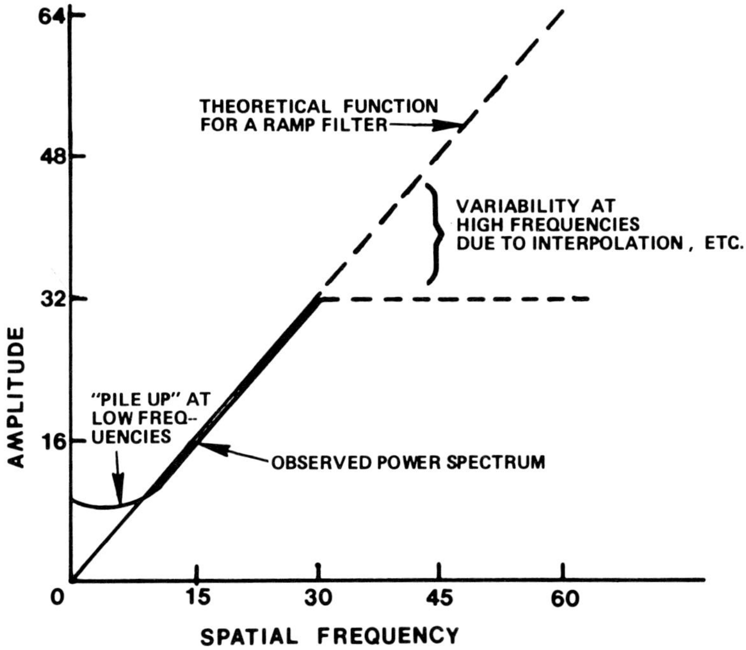

FIGURE 10. The noise power shown as a function of frequency, indicating that the noise power spectrum is filter function in shape.

C. Interpolation

When performing the backprojection, two basic and distinct algorithms are normally employed. The first, described above, may be called projection-driven. Each point on the projection line is placed with an appropriate weight into pixels along the ray line. The second commonly used algorithm is termed "pixel driven". Here, the algorithm proceeds as follows.

```
For each angle θ and PROJECTION line DO [
  FOR each pixel (I,J) in the IMAGE DO [
  CALCULATE K the distance from the pixel to the
    perpendicular from the projection to the axis of
    rotation;
    IMAGE (I,J): = IMAGE (I,J) + PROJECTION (K,θ)
  ]]
```

This has a considerable advantage over the projection-driven approach in that no weights dependent on position or angle need to be computed. The distance K is real, however, while the data on the projection line are discrete. Therefore, some method of matching the two is required. This generally is termed the interpolation problem.

The two simplest solutions are called the nearest-neighbor algorithm and the linear interpolation algorithm. For the former, the real value K is rounded to the nearest integer value and the corresponding element of data on the projection is used. The latter simply interpolates linearly between the two elements of data on the projection corresponding to the integer value below and above the computed value of K. These two approaches are illustrated in Figure 11. More complex interpolation schemes, for example, exponentially weighted sums and interpolation between angles, also have been used.[47,48] The reason for taking care in this area is that this interpolation is in fact a filtering operation acting on the high frequencies. The nearest neighbor algorithm is equivalent to a SINC window, while linear interpolation is equivalent to a $SINC^2$ window.

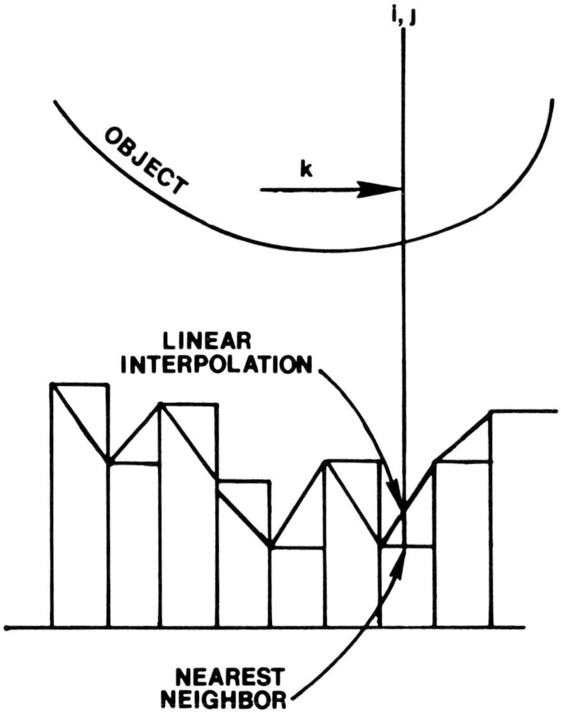

FIGURE 11. A diagram indicating the need for interpolation in tomographic reconstruction. For a point i,j in the reconstructed plane a value on the projection line must be found which will not normally fall exactly on a projection point. Two common algorithms are employed to choose the value to use in the reconstruction, indicated here as linear interpolation and nearest neighbor.

D. Pre- and Postprocessing Filters

The basic windowing filters suggested above are preprocessing filters. They are applied to the projections in 1-D before reconstruction. Since the filtering operation is linear, however, they may be equally well applied in 2-D to the same data after reconstruction. In this case they may be called postprocessing filters. Computationally, there is an advantage to their use as preprocessors; however, there may be an advantage to using them as postprocessing filters if the data are required to be reconstructed many times with different filters.

Other operations have been performed both before and after reconstruction. Median filters serve to reduce noise but in a nonlinear manner. The basic median filter applied to the projection data is expressed as

$$p'(\xi,\theta) = \text{Median}\ |p(k,\theta)|\begin{matrix} k = \xi + k' \\ k = \xi - k' \end{matrix} \tag{60}$$

where k′ defines the window to be used. A typical value is 2, the median being determined over a group of 5 values. The median filter can be applied also in 2-D before and after reconstruction.

When 2-D filters are applied as preprocessors, they may be applied such that the two dimensions correspond to x and y in a projection image, that is, a projection image comprised of data from many slices obtained for a single unique value of θ. Alternatively they may be applied in x (along the projection line) and θ, using projections from neighboring angles.

When such filters are used as postprocessors, they may be applied in 3-D to the complete 3-D set of reconstructions. There appear to be considerable gains in doing this, notably in terms of reducing the overall signal to noise ratio compared to 2-D filtering (equivalent to 1-D preprocessing).

VI. OTHER RECONSTRUCTION METHODS

A number of other reconstruction methods are also becoming of increasing importance, now that hardware suitable for implementing the corresponding algorithms is becoming available.

A. Maximum Likelihood and Entropy

As before, let **p** be the set of the n observed projection values and let **f** be the set of m values of the image which we are trying to reconstruct. We can reduce the problem from a two-dimensional problem to a one-dimensional problem simply by taking all the points i,j and turning it into a list of points m, and likewise taking the set of projection values ξ,θ and turning it into a list of points n. Now, let PROB (n,m) be the probability of detecting an event from m at a point n on a projection. Thus PROB (n,m) is a generalization of the system-response function. For a given point n, it represents the response function of the system for the set of values of m. Note that in general this matrix PROB (n,m) is very large, but sparse in that many elements are zero and repetitive since the transfer function does not change much with n.

One approach suggested by Shepp and Vardi[49] is to perform the iteration

$$f^{k+1}(m) = f^k(m) \sum_n \frac{p(n)\ \mathrm{PROB}(n,m)}{\sum_{m'} f^k(m')\ \mathrm{PROB}(n,m')} \tag{61}$$

which they stated to be a maximum likelihood estimator of $\hat{\mathbf{f}}$ (m), the "true" solution, from the observations p (n) (see also Reference 50).

The basic formulation of the maximum entropy approach[51] is that:

$$p(n) = \sum_m [\mathrm{PROB}(n,m)\ f(m)] + \mathrm{noise}(n) \tag{62}$$

Thus, if a solution $\hat{\mathbf{f}}$ exists, we would like to minimize the difference between p and $\mathbf{PROB.f}^k$ (which will be called **p′**), where $\mathbf{f}^f$ is the kth estimate. Again iterative algorithms may be chosen, the best known of which is Minerbo's.[52] Kemp and Skilling[34] have worked on such a method using a χ-square statistic, which is essentially the same as that previously described, replacing the forward projection operator by the more general function **PROB** to give

$$\chi^2 = \sum_n \left[\left(\sum_m [\mathrm{PROB}(n,m)\ f^k(m)] - p(n) \right) / \mathrm{VAR}(n) \right] \tag{63}$$

where VAR(n) is the estimate of the variance of **p′** at the point n. The desired solution will minimize this statistic or rather reduce it below some threshold. Many such solutions will exist. The solution actually chosen is suggested as that which has maximum entropy, or maximizes H such that

$$H = -\Sigma[\mathrm{pr}(m) \log \mathrm{pr}(m)] \tag{64}$$

$$\mathrm{pr}(m) = f(m)/\sum_m f(m) \tag{65}$$

It should be noted, however, that some authors have maximized only Σ log pr(m).

Some satisfying results have been published for all these techniques. In particular, the maximum entropy images from a single-slice ring system have shown striking improvement over conventional filtered backprojection reconstruction, since such a reconstruction process is less sensitive to errors caused by the angular undersampling of such systems.

The strength of these types of techniques is their use of a spatially varying function PROB(m,n) incorporating variations in sensitivity and resolution as a function of distance from the detector. Such methods will also tend to be more stable in the presence of noise and undersampling. Their major drawback is the considerable computation involved and the lack of any mathematical certainty (as far as the author is aware at present) as to their convergence. Various other linear programming techniques could be used.

This is by no means a complete review of all possible methods for reconstructing an image. Decomposition into suitable polynomials[53,55] is an alternative but associated technique. Likewise, it is suggested[47] that there may be better ways of combining sample from different angles. Reference 23 is recommended for further specialized reading.

B. Steepest Descent and Conjugate Gradient Algorithms

In general, there is a class of algorithms which attempts to minimize the χ^2 statistic described previously. One additional factor that may be used to improve convergence is the so-called "direction" and amplitude of the iterative step, that is, which values are to be changed and by how much, in each step of the iterative process

$$f^{n+1} = f^n + a_n d^n \tag{66}$$

where $\mathbf{f}^n$ is the nth estimate of the object $\mathbf{f}$, $\mathbf{d}^n$ is the direction of the nth step, and $\mathbf{a}_n$ is a suitable factor (set of weights). We would like to minimize the value of χ^2 (n + 1), the value of the χ squared statistic after the iteration. Thus, it is suggested that the derivative of $\chi^2(n+1)$, with respect to $\mathbf{a}_n$, be set to zero and that we solve for $\mathbf{a}_n$. The solution given by Huesman et al.[26] is

$$\mathbf{a}_n = (\mathbf{d}^n \cdot \alpha^n)/(\mathbf{d}^n + d\,\mathbf{M}\mathbf{d}^n) \tag{67}$$

where $\mathbf{M}$ is a matrix such that the i,jth element is given by

$$M(i,j) = \sum_k [PROB(k,i)\ PROB(k,j)/Var(k)] \tag{68}$$

where PROB(i,j) is the fraction of events at position j that is mapped onto the projection at position i, essentially as discussed in Section VI.A. The vector $\boldsymbol{\alpha}^n$ is proportional to the gradient of $\boldsymbol{\chi}^2(\mathbf{n})$, such that

$$\boldsymbol{\alpha}^n = \mathbf{v} - \mathbf{M}\,\mathbf{f}^n \tag{69}$$

where

$$v(i) = \sum_k [(PROB(k,i)\ p(k))/Var(k)] \tag{70}$$

In the method of steepest descent, the step direction is chosen as that direction in which $\chi^2(n)$ decreases most rapidly, e.g., $\mathbf{d}^n = \boldsymbol{\alpha}^n$. In the conjugate gradient method,[57] the step direction is chosen for step n so that it is forced to be orthogonal to all previous steps, where the first step is chosen as for the steepest gradient. Thus,

$$d^n = \alpha^n - b_n d^{n-1} \tag{71}$$

where $\mathbf{b_n}$ is a function chosen to assure orthogonality of successive steps. A discussion on convergence is given in Reference 58.

C. Regularization

Consider the solution of the familiar equation

$$A x = y \tag{72}$$

Regularization may be considered to be the finding of a suitable value of a positive numerical parameter α and the identity operator **E** where

$$\begin{aligned}(A + \alpha \mathbf{E})\mathbf{x} &= \mathbf{A\ x} + \alpha\ \mathbf{x} \\ &= \mathbf{y}\end{aligned} \tag{73}$$

where α is a positive numerical parameter, such that

$$\mathbf{x}_\alpha = (\mathbf{A} + \alpha\ \mathbf{E})^{-1}\ \mathbf{y} \tag{74}$$

is an approximate but well-posed solution of the previous equation.

There is extensive literature on the subject, see for example Tikhonov and Arsenin,[30] Bertero,[31] and Groetsch,[59] among others. In simplistic terms, the idea of regularization is that, instead of trying to find a solution using $\mathbf{A}^{-1}$ directly which will be unstable, we transform the problem, finding the solution for a smaller but more stable function $(\mathbf{A} + \alpha\ \mathbf{E})^{-1}$. This normally implies multiplication by a regularizing function which may be thought of crudely as a multiplication by a "window" function. It should be noted that in such methods the spectrum of singular values gives an idea of the stability of the process, and can be controlled by a suitable choice of α and **E**. For a more detailed discussion of the method, see the references previously cited. It must be stressed that such methods are of considerable practical importance, particularly as the reconstruction problem becomes more ill-posed (for example, in limited angle tomography).

VII. ATTENUATION CORRECTION IN ECT

Attenuation correction is a rather complex area in reconstruction algorithms and is still the subject of considerable research. It is essential, if any reconstructed data are to be quantitated in ECT, otherwise considerable errors in the estimations of activity/unit volume will be made. The basic variants in the different methods employed are those of preprocessing, those based on some analytical modification of the reconstruction process (here called inverse attenuated radon transform methods), modifications of iterative processes, and postprocessing corrections.

All such techniques must be considered first from the mathematical point of view, that is, what underlying assumptions have been made, and then from a practical point of view, that is, do they accurately represent the physical situation?, do they work?, how fast are they?, etc.

A. Preprocessing

The basic widely used preprocessing method for attenuation correction is to form some combination of opposed views, for example, the geometrical mean.[19] The arithmetic mean of opposed views is equivalent and identical to performing a normal reconstruction over

360° without attenuation correction. The use of the geometrical mean does have the apparent affect of reducing the observed attenuation of a point source in scattering material as a function of depth. It also introduces artefacts, however (as a result of ill-behaved cross-product terms). Neither method corrects properly for attenuation.

It is sometimes possible to measure the attenuation through the object to be reconstructed by using an external source and measuring a correction term

$$C(\xi,\theta) = \exp\left(-\int_{L(\xi,\theta)} \mu_{L'}\, dL'\right) \tag{75}$$

for every path $L(\xi,\theta)$, for every projection point ξ,θ where $\mu_{L'}$ is the linear attenuation coefficient at a point L′ on that path. This correction term also may be calculated from a knowledge of the contour of the object and assuming some value for μ. Thus, a corrected projection $p'(\xi,\theta)$ may be obtained

$$p'(\xi,\theta) = p(\xi,\theta)/C(\xi,\theta) \tag{76}$$

Unfortunately, this technique does not correct for attenuation except for sources of uniform activity.

When an implicit assumption is made that the object is uniformly distributed within the attenuating material and assuming a constant value for the attenuation coefficient μ, another preprocessing correction factor which has been widely employed[9] (or slightly modified[60]) is

$$p'(\xi,\theta) = \frac{p_g(\xi,\theta)\ \mu\ L(\xi,\theta)}{[1 - \exp(-(\mu\ L(\xi,\theta))]} \tag{77}$$

where $p_g(\xi,\theta)$ refers to the geometric mean,

$$p_g(\xi,\theta) = [p(\xi,\theta)^2 + p(\xi,\theta+\pi)^2]^{1/2} \tag{78}$$

and $L(\xi,\theta)$ is the length of the projection ray through the object for the point ξ,θ on the projection.

Again, this technique does not correct for attenuation except for sources of uniform activity and constant μ. The errors can be quite considerable for real objects.

B. Attenuated Inverse Radon Transform

The attenuated inverse Radon transform has been described by several groups, notably Gullberg[61] and Bellini.[62] The basic operation (following Bellini) may be divided into a number of steps.

Basically, Bellini suggests using a change of variables from the conventional polar coordinates r,θ into the variables r',θ' given by

$$r' = (r^2 + \mu^2/4\pi^2)^{1/2} \tag{79}$$

and

$$\theta' = \theta + i \sinh^{-1}(\mu/2\pi R) \tag{80}$$

where R is a constant.

Only after this transformation is the central-slice theory true for the attenuated data. This operation has thus been suggested as a preprocessing method before conventional filtered

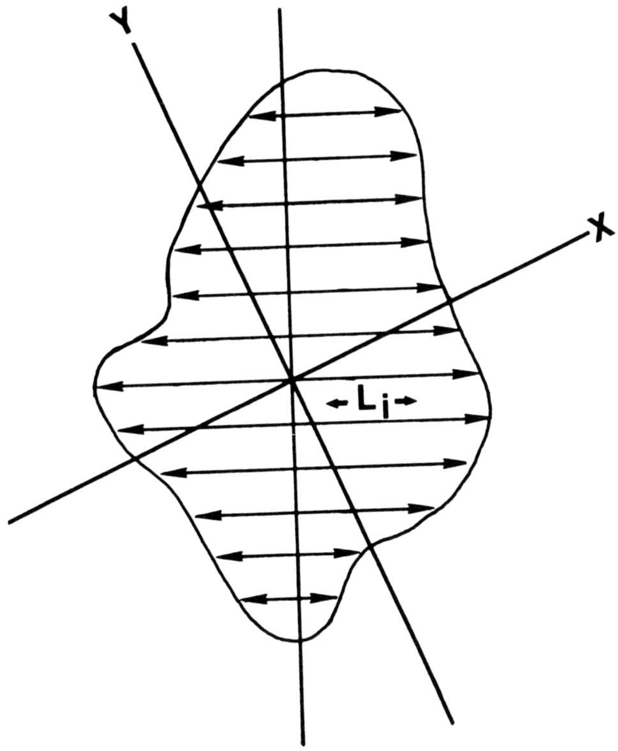

FIGURE 12. The initial correction used in the Bellini/Gullberg attenuation correction, using the path lengths through the object at various angles θ, in order to recenter to reconstruction in the Radon domain.

backprojection. The first step for performing this can be thought of as a recentering of the Radon transform domain and requires a multiplication by a set of coefficients exp $[\mu L(\xi,\theta)]$ as shown in Figure 12. This is followed by taking the arithmetic mean of opposed projections and obtaining the Fourier transform of the sum. The third step is to perform a frequency shift by replacing r by r′ as defined above, and an angular rotation replacing θ by θ′. This calculation requires appropriate interpolation. Note also that this transformation is dependent on the value of μ, here assumed to be constant.

Gullberg has treated the process as a recentering and has illustrated the coordinate transformation as a modification of the basic ramp reconstruction filter, effectively truncating the low frequencies (see also Reference 63).

C. Postprocessing Correction

The simplest of the postprocessing methods is the so-called Chang technique.[64] As illustrated in Figure 13, for a given point i,j within the object a series of lines of length L(θ,i,j) can be defined between the point and the edge of the object. For a constant value of μ, a correction factor C(i,j) can be defined as

$$C(i,j) = K \sum_{\theta} \exp(\mu\ L(\theta,i,j)) \tag{81}$$

where K is a suitable scaling factor which can be determined afterward (e.g., a fudge factor). This method seems to work surprisingly well. It can be modified to work with variable μ, and can be iterated. The sampling of the angles may be quite coarse, but different sampling methods can cause subtle variations in the accuracy of the results.

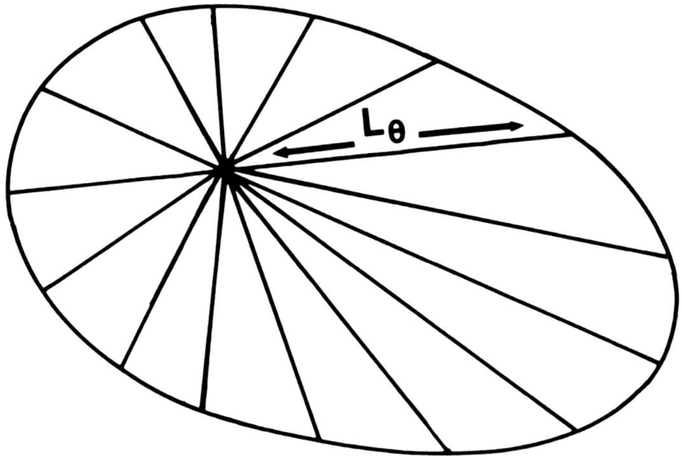

FIGURE 13. As illustrated diagrammatically here, the Chang attenuation correction algorithm uses the weighted sum of attenuation estimates at equal angular increments for each point in the reconstructed object.

D. Iterative Methods

Let us create a forward projection operator $\mathbf{F}_a$ which includes in the weights associated with each pixel a term estimating attenuation, for example, exp ($\mu L(i,j,\theta)$) where $L(i,j,\theta)$ is the distance from the pixel i,j to the edge of the object at angle θ. Supposed to have been constant, μ could also be variable. A relatively simple iterative procedure can be imagined such that the attenuated forward-projection operator is substituted in the normal ART type of iterative reconstruction.[65] Since the observed projections are attenuated, if the estimation of attenuation included in $\mathbf{F}_a$ is correct, the solution should be the object without attenuation. This simple iterative technique usually is modified by changing the backprojection operator such that it too incorporates weights associated with attenuation such that the error terms are backprojected with increased weight associated with nearer values. This same process can be included into a variety of other, more complex iterative procedures, notably those of the form of the steepest descent or conjugate gradient described previously.

The problem with such methods is establishing convergence since the inclusion of the exponential-type weighting factors make instability much greater. Such methods then usually are relaxed by incorporation of a suitable relaxation weight, λ, to reduce the speed of convergence and reduce the likelihood of oscillation. The use of more powerful stabilization methods such as regularization is likely to be of considerable help[66] in this type of iterative approach.

An alternative approach has been proposed[68] which attempts to reconstruct both emission and attenuation as single processes. Such a method might likely require a very high signal-to-noise ratio since this problem is much more unstable (ill-posed) than for emission alone.

E. Scatter Correction

Applying attenuation correction using the attenuation coefficient determined for narrow-beam (idealized) measurements directly to SPECT data is invalid without performing a scatter correction.[69] For this reason, attenuation correction normally is employed using lower values for μ than normally found in the literature in order to compensate for scatter. For example, a value of 0.12 cm^{-1} for μ for ^{99m}Tc normally is found to be more appropriate rather than the narrow-beam value of 0.15 cm^{-1}. However, it is likely that attenuation is object-dependent and any attenuation correction procedure which does not take this into account may well result in considerable error.[70]

The complete analytical form of the inverse problem, including scatter, attenuation, and spatially variable response function, is highly unwieldy.[71] One approach[69] is to adopt the following simplification. Let the point-spread function at an energy i be called PSF_i, such that at the photopeak (principal gamma-photon energy) we may observe PSF_p, and at the Compton window we may observe PSF_c. It is thus possible to define a general filtering operation as:

$$p'(\xi,\theta) = \sum_j p_j(x,\theta) * FILT_j \tag{82}$$

where $p_j(x,\theta)$ is the projection data acquired at the jth window, $FILT_j$ is some corresponding filter function, and * indicates a convolution. The operation can be extended into two dimensions, filtering the whole of the acquired projection image.

While it is not possible to achieve complete stationarity since various approximations have been made, we would like to choose the values of $FILT_j$ such that the resulting PSF′ after filtering is, to a first approximation, object-independent. The aim of such scatter-correction technique, therefore, is not to eliminate scatter completely, but to reduce it considerably. The PSFs for the various energy windows can be established both from a model and from experimental measurements. One estimate of $FILT_j$ is

$$FILT_j = \mathbf{F}^{-1} \{\mathbf{F}\{PSE_p(\xi)\}/\mathbf{F}\{PSE_n j(\xi)\}\} \tag{83}$$

where **F**{ } and $\mathbf{F}^{-1}${ } represent the Fourier and inverse Fourier transforms. The corrected PSF is then an estimate of the PSF of the unscattered events alone in the photopeak window. The next problem is to estimate a suitable overall weighting function (i.e., integral of the filter). This seems best performed by using a model.

F. Models

Monte Carlo simulations have been used by a number of authors, for example by O Ying Lie,[71] who simulated a point source in the center of a circularly symmetrical attenuating medium. From such data it has been found that the PSF of a system can be modeled as the sum of two Gaussian functions:

$$PSE(x) = C1 \exp(-C2\, x^2) + C3 \exp(-C4\, x^2) \tag{84}$$

where C1 to C4 are constants which depend on the energy window, collimator response function, the activity distribution, and attenuation. It may also be observed that there is a considerable difference between the PSF obtained for single scattered events and for multiple scattered events. In the latter case, the PSF is very flat, and a simple background subtraction should suffice as a correction technique. In particular, O Ying Lie found that the PSF for the photopeak energy was found to have a "narrow" component where C1 and C2 were object-independent and a "broad" component where C3 and C4 were object-dependent. Note that the effects of scatter in a projection are essentially a linear summation of scattered and unscattered events.

G. Inverse Monte Carlo Methods

Inverse Monte Carlo[72] (as it has been called) is a general technique which may be used for a number of inverse problems. Workers at Duke University in North Carolina have developed Monte Carlo-based reconstruction techniques incorporating attenuation and scatter correction.[73,74] As usual, we must to solve for f(m) in

$$p(n) = \sum_{m} [PROB(n,m)\ f(m)] + noise(n) \qquad (85)$$

which may be performed by a variety of methods, for example, using the EM (maximum likelihood) algorithm. One problem with such a method is establishing values for PROB(n,m). Floyd et al.[73] have described a Monte Carlo technique which may be used. For a given point m, solutions of the transport equations with appropriate boundary conditions may be implemented using Monte Carlo methods, that is, by following individual events on a probabilistic basis. Thus, effectively a point source is simulated in a scattering medium of known form (e.g., the patient) and the response at all projection points n may be determined. Repeating this procedure for all points m within the object then fully determines PROB(n,m), after which knowing **p** we can find **f** by conventional methods. This technique therefore includes both scatter and attenuation in the determination of the matrix **PROB** and the solution therefore should correct for these effects. Likewise, the effects of collimator PSF also can be incorporated; however, the technique assumes that the boundary conditions, that is, the distribution of tissue, are accurately known. Initial results are very promising. A very interesting observation is that, with scatter, the matrix **PROB** is no longer very sparse.

Estimation of the effect of the point spread function itself on sampling is another important area to correct for the apparent loss of signal with decreasing object size.[38] This effect should be distinguished from the so-called ''partial volume'' effect, where the apparent signal is reduced when the object is smaller in thickness than the slice width.

VIII. 3-D RECONSTRUCTION

The forms discussed above can be extended into 3-D with some additional complexity. By this is meant the idea of using angles other than those parallel to the transverse axial plane, data which are normally either not available (with, for example, a parallel hole collimator) or are discarded (for example, with many positron systems).

In many ways 3-D reconstruction can be considered as a simple extension of 2-D reconstruction but with some significant gains in performance and costs in terms of difficulty. The generalized inverse may be stated simply in 3-D. The result is a very sparse matrix and theoretically could be solved. Likewise, the inverse Radon transform can be extended into 3-D (and higher dimensions) where it normally is called the inverse X-ray transform; however, practical numerical solutions are required.

The simplest practical approach to this problem has been presented by Gullberg.[75] Reconstruction using conventional filtered backprojection is performed, as before, slice by slice; however, a noise reducing filtering operation is performed in 3-D by using a filter which resembles a sphere in 3-D Fourier space. This approach is said to give an improved signal-to-noise ratio (by a factor of about 1.3) by comparison with the equivalent 2-D method.

Information, however, at angles other than parallel to the transverse plane can be included directly in the reconstruction method by extending fan beam methods to include cone beam. A direct approach utilizing the sparsity of the matrix has been tried by Altschuler.[76] Cone beam methods are described in References 77 and 78, among others. Cho et al.[79] have attempted to generalize the problem to the extent of using all possible oblique angles. It should be recalled that here again a limited angle problem is found in that complete spherical sampling is not available. Methods appropriate for conventional single-plane, limited-angle tomography can be extended into three dimensions, noting that great care to stabilize the algorithm, for example, by using regularizing methods, needs to be employed; however, in some respects, the kernel of the integral equation in 3-D is better behaved than in 2-D and direct 3-D reconstruction methods have distinct advantages with respect to the quality of the reconstruction, although requiring greater computational resources. Such methods are also important when using collimators other than parallel hole, for example, cone beam and fan beam collimators.

IX. SUMMARY AND CONCLUSIONS

Various methods for reconstructing tomographic data have been presented, ranging from the simple methods, such as ART, to the more complex methods, such as the use of the inverse attenuated Radon transform and the inverse Monte Carlo method. In SPECT, a basic problem is the need to incorporate scatter and attenuation. Iterative schemes are basically more attractive for SPECT and to some extent PET since such effects can be incorporated within them. Such iterative methods are, however, much slower than direct analytical methods. To date such sophisticated methods have been little employed, as a result of the time required, and almost all data have been evaluated on a qualitative basis rather than from a quantitative point of view. While distorted data can be used and made to give reliable clinical information, possibly with some considerable sacrifice in accuracy, it may be that the full potential of SPECT can be realized only via the use of computers of sufficient power to implement better algorithms. It must be noted also that, since such algorithms require input data of good quality (where artefacts are absent), much greater care must be taken to ensure the reliability of such data. While such methods are standard in, for example, NMR, it remains to be proven that the increase in accuracy of the reconstruction in SPECT is clinically worth the extra cost.

REFERENCES

1. **Cormack, A. M.,** Representation of a function by its integrals with some radiological applications, *J. Appl. Phys.*, 34, 2722, 1963.
2. **Hounsfield, G. N.,** A Method of and Apparatus for Examination of a Body by Radiation such as X or Gamma Radiation, The Patent Office, London, Patent Spec. 1283915, 1972.
3. **Korenblyum, B. I., Tetel'baum, S. I., and Tyutin, A. A.,** About one scheme of tomography, *Bull. Inst. Higher Ed. Radiophys. (Gorky University),* 1 (3), 151, 1958.
4. **Lauterbur, P. C.,** Image formation by induced local interactions: examples employing nuclear magnetic resonance, *Nature,* 242, 190, 1973.
5. **Kumar, A., Welti, D., and Ernst, R.,** NMR Fourier zeugmatography, *J. Magn. Reson.*, 18, 69, 1975.
6. **Price, L. R.,** Electrical impedance computed tomography (ICT): a new CT imaging technique, *IEEE Trans. Nucl. Sci.*, NS-26, 2736, 1979.
7. **Greenleaf, J. F., Johnson, S. A., Lee, S. L., Herman, G. T., and Wood, E. M.,** Algebraic reconstruction of spatial distributions of acoustic absorption within tissue from their two-dimensional acoustic projections, *Acous. Hologr.*, 5, 591, 1974.
8. **Kuhl, D. E. and Edwards, R. Q.,** Image separation radioisotope scanning, *Radiology,* 80, 653, 1963.
9. **Larsson, S. A.,** Gamma camera emission tomography — development and properties of a multi-sectional emission computed tomography system, *Acta Radiol. Suppl.*, 363, 1980.
10. **Kuhl, D. E., Edwards, R. Q., Ricci, A. R., and Reivich, M.,** Quantitative section scanning using orthogonal tangent correction, *J. Nucl. Med.*, 14, 196, 1973.
11. **Moore, S. C., Brunelle, J. A., and Kirsch, C. M.,** Quantitative multi-detector emission computerized tomography using iterative compensation, *J. Nucl. Med.*, 23, 706, 1982.
12. **Ter-Pogossian, M. M., Mullani, N. A., Ficke, D. C., Markam, J., and Snyder, D. L.,** Photon time-of-flight positron emission tomography, *J. Comput. Assist. Tomogr.*, 5, 227, 1981.
13. **Tomitani, T.,** Image reconstruction and noise evaluation in photon time-of-flight assisted positron emission tomography, *IEEE Trans. Nucl. Sci.*, NS-28, 4582, 1981.
14. **Bracewell, R. N. and Riddle, A. C.,** Inversion of fan-beam scans in radio astronomy, *Astrophys. J.*, 150, 427, 1967.
15. **Gordon, R., Bender, R., and Herman, G. T.,** Algebraic reconstruction techniques (ART) for three-dimensional electron microscopy pictures and x-ray photography, *J. Theor. Biol.*, 29, 471, 1970.
16. **Crowther, R. A., DeRosier, D. J., and Klug, A.,** The reconstruction of a three-dimensional structure from projections and its application to electron microscopy, *Proc. R. Soc. London, Ser. A:,* 317, 319, 1970.
17. **Gilbert, P. F. C.,** The reconstruction of a three dimensional object from its projections and its application to electron microscopy II, direct methods, *Proc. R. Soc. London Ser. B:,* 182, 89, 1972.

18. **Brooks, R. A. and Di Chiro, G.,** Principles of computer assisted tomography (CAT) in radiographic and radioisotope imaging, *Phys. Med. Biol.,* 5, 689, 1976.
19. **Snyder, D. L. and Cox, J. R., Jr.,** An Overview of Reconstructive Tomography and Limitations Imposed by a Finite Number of Projections, in Reconstruction Tomography in Diagnostic Radiology and Nuclear Medicine, Ter-Pogossian, M. M., Phelps, M. E., Brownell, G. L., et al, Eds., Johns Hopkins University Press, Baltimore, 1977, 3.
20. **Budinger, T. F., Gullberg, G. T., and Huesman, R. H.,** *Emission Computed Tomography, in Image Reconstruction from Projections: Implementation and Applications,* Herman, G. T., Ed., Springer-Verlag, New York, 1979, 147.
21. **Youla, D. C. and Webb, H.,** Image restoration by the method of convex projections: part I - theory, *IEEE Trans.,* MI-1, 81, 1982.
22. **Herman, G. T. and Natterer F., Eds.,** *Mathematical Aspects of Computed Tomography, Lecture Notes in Medical Informatics,* 8, Springer-Verlag, Berlin, 1981.
23. **Barrett, H. H.,** The Radon transform and its applications, in *Progress on Optics XXI,* Wolf, E., Ed., Elsevier, Amsterdam, 1984, 218.
24. **Deans, S. R.,** *The Radon Transform and Some of its Applications,* John Wiley & Sons, New York, 1983.
25. **Herman, G. T. and Naparstek, A.,** Fast image reconstruction based on a Radon inversion formula appropriate for rapidly collected data, SIAM *J. Appl. Math.,* 33, 511, 1977.
26. **Huesman, R. H., Gullberg, G. T., Greenberg, W. L., and Budinger, T. F.,** RECLBL Library Users Manual — Donner Algorithms for Reconstruction Tomography, Rep. No. PUB-214, Lawrence-Berkeley Lab, University of California, 1977.
27. **Gordon, R. and Herman, G. T.,** Three dimensional reconstruction from projections: a review of algorithms, *Int. Rev. Cytol.,* 38, 111, 1974.
28. **Radon, J.,** Uber die Bestimmung von Funktionen durch ihre Integralwarte langs Gewisser Mannigfaltigkeiten, *Ber. Saechsisch Akad. Wiss.,* 69, 262, 1917.
29. **Ben-Israel A. and Greville, T. N. E.,** *Generalized Inverses — Theory and Applications,* John Wiley & Sons, New York, 1974.
30. **Tikhonov, A. N. and Arsenin, V. Y.,** Solutions to ill-posed problems, Winston VH, Washington, D.C., 1977.
31. **Bertero, M. and Dovi, V.,** Regularized and positive-constrained inverse methods in the problem of object restoration, *Opt. Acta,* 28, 1635, 1981.
32. **Gordon, R.,** A tutorial on ART (Algebraic Reconstruction Techniques), *IEEE Trans,* NS-21, 78, 1974.
33. **Schmidlin, P.,** Iterative separation of sections in tomographic scintigrams, *Nucl. Med. (Stuttgart),* 11, 1, 1972.
34. **Kemp, M. S. and Skilling, J.,** Image reconstruction by maximum entropy. *Proc. IEEE,* 6, 63, 1982.
35. **Baker, C. T. H. and Miller, G. F., Eds.,** *Treatment of Integral Equations by Numerical Methods,* Academic Press, London, 1982.
36. **Gilbert, P.,** Iterative methods for the reconstruction of three-dimensional objects from projections, *J. Theor. Biol.,* 36, 105, 1972.
37. **Horn, B. K.,** Density reconstruction using arbitrary ray-sampling schemes, *Proc. IEEE,* 66, 551, 1978.
38. **Ying-Lie, O.,** A Single-Photon ECAT Reconstruction Procedure Based on a PSF Model, Ph.D. thesis, Delft University Press, Delft, The Netherlands, 1984.
39. **Smith, P. R., Peters, T. M., and Bates, R. H. T.,** Image reconstruction from finite numbers of projections, *J. Phys. A: Math., Nucl. Gen.,* 6, 361, 1973.
40. **Shepp, L. A. and Logan, B. F.,** The Fourier reconstruction of a head section, *IEEE Trans. Nucl. Sci.,* NS-21, 21, 1974.
41. **Ramachandran, G. N. and Lakshminarayanan, A. V.,** Three dimensional reconstruction from radiographs and electron micrographs: applications of convolutions instead of Fourier transforms, *Proc. Natl. Acad. Sci. U.S.A.,* 68, 2236, 1970.
42. **Hamming, R. W.,** *Digital Filters,* Prentice-Hall, Englewood Cliffs, NJ, 1977.
43. **Reiderer, S. J., Pelc, N. J., and Chesler, D. A.,** The noise power spectrum in computer x-ray tomography, *Phys. Med. Biol.,* 23, 446, 1978.
44. **Budinger, T. F., Derenzo, S. E., Greenberg, W. L., Gullberg, G. T., and Huesman, R. H.,** Quantitative potentials of dynamic emission computed tomography, *J. Nucl. Med.,* 19, 309, 1979.
45. **Alpert, N. M., Chesler, D. A., Correia, J. A., et al.,** Estimation of the local statistical error in emission computer tomography, *IEEE Trans.,* MI-1, 142, 1982.
46. **Huesman, R. H.,** A new fast algorithm for the evaluation of regions of interest and statistical uncertainty in computed tomography, *Phys. Med. Biol.,* 29, 543, 1984.
47. **Brooks, R. A., Weiss, G. H., and Talbert, A. J.,** A new approach to interpolation in computer tomography, *J. Comput. Assist. Tomogr.,* 2, 577, 1978.
48. **Mersereau, R. M.,** Recovering multidimensional signals from their projections, *Comput. Graph. Image Process.,* 2, 179, 1973.

49. **Shepp, L. A. and Vardi, Y.,** Maximum likelihood reconstruction for emission tomography, *IEEE Trans.*, MI-1, 113, 1982.
50. **Lange, K. and Carson, R.,** EM reconstruction algorithms for emission and transmission tomography, *J. Comput. Assist. Tomogr.*, 8, 306, 1982.
51. **Kemp, M. C.,** Maximum entropy reconstruction in emission tomography, in *Medical Radionuclide Imaging*, International Atomic Energy Association, Vienna, 1981, 313.
52. **Minerbo, G. N.,** Convolutional reconstruction from cone-beam projection data, *IEEE Trans.*, NS-26, 2682, 1979.
53. **Marr, R. B.,** On the reconstruction of a function on a circular domain from a sampling of its line integrals, *J. Math. Anal. Appl.*, 45, 357, 1974.
54. **Hansen, E. W.,** Theory of circular harmonic image reconstruction, *J. Opt. Soc. Am.*, 71, 304, 1981.
55. **Verly, J. G.,** Circular and extended circular harmonic transforms and their relevance to image reconstruction from line integrals, *J. Opt. Soc. Am.*, 71, 825, 1981.
56. **Keyes, W. I.,** The fan-beam gamma camera, *Phys. Med. Biol.*, 20, 489, 1975.
57. **Hestenes, M. R. and Stiefel E.,** Methods of conjugate gradients for solving linear systems, *J. Res. Natl. Bur. Standards Sect. B.*, 49, 409, 1952.
58. **Kammerer, W. J. and Nashed, M. Z.,** On the convergence of the conjugate gradient method for singular linear operator equations, *SIAM J. Numer. Anal.*, 9, 165, 1972.
59. **Groetsch, C. W.,** The theory of Tikhonov regularization for Fredholm equations of the first kinds in *Research Notes in Mathematics,* Pitman Publishing, Boston, 1984.
60. **Kay, D. B. and Keyes, J. W.,** First-order corrections for absorption and resolution compensation in radionuclide Fourier tomography, *J. Nucl. Med.*, 16, 540, 1975.
61. **Gullberg, G. T.,** The Attenuated Radon Transform: Theory and Application in Medicine and Biology, Ph.D. thesis, University of California, Berkeley, LB1-7486, 1979.
62. **Bellini, S., Piacentini, M., Cafforio, C., and Rocca, F.,** Compensation of tissue absorption in emission tomography, *IEEE Trans.*, ASSP-27, 213, 1979.
63. **Tretiak, O. J. and Metz, C. E.,** The exponential Radon transform, *SIAM J. Appl. Math.*, 39, 341, 1980.
64. **Chang, L. T.,** A method for attenuation correction in radionuclide tomography, *IEEE Trans.*, NS-25, 638, 1978.
65. **Walters, T. E., Simon, W., Chesler, D. A., and Correia, J. A.,** Attenuation correction in gamma emission computed tomography, *J. Comput. Assist. Tomogr.*, 5, 89, 1981.
66. **Soussaline, F. and Le Coq, G.,** A regularizing method for quantitative SPECT reconstruction, *IEEE Trans.*, MI-2, 24, 1983.
67. **Moore, S. C.,** Attenuation compensation, in *Computed Emission Tomography,* Ell, P. J. and Holman, B. L., Eds., 1982, chap. 11.
68. **Censor, Y., Gustafson, D. E., Lent, A., and Tuy, H.,** A new approach to the emission computerized tomography problem: simultaneous calculation of attenuation and activity coefficients, *IEEE Trans.*, NS-26, 2775, 1979.
69. **Todd-Pokropek, A., Clarke, G., and Marsh, R.,** Preprocessing of SPECT data as a precursor for attenuation correction, in *Information Processing in Medical Imaging,* Deconinck, F., Ed., Martinus Nijhoff, Boston, 1984, 130.
70. **Pang, S. C. and Genna, S.,** The effect of Compton scattered photons on emission computerized transaxial tomography, *IEEE Trans.*, NS-26, 2772, 1980.
71. **Dunn, W. L.,** Inverse Monte Carlo analysis. *J. Comput. Phys.*, 41, 154, 1981.
72. **Beck, J. W., Jaszczak, R. J., Coleman, R. E., Starmer, C. F., and Nolte, L. W.,** Analysis of SPECT including scatter and attenuation using sophisticated Monte Carlo modeling methods, *IEEE Trans.*, NS-29, 506, 1982.
73. **Floyd, C. E., Jaszczak, R. J., and Coleman, R. E.,** Inverse Monte Carlo: a unified reconstruction algorithm for SPECT, *IEEE Trans.*, NS-32, 779, 1985.
74. **Ying-Lie, O.,** An ECAT reconstruction method which corrects for attenuation and detector response, *IEEE Trans.*, NS-30, 632, 1983.
75. **Gullberg, G. T.,** True three-dimensional reconstruction in single photon emission computed tomography, *J. Nucl. Med.*, 24, 81, 1983.
76. **Altschuler, M. D. and Herman, G. T.,** Fully three-dimensional image reconstruction using series expansion methods, in Information Processing in Medical Imaging, ORNL/BCTIC-2, Oak Ridge National Laboratories, Oak Ridge, TN, 1977, 125.
77. **Nalcioglu, O. and Cho, Z. H.** Reconstruction of 3-D objects from cone-beam projections, *Proc. IEEE,* 66, 1584, 1978.
78. **Pelc, N. J. and Chesler, D. A.,** Utilization of cross-plane rays for three-dimensional reconstruction by filtered backprojection, *J. Comput. Assist. Tomogr.*, 3, 385, 1979.
79. **Cho, Z. H., Ra, J. B., and Hilal, S. K.,** True three-dimensional reconstruction- application of algorithm towards full utilization of oblique rays, *IEEE Trans. Med. Imaging,* MI-2, 6, 1983.

Chapter 3

COMPUTER AND HARDWARE REQUIREMENTS FOR SINGLE-PHOTON EMISSION COMPUTED TOMOGRAPHY (SPECT)

Michael King

TABLE OF CONTENTS

I. INTRODUCTION

In order to do computed tomography in nuclear medicine, one needs a computer with sufficient memory to hold the reconstruction software and slice being reconstructed, storage space for the acquisition data and reconstructed images, and a method of displaying the images. In addition, a set of analog-to-digital converters (ADCs) are needed to transfer data from the acquisition device(s) to the computer, and hardware may be required to control the motion of the detector(s). With appropriate software, all presently available nuclear medicine computer systems can reconstruct tomographic images. For best performance, however, a system may need tailoring to meet the demands of tomographic imaging.[1,2] This may mean the addition of more or faster memory, hardware for faster arithmetic computation, larger disk drives, improved image displays, or a better set of ADCs. The following sections discuss each of these various hardware components which may be required for improving the performance of a computer system used for tomography. In these discussions it is assumed that the reader is familiar with the basics of computers. A number of good sources exist for those who may wish a review of this material.[3-7]

II. CENTRAL PROCESSING UNIT (CPU)

The hardware portion of computer systems can be divided up into the CPU, which is the "brain" of the system and the peripheral devices such as terminals, disk drives, video displays, and ADCs. The latter collectively are called input and output devices and are linked with the CPU by bus cables as shown in Figure 1. The CPU itself can, in turn, be broken up into three functional units as shown in Figure 1: the control unit, the main memory, and the ALU.

A. Control Unit

The control unit is the portion of the CPU that transfers data and instructions, decodes instructions, and supervises the sequence of operations. The design and cycle time (speed of execution) of the control unit will influence the speed with which processing is carried out; the operating system (system software) and application software, however, will also affect program execution time.[4] Thus, comparing CPUs alone may be misleading.

The number of bits (binary digits) which can be handled by the registers (special temporary storage areas) and the bus of the control unit are called the word length. At one time, CPUs were classified as being either microcomputers, minicomputers, or mainframes, according to their word length. This distinction has since been lost and there are now, for instance, 32-bit microcomputers. The word length is important, however, because it determines the number of bits which can be moved along the bus in parallel at one time (i.e., the number of wires carrying data in the bus cable) and the amount of memory which can be directly addressed.

B. Main Memory

The main memory of a computer system is an integral part of the CPU. Its function is to provide "fast" storage for data and instructions. These are usually intermixed with only the current software able to decipher which is which. With each memory location (word) an address is associated by which the control unit can access the contents of that location.

There are a number of different types of memory.[3-7] The type which is typically used in tomographic computer systems is solid-state memory because it is inexpensive to manufacture. Solid-state memory can be either bipolar, which stores data in terms of voltage state, or metal oxide semiconductor (MOS), which uses the presence or absence of an electrical charge to store data. Solid-state memory is volatile, which means that its contents are lost when power is removed.

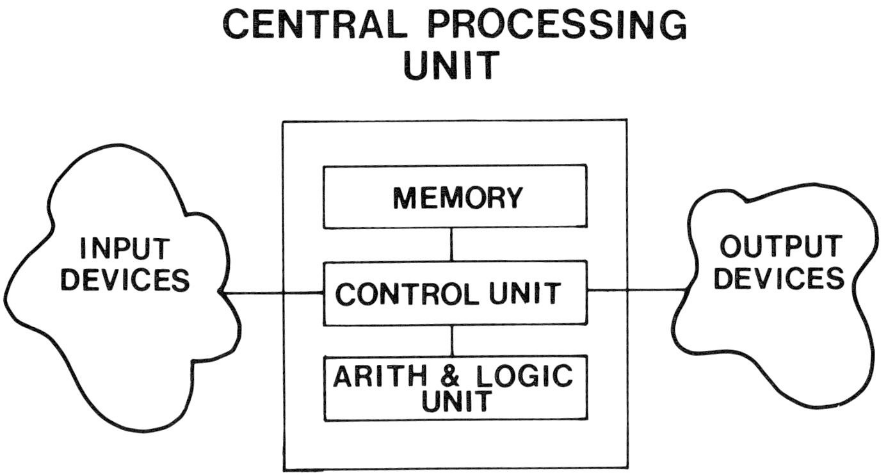

FIGURE 1. Block diagram showing major functional units of CPU. The presence of various input and output devices is also indicated.

To speed processing of tomographic studies, it may be desirable to add a special "very fast" auxillary memory device known as *cache memory*. Cache memory contains a duplicate copy of the data and instructions stored in a portion of main memory. Whenever information is requested from main memory, cache memory is also queried. If the information also resides in cache, then it will be returned faster than if it were only present in main memory. The problem is that only a portion of main memory is duplicated by cache memory since cache is much more expensive. Thus, the most frequently used contents of main memory should be stored in cache. This is done by copying the contents of any address of main memory, when referenced by the program, to cache unless it is already there. Thus, addresses which are frequently used stay in cache and those that are not are replaced by those more frequently addressed.

Tomographic image processing typically makes large demands on main memory. This is especially true if a system is desired which can do "simultaneous" acquisition and reconstruction. A 16-bit word length minicomputer is restricted to 32 k of byte mode, directly addressable, main memory. Either a longer word length processor, or a 16-bit CPU with a *memory management* or memory relocation unit should, therefore, be sought. Memory management allows the mapping of the 16-bit address used by the control unit into an 18- or 22-bit physical address for memory. Thus, the amount of physically addressable memory is increased. One is typically limited to working with 32 k word segments at any one time, and it requires time to generate these physical addresses, thereby increasing program execution time. These drawbacks are not present in a 32-bit CPU; hence, it appears likely that as their cost decreases they will become the standard CPUs of the future for medical imaging.

Another way to increase the apparent size of main memory is through the use of *virtual memory*. With this technique, information is stored on secondary storage and "swapped" into main memory, replacing part of the information contained there. Unlike using *overlaying*, where the programmer breaks the program into segments which can swap back and forth to disk, with virtual memory the programmer is "freed" from this task by having the system automatically break the program into segments. The problem with using virtual memory is that it can increase program execution time due to disk input/output (I/O).

C. Arithmetic and Logic Unit (ALU)

The ALU is the part of the CPU which performs all of the arithmetic and logical operations. In a standard nuclear medicine computer system this unit is designed to work with *integer*

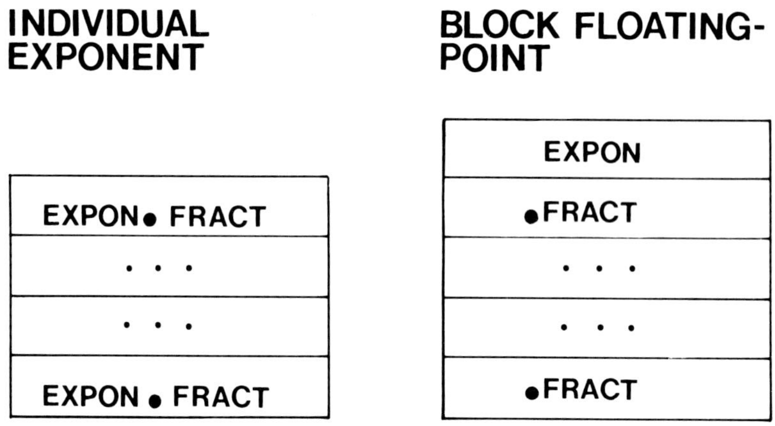

FIGURE 2. Individual exponent and block floating-point formats used to store floating-point numbers in an array processor as a combination of binary exponents (expon) and fractions (fract).

(whole number) data. The standard format for integer data is a two complement binary number 16 bits long which is the word length for most nuclear medicine systems.

In many cases, other than whole numbers are needed for calculations. *Floating-point* (for numbers with a decimal point) is used to represent numbers which may have a fractional part. These numbers are typically stored in two or four words of memory with a sign bit, followed by an exponent, and a binary fraction as illustrated in the left-hand format of Figure 2. Arithmetic and logical operations with such numbers are carried out with software when the standard ALU is used. Thus, several ''integer'' operations are required to carry out a single floating-point operation. This becomes a significant problem in image reconstruction because of the large number of the floating-point operations required. It is very desirable, therefore, to augment the ALU of a nuclear medicine computer system with special hardware to allow fast reconstruction.

III. SPECIAL ARITHMETIC HARDWARE

A. Floating Point ALU

The least expensive and most common special arithmetic hardware added to nuclear medicine computer systems is a *floating-point ALU*. This device is designed to carry out operations with the 32- to 64-bit representations of floating-point numbers which are commonly used. Because the operations are carried out by hardware instead of multiple software instructions, execution speed for floating-point operations can be enhanced significantly. For example, the time to reconstruct a 64 × 64 slice from 64 views is decreased from 1 min to about 15 s with the addition of floating-point hardware and appropriate software to a standard minicomputer.[2]

B. Array Processors

The other major type of special arithmetic hardware typically employed with emission tomographic systems is an *array processor*.[8-11] An array processor is a programmable high-speed arithmetic computation unit designed to be operated in conjunction with a general purpose computer. It is composed of a set of identical ALU pathways which operates synchronously under a common control unit. Array processors achieve their speed by using fast hardware in *parallel* so that a number of pieces of data can be processed at one time. There is usually also a *pipeline* structure to the ALU. That is, the ALU is partitioned into

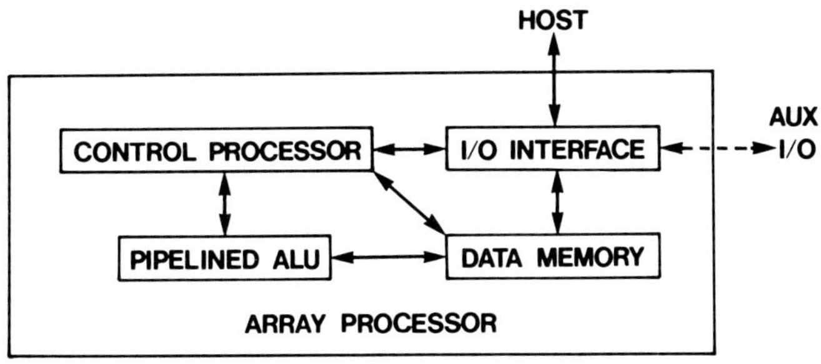

FIGURE 3. Four basic functional units of array processor and its internal buses. (Reproduced with permission from King, M. A., Doherty, P. W., Rosenberg, R. J., and Cool, S. L., *J. Nucl. Med.*, 24, 1072, 1983.)

several stages, and new data are introduced to the first stage when the previous data move to the second stage, etc., analogous to the way oil flows through a pipeline. Pipelining thus results in saving time by keeping all of the hardware busy most of the time.

The hardware of an array processor can generally be divided into four functional units as illustrated in Figure 3. The *I/O interface* serves to provide for transfer of data and commands between the host and the array processor. Array processors also have their own *control processor* which allows them to run independently of the host. This allows for *distributive processing* techniques that share the processing load between the host and the array processor so that each can perform separate tasks simultaneously.

Array processors usually have their own *data memory* which is used to store data in arrays. By having a separate high-speed data memory, the array processor can perform operations on data without tying up the host's bus or being limited by the host's data-retrieval time. The amount of data memory is very important. For best performance it is necessary to have enough data memory so that I/O with the host is kept to a minimum. More than an order of magnitude increase in execution time can occur with an insufficient amount of data memory.[11] Besides the amount of data memory, the number of bits in each word and storage format is also important as it determines the precision with which numbers are expressed. Some of the less expensive array processors (or pipeline processors) use an integer or fixed-point word format. This saves on hardware costs but limits the dynamic range of the data and calculations which can be handled. The two types of floating-point word formats which are used to store arrays in data memory are illustrated in Figure 2. With the *individual exponent floating-point* format, each piece of data is stored with its own exponent. With the *block floating-point* format, a single exponent is used for the entire block of data (fractions). For example, a 64 × 64-pixel image would be stored with a single exponent first and then 4096 fractions (i.e., one for each pixel) in block floating-point format. The latter saves time when one is working with an array of data, since only one exponent per block of data need be dealt with. It does limit the range and precision of the data, however.

The last functional unit of an array processor is the *pipeline arithmetic unit*. This provides the "number crunching" muscle of the array processor as described before. It contains parallel hardware operating in a pipeline fashion.

In emission tomographic computing systems, array processors can reduce reconstruction time by more than an order of magnitude compared to floating-point hardware[2] and allow the implementation of other reconstruction algorithms besides filtered backprojection in clinically acceptable time frames.[12] They can also be used for speeding up attenuation correction, uniformity correction, and reconstruction of sagittal and coronal slices.

Another important application of array processors is the speeding up of two-dimensional preconstruction filtering of emission images. One-dimensional filtering has generally been used in emission tomography, probably because much of the work on tomographic reconstruction was done in transmission tomography where data are typically collected from only one slice at a time. In the case of SPECT where a two-dimensional image is acquired, the use of two-dimensional filtering of the images before backprojection seems a natural. It would allow the use of a larger statistical sample to determine the value supplied to the backprojector at each point. This is very important since SPECT imaging is photon limited and the additional information contained in adjoining slices can help in reducing noise and increasing contrast.[13] The main problem with two-dimensional prereconstruction filtering has been the added processing time. With an array processor, 64 acquisition frames of 64 × 64 pixels each can be two-dimensionally deconvolved in 18 s.[13] This is less time than it would take to similarly process a single frame using floating-point hardware.

IV. STORAGE DEVICES

Emission computed tomography involves working with very large data sets. For example, SPECT acquisitions may consist of anywhere from 32 frames of 64 × 64 pixels each (256 kbytes), to 128 frames of 128 × 128 pixels each (4096 kbytes). Space is also required for the reconstructed slices. Thus, the amount and type of secondary storage are important on a tomographic computer system.

Enough fast secondary storage should be provided to hold the required software and at least several days worth of acquisition data and reconstructed images. This type of storage is usually done on magnetic disks. The two most commonly used disk types are *cartridge* and *Winchester* disks. Cartridge disks are removable, which is their advantage as they can be used for "backing up" system disks and long-term storage of studies. Their cost, however, limits their attractiveness for the latter except for special studies. Winchester disks are nonremovable, hermetically sealed units which contain the read/write head mechanism as well as the disk platter. Because they are a sealed unit, they can provide much denser data packing capabilities. This results in a device with larger storage capacity for its size and faster retrieval time for data than removable disks. They therefore make an attractive device for short-term storage of patient data. If they are used as a system device, however, a means should be provided to "back up" software in case of disk failure.

For long-term storage of tomographic images and data, either *magnetic tape* or *floppy disks* should be provided. The media cost of storing studies on magnetic tape is less than that of floppy disks. The access time for studies on magnetic tape can be considerable, however. The drawback to floppy disks has been their storage capacity. Dual-sided, dual-density floppies are now available which can store over 1 Mbyte of data. This is quite suitable for 64 × 64-pixel acquisitions. The new quad-density floppy drives should provide a medium capable of storing most tomographic acquisitions.

A new form of disk storage which appears to be quite attractive for storing tomographic studies is the *optical disk*.[7,14] It has tremendous storage capacity (greater than 1 Gbyte) and long-term storage stability, but has the disadvantage of not being able to rewrite information to the disk, and it lacks industrial standards.

V. IMAGE DISPLAY

Emission tomography provides the clinician with a wealth of information. The best way to display these data remains to be defined.[15] For the present, image display systems should provide the user with a large amount of image memory to hold slices and acquisition images and should provide flexibility in terms of apportioning the display of the memory contents. The system should provide at least 64 shades of gray[16] and should be capable of color display. In SPECT, use of a rotating cinematic display of acquisition frames has proved useful and should be provided.[15] The provision of software which makes use of three-dimensional edge detection, hidden-edge removal, and shading- or contour-line generation to display three-dimensional surfaces on a two-dimensional display is also desirable.[15,17,18] In the future, "true" three-dimensional displays may become an integral part of tomographic systems.[18] Much work still remains to be done in this area, and costs are still too high for widespread clinical use of these systems.

VI. ANALOG-TO-DIGITAL CONVERTORS

The ADCs of a standard computer system may need replacement or upgrading when acquisition of tomographic images is added to its functions. This is because a very small differential nonlinearity which would go unnoticed in a planar clinical study will be amplified to a significant defect by the backprojection process.[2,19] This effect is most pronounced when the nonlinearity occurs near the center of rotation. Due to this effect, much stricter requirements should be placed on acceptance testing and quality control of the differential linearity of ADCs used with tomography.

For SPECT, a set of ADCs which allows for at least dual-energy window selection is quite useful. This can allow the acquisition of dual radionuclide studies for comparison of localization, the subtraction of scatter from the primary image,[20] and the use of a scatter image to define the patient's body outline for attenuation correction.

REFERENCES

1. **Keys, J. W., Jr.,** Perspectives on tomography, *J. Nucl. Med.,* 23, 633, 1982.
2. **Larsson, S. and Israelsson, A.,** Considerations on system design, implementation and computer processing of SPECT, *IEEE Trans. Nucl. Sci.,* 29, 1331, 1982.
3. **Lieberman, D. E.,** *Computer Methods: The Fundamentals of Digital Nuclear Medicine,* C. V. Mosby, St. Louis, 1977.
4. **Erickson, J. J. and Rollo, F. D.,** *Digital Nuclear Medicine,* Lippincott, Philadelphia, 1983.
5. **Cradduck, T. D. and Knowles, L. G.,** Computers in nuclear medicine, in *Nuclear Medicine Physics, Instrumentation, and Agents,* Rollo, F. D., Ed., C. V. Mosby, St. Louis, 1977, 453.
6. **Holman, B. L. and Parker, J. A.,** *Computer-Assisted Cardiac Nuclear Medicine,* Little, Brown, Boston, 1981.
7. **Froelich, J. W.,** Computer hardware designed for medical imaging, *RNM Images,* 14, 46, 1984.
8. **Berhnard, R.,** Giants in small packages, *IEEE Spect.,* 19, 39, 1982.
9. **Alexander, P.,** Array processors in medical imaging, *IEEE Computer,* 16, 17, 1983.
10. **Lewis, R.,** Architectural considerations in array processing, *Elect. Imaging,* 2, 70, 1984.
11. **King, M. A., Doherty, P. W., Rosenberg, R. J., and Cool, S. L.,** Array processors: an introduction to their architecture, software, and applications in nuclear medicine, *J. Nucl. Med.,* 24, 1072, 1983.
12. **Arthaud, N. and Ammirati, J. L.,** Comparison of SPECT techniques on high-speed digital array processor, in *Emission Computed Tomography Current Trends,* Esser, P. D., Ed., Society of Nuclear Medicine, New York, 1983, 193.
13. **King, M. A., Schwinger, R. B., Doherty, P. W., and Penney, B. C.,** Two-dimensional filtering of SPECT images using the Metz and Wiener filters, *J. Nucl. Med.,* in press.
14. **Frattarola, J. R.,** Optical mass memory, in *Digital Imaging: Clinical Advances in Nuclear Medicine,* Esser, P. D., Ed., Society of Nuclear Medicine, New York, 1982, 31.
15. **Keyes, J. W., Jr.,** Display of three-dimensional tomographic images, in *Functional Mapping of Organ Systems and Other Computer Topics,* Esser, P. D., Ed., Society of Nuclear Medicine, New York, 1981, 219.
16. **Todd-Pokropek, A. E. and Pizer, S. M.,** Displays in scintigraphy, in *Medical Radionuclide Imaging,* Vol. 1, International Atomic Energy Agency, Vienna, 1977, 505.
17. **Cook, L. T., Dwyer, S. J., Batnitzky, S., and Lee, K. R.,** A three-dimensional display system for diagnostic imaging applications, *IEEE Comp. Graphics Appl.,* 3, 13, 1983.

18. **Budinger, T. F.,** 3D image displays bring scans to life, *Diag. Imag.,* 5, 54, 1983.
19. **Rogers, W. L., Clinthorne, N. H., Harkness, B. A., Koral, K. F., and Keyes, J. W., Jr.,** Field-flood requirements for emission computed tomography with an Anger camera, *J. Nucl. Med.,* 23, 162, 1982.
20. **Jaszczak, R. J., Coleman, R. E., and Greer, K. L.,** The subtraction of scattered events from SPECT photopeak events, *J. Nucl. Med.,* 24, 82, 1983.

Chapter 4

SINGLE-PHOTON EMISSION COMPUTED TOMOGRAPHY (SPECT) IMAGING SYSTEM AND QUALITY CONTROL

B. Ahluwalia

TABLE OF CONTENTS

I. SPECT IMAGING SYSTEM

Single-photon emission computed tomography (SPECT) is not new in nuclear medicine. Use of tomographic procedures in nuclear medicine was first applied by Kuhl in the early 1960s.[1,2]

A. Introduction

SPECT cameras can accumulate data for transverse and longitudinal sections simultaneously during a single revolution. A SPECT system gives a total image, has the ability to eliminate under- and overlying activity, increases contrast relative to planar imaging, and has capability for quantitative measurement of radiopharmaceutical volume and concentration. The last characteristic when employed with newly developed single-photon radiopharmaceuticals and appropriate biological models, has resulted in the ability to quantitatively measure *in vivo* parameters, such as regional blood flow, noninvasively. During the last 15 years there has been marked development in both instrumentation and radiopharmaceuticals. Basically, there are two types of SPECT instruments, longitudinal and transverse section devices. Longitudinal planar system, rotating slant hole, and multipinhole belong to the first category. These devices are described in Chapters 7, 8, and 9, respectively. Longitudinal devices provide only longitudinal sections and collect data through limited angles, while the transverse section devices collect data at all angles.

B. Kuhl's SPECT Systems

The instruments developed by Kuhl and co-workers[1,2] in the early 1960s performed longitudinal and transverse section images. This system had a dual probe with rectilinear as well as circular motion. The probes rotated 7.5° between images and 24 sets of linear data were accumulated in 180° rotation.

During 1970, a modified system, the Mark III, was designed for head imaging by Kuhl. The earlier brain scanner consisted of four 2 × 0.5 in. thick NaI (Tl) crystal detectors, with a special collimator to visualize the activity with consistent resolution at different depths. Later Mark IV was developed by Kuhl.[3] In the Mark IV system, the single crystals of Mark III were replaced by a linear array of eight crystals of 3 × 1 × 1 in. There were 32 crystals overall. The system moved 7.5° in successive increments. Data were accumulated at each angle through a 360° rotation. For satisfactory statistics, a set of 5 revolutions was performed for cross-sectional imaging; rotation time for each revolution was 50 s. This system has been used extensively for single photon as well as positron emission cross sectional imaging.

C. Planar SPECT Systems

SPECT imaging systems are modifications of an Anger camera. In general, SPECT cameras consist of a single or dual large field of view crystal head mounted on a rotatable gantry. SPECT systems also require a sophisticated computer and reconstruction algorithms. Besides specialized SPECT imaging, the system can be used for planar imaging.

Since early 1980, a variety of single head or dual head Anger type camera systems have been used for SPECT. Systems developed by Kuhl could provide only a few slices at a time. With an Anger camera, however, the projection images of the entire organ and the distributed radioactivity are taken. The SPECT instruments are programmed with a microprocessor which rotates around the patient. The cross-sectional images can be constructed in a manner similar to the technique used in transmission computed tomography. A full 360° or 180° rotation is used in different protocols.

The SPECT Anger system consists of the basic components of a gamma camera, with extra mechanical motion of the gantry, and a large number of computer controlled operations. Basic elements of a SPECT system are described below.

1. Detector Head

The detector material is a thallium-activated sodium iodide NaI(Tl) crystal with a thickness of 0.375 to 0.5 in. For this range of thickness, the range for energy detection is 100 to 250 KeV. In general, the crystal diameter is about 15 to 22 in. The crystal is properly shielded with lead and iron and is packed in a metal housing, which has an overall diameter of generally 21 to 26 in. The peripheral section around the active area is shielded. The crystal packaging and coupling to a photomultiplier (PM) tube are described in detail by Williams.[4] Most of the systems have 37 PM tubes, some have 91 PM tubes, and they are arranged in a hexagonal packing. The overall field-of-view of the system is hexagonal, circular, or square.

2. Collimators

As in planar imaging, there is a variety of collimator systems for SPECT imaging, with parallel hole collimators, convergent collimators, and parallel angulated collimators used most commonly. Angulated collimators help to reduce the actual distance between the organ and the crystal. Angulated (30°) collimators are used for brain and heart imaging. Low energy collimators cover energies up to about 200 KeV and medium energy collimators may be a high resolution, high sensitivity, or an all-purpose type.

3. Gantry

The gantry which is mounted rigidly on the floor, holds the camera head (or heads) and provides specific rotation around the patient. The camera head has a range of motion, inward to outward relative to the axis of rotation (AOR), so that the position of the camera face can be adjusted. The head can swivel about the rigid gantry arms so that the collimator angle to the organ can be adjusted. The gantry arm should be rigid and no sagging should occur at any angular location. Any sagging would cause shift and thus would result in shifting of the image relative to the AOR and would cause artifacts or produce unacceptable images.

In General Electric cameras, the gantry arm is pivoted and moves around a circle. The gantry arm has a gamma camera head on one end and a counter weight on the opposite end. The camera motion can be controlled manually or with the computer. The gantry arm length on the camera side can be adjusted; likewise, the counter weight location can be adjusted. In the Raytheon camera design no counter weight is used. In the Raytheon system camera, the head is pivoted at the end of the gantry arm. The gantry arm of fixed length, is affixed to the circle of rotation and can raise or lower the camera. The gantry arms are held at 90° to the orbit of rotation.

In all the SPECT cameras, the motion of the gantry around the patient is controlled and the speed can be adjusted. The motion can be continuous or can be programmed for angular incremental stops. A Raytheon SPECT system spectrum 150-DT is shown in Figure 1. This system moves on rails affixed to the floor and can be locked.

4. Patient Table

The patient table is rigid and is made of a material with a low atomic number so that gamma attenuation is minimum. The table is cantilevered so that the camera can be rotated around the patient. The table should have a Velcro belt to wrap around both patient and table to immobilize the patient during imaging. The table is generally narrow in width to minimize detector patient spacing and thus allow contour following.

Similar to the gantry, the patient table is generally either fixed or moves on rails. The position of the table can be adjusted with reference to the floor. The table should also have motion controls in longitudinal and lateral directions. Some systems have the table movements controlled by computer during imaging.

5. Gantry, Table Movements, and Body Contour Following

The SPECT gantries which have a fixed radius of rotation yield unsatisfactory images.

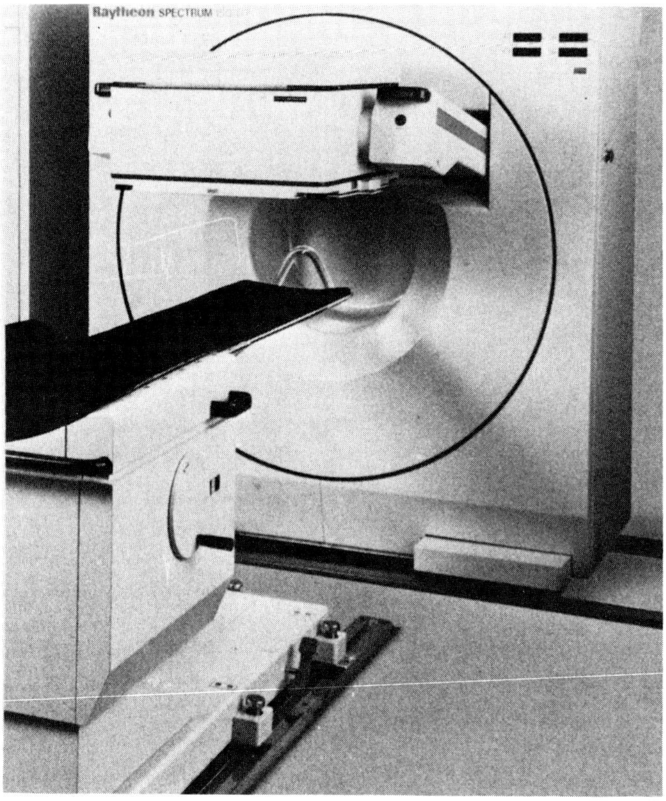

FIGURE 1. Raytheon SPECT imaging system Spectrum 150-DT.

Resolution is not optimum, because the collimator is not close to the patient. Unless the axis coincides with the body axis, certain portions of the organ may be outside the field of view for more of the rotation period than is necessary. In body contour following, the radius of rotation is continuously adjusted by automatic processes during rotation around the patient to minimize the distance between the collimator and patient.

A system which automatically adjusts the radius of rotation for minimizing detector-to-patient space during rotation has been devised by Blum.[5] The axis of rotation is fixed within the body for the entire organ imaging without affecting detector-to-patient distance. The radius of rotation may be adjusted during rotation without disturbing computer reconstruction, provided certain conditions are met: (1) the AOR remains fixed within the body; (2) the face of the detector is maintained parallel to the AOR and a line in that face remains tangential to any cylinders generated by rotation of the detector; (3) angular rotation is uniform; (4) there is no longitudinal shift of the field of view. If there is any nonuniform motion or shift in the field of view, the computer program will make the required corrections.

In the body contour following technique, the operator manually adjusts the distance between the body and the detector in a preliminary rotation. Position indicators send the angle position and the detector-to-patient distance to the computer. During actual collection of the data, the position sensors reproduce the stored contour. The detector tilt is automatically adjusted during rotation.

In some SPECT systems, the table stays stationary and all the adjustments are performed by the head. In others, table motion is used to achieve the body contour following. The radius of motion for the detector is fixed for such systems.

II. EQUIPMENT EVALUATION AND QUALITY CONTROL

SPECT systems are complex and include very specialized electronic devices and computers. There are many parameters which should be routinely evaluated and controlled for optimum performance for patient throughput and image quality. It is imperative to carry out a quality control program for image quality. Quality control should involve performance and evaluation of all components, i.e., camera head, computer, image quality, gantry motion, patient couch motion, mechanical safety evaluations, emergency motion stop switches, and mechanical alignments. Imaging protocols should also be reviewed for optimization of clinical information and patient comfort.

Certain quality control test procedures, such as field uniformity, sensitivity, linearity, spatial resolution, and energy resolution, are similar to those used for planar imaging. The requirements in SPECT imaging, however, are stringent. Certain tests such as center of rotation (COR), pixel size, gamma camera and table alignment, gamma camera and AOR alignment, and x-y gain are specific requirements for SPECT Systems.

A. Overall Gamma Camera Performance

The most important component in SPECT imaging is the gamma camera. Most of the imaging systems have some sort of uniformity correction. The Picker Z system produces shift in the pulse-height analysis window from higher to lower and it also skims counts to achieve correction for uniformity. The nonuniformity is corrected by Elscint and Siemens systems by shifting the event by a predetermined amount. Shifting is managed up to 0.04 mm. The correction factor for planar images is stored in memory and the correction is performed through hardware interpolation. A single set of linearity correction coefficients achieves integral uniformity of less than 5%. A higher degree of accuracy of correction is required in rotating emission cameras. Siemens has special cameras with ZLC modifications, where ZLC stands for "Z map and linearity corrections". Z map is the intensity map which is stored for linearity correction. The Siemens cameras also have fast electronics and dual integrator. The fast electronics circuitry increases the count rate sensitivity without loss of image quality, 70 Kcps in normal count rate and 127 Kcps in high count rate mode. A dual integrator consists of two identical integrators; the time-share and the input/output. If one integrator is busy processing an input pulse, and a second input pulse occurs, the other integrator is available to process. Thus, with a dual integrator the count losses are minimum. Similar to the Z map for uniformity, Elscint has included an array microprocessor which allows for the storage of an energy correction map.

Basic requirements for a SPECT camera are a system with spatial resolution of 3 to 4 mm, an absolute linearity deviation of less than 1 mm, and an integral uniformity of less than 10% across the useful field of view. An integral uniformity of 10% corresponds to a uniformity deviation of approximately 7% across the useful field of view. The system should also have good energy resolution so that scatter contribution is minimum. Energy resolution on the order of 10 to 12% is satisfactory.

The tests related to the uniformity, linearity, energy and spatial resolution, and deadtime should be performed at the time of acceptance and at regular intervals. Procedures of NEMA[7] (National Electrical Manufacturers Association) should be followed. Gamma camera quality tests for Anger cameras have been outlined by Graham.[8] When the camera is used for SPECT imaging, additional tests are considered for quality control. Recent publications[9,10] have reviewed the acceptance and quality control procedures for SPECT. Basic aspects of these are outlined in this section.

B. Uniformity and Sensitivity Correction

Each planar image is corrected for uniformity before being used in image reconstruction. The variation is regional sensitivity and uniformity are due to intrinsic crystal response, nonlinearities of the crystal and collimator, improper light guide coupling, or variation in the photocathode yield with time. An asymmetric window setting also could contribute to nonuniformity. Todd-Pokropek[11] has pointed out that nonuniformities are very energy dependent. Changes on the order of 5 KeV in the location of the energy window can create large changes in apparent contrast and can produce "crescent" artifacts. Greer et al.[12] recommend that the centering of the window on the photopeak be performed with auto routines. Due to these types of fluctuations, it is imperative that the uniformity correction be evaluated on a regular basis.

Each image is corrected with a flood image which reflects corrections. For a uniformity variation of 2% in each angular view, there is about 12% error in the reconstructed slice. A 2% error or variation is for a maximum 2500 counts per pixel. A regional nonuniformity spreads out during processing, which results in rings of increased or decreased intensity. Studies of Roger et al.[13] have shown that flood correction is essential for artifact suppression. For the acquisition of uniformity correction, an image of a flood phantom should be taken for the camera and specific collimator. A new flood is required whenever a different collimator is used. A flood image with over 30 million counts should be obtained using a 64 × 64 matrix and 5 and 6 mCi of ^{99m}Tc pertechnitate. Activity should be limited so as not to have count losses due to deadtime. Count rate should be on the order of 30,000 counts per second. The counts per pixel will be 10,000 counts and the flood image will be accurate to within 1%. Similarly, for collection on an image matrix of 128 × 128, 120 million counts are required. The flood should be placed on a flat surface and all the air bubbles be taken out. Extreme care should be taken in the collection of the flood correction image. An improper flood could introduce additional artifacts.

A reference flood for the collimators should be accumulated weekly. Water filled phantoms are manufactured specially with 0.5 in. thick lucite so that there is an insignificant tendency of bulge at the center of the phantom. Lightweight plastic flood sources of ^{57}Co are also used instead of water-filled phantoms. ^{57}Co flood images are often used for corrections for studies involving ^{99m}Tc, ^{123}I, ^{201}Tl, and ^{67}Ga. The flood images should not be smoothed, as the nonuniformity feature will be lost in the process. Flood correction programs are provided by the SPECT manufacturers; these calculate the correction factors for each pixel. These correction factors are stored.

Uniformity and sensitivity must remain constant as the detector rotates. It is assumed that the camera response is not affected by gravity and the photomultiplier tubes are mounted rigidly with proper magnetic shielding. Variation in sensitivity should be less than 1% over a 360° rotation. Rotational sensitivity and uniformity should be evaluated at initial acceptance and yearly thereafter. The rotational sensitivity test is performed with a ^{57}Co flood source, which should be rigidly attached to the camera. The images are taken at different angles. Total image counts are plotted for each angle. At least 1 million counts must be acquired per angle so as to reflect 2% variation in sensitivity.

Similarly, the rotational uniformity is evaluated by analyzing the different angular views.

C. Center of Rotation (COR)

In the tomographic reconstruction process, the reconstructed image is placed in a pixel array and it is required to provide the pixel value of COR. A shift in the COR will result in a loss of resolution and an introduction of artifacts.

COR acquisition must be performed weekly. The COR value may be different for different collimators. The COR is determined with the use of a point source. A set of 32 rotational images is taken over 360°. The point source images will shift left to right. The COR correction corresponds midway between maximum and minimum point source deviation. The plot of image location with reference to the gantry angle will be a sinusoidal wave. Some software display the values of the COR. Figure 2 shows these values generated by ADAC software.

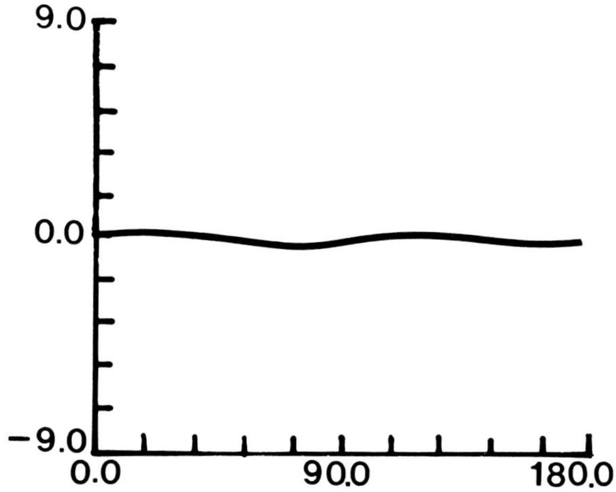

FIGURE 2. Values of the center of rotation expressed in terms of pixel width are given along y-axis and the corresponding gantry location is given in degrees along x-axis.

The x-axis is the angle and corresponding COR values are plotted along the y-axis. The system also displays information about values of correct axis of rotation (AOR), mean AOR, error in AOR, and maximum and minimum error in AOR. Harkness et al.[14] determine COR value from two projections 180° apart.

The camera manufacturers provide pertinent procedures for COR correction for their software. An error of one pixel in the COR value causes significant distortions in the image. This will also result in errors when quantitative evaluations are performed with the image. The COR value is affected by a change in voltage offsets, x,y gains of the analog to digital converter. Precise COR location should be determined within 1/10th of pixel width.

D. Alignment of Camera and Table with the Axis of Rotation (AOR)

SPECT system performance is unsatisfactory unless a proper alignment of the detector gantry and the patient table is done with reference to the axis of rotation (AOR). The gantry stand should be leveled perpendicular to the floor. The face of the detector must remain parallel with the detector AOR throughout a 360° rotation. The detector head is leveled at the highest point with a bubble level, the head is rotated through 180° and an angle subtended with the horizontal plane is measured. The angle subtended should not be more than 1°. Improper alignment of the camera head with the AOR will result in loss of resolution similar to misalignment of the COR. Similarly, the patient table should be centered and parallel to the AOR. Alignments of the table, gantry stand, and the camera with the AOR should be checked periodically.

E. Pixel Size Calibrations

Pixel size refers to dimensions and should be calibrated. Pixel size changes with a gain. The gains in x and y directions should be matched so that the pixel cross-sections are perfect squares. Precise size measurement of the pixel is measured by imaging finite size line sources in the x and y directions. The sources are separated by a known distance. The number of pixels in between the peaks of the count profiles of the image, for x and y directions, corresponding to the actual distance in the line sources. This calibration should be performed weekly. Manufacturers have software which automates this calibration.

F. SPECT Phantoms and Quality Control Routines

Quality control should be carried out on a routine basis. These tests can be performed

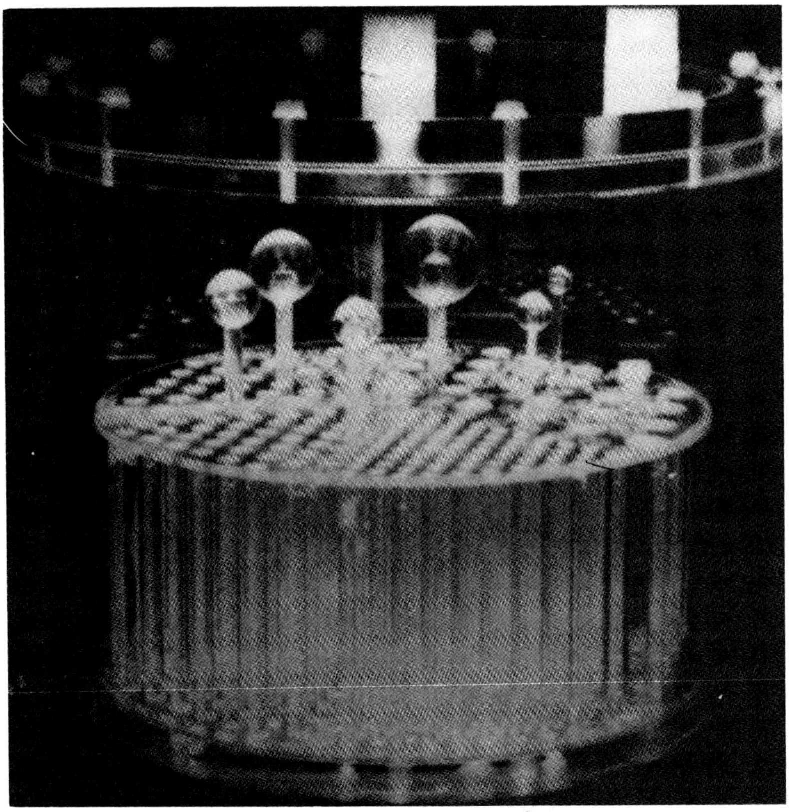

FIGURE 3. A standard SPECT phantom of Data Spectrum Corporation, Chapel Hill, NC.

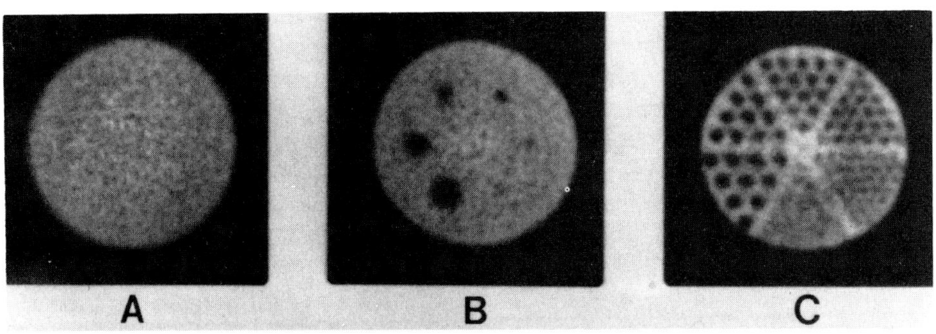

FIGURE 4. These transverse section slices have been obtained with the phantom of Data Spectrum Corporation. (A) slice showing the system uniformity; (B) slice through the cold spot spherical inserts for evaluation of system resolution; (C) slice through lucite rods of different diameters for evaluation of system resolution. (Courtesy of Data Spectrum Corporation, Chapel Hill, NC.)

easily with some specialized SPECT phantoms commercially available. Figure 3 shows a SPECT phantom of Data Spectrum Corporation, Chapel Hill, NC. This phantom consists of a lucite water-filled cylinder having inserts for evaluation of hot-spot/cold-spot resolution, tomographic linearity, volume sensitivity, uniformity, and spatial resolution in the transverse section images. Figure 4 is a slice showing systems uniformity, size of cold spheres which are resolved, and line resolution cut through lucite rods of different diameters. These images are taken with a SPECT phantom filled with 10 to 15 mCi of ^{99m}Tc. The phantom is placed on the pallet. The axis of the phantom is parallel to the AOR. Angular views with 50,000 counts each are acquired on a 64 × 64 matrix for analysis. Frequency of the quality control routines is described below.

Gamma camera planar imaging — Gamma camera extrinsic flood uniformity should be performed daily. Gamma camera intrinsic uniformity, spatial resolution, and linearity tests should be performed weekly. Gamma camera energy resolution and count rate performance should be evaluated every 6 months.

SPECT system evaluation — Flood correction images, center of rotation, and pixel calibration should be evaluated weekly. Computer assisted routines should be followed for consistency in operation. System sensitivity and uniformity in rotational cuts should be evaluated quarterly. Mechanical alignments of AOR, camera gantry, gantry stand, camera head orientation during rotation, and table alignment checked quarterly. In general, the SPECT system total performance should be evaluated quarterly.

III. ARTIFACTS

Artifacts are due to errors in the alignment processes, collection of images, and improper parameters used in reconstruction.[14]

Concentric ring artifacts are due to nonuniformities. When the camera head is not properly leveled, it can cause image blurring. When an improper value of COR is used, inappropriate placing of the images occurs and results in loss of resolution. It is suggested that the COR calibration be performed more frequently than weekly and the images be evaluated for improvement in quality. Insufficient count density causes image noise. This artifact can be eliminated by giving a larger dose of the radionuclide or by collecting for longer durations. Patient motion during imaging also causes blurring and loss of resolution. Reconstruction parameters introduce errors and artifacts which can be altered by altering the reconstruction parameters. The artifacts due to reconstruction processes are blurring, image noise, and ring at the organ boundaries. A filter which oversmooths will result in loss of resolution.

REFERENCES

1. **Kuhl, D. E. and Edwards, R. Q.,** Image separation radioisotope scanning, *Radiology,* 80, 653, 1963.
2. **Kuhl, D. E. and Edwards, R. Q.,** Cylindrical and section radioisotope scanning of the liver and brain, *Radiology,* 83, 926, 1964.
3. **Kuhl, D. E. et al.,** The Mark IV System for radionuclide computed tomography of the brain, *Radiology,* 121, 405, 1976.
4. **Williams, L.,** *Nuclear Medical Physics,* CRC Press, Boca Raton, FL, 1987.
5. **Blum, A. S.,** Photon Emission Tomographic Apparatus and Method, U.S. Patent 4,368,389, January 1983.
6. **Blum, A. S.,** Improving SPECT image quality by body contour following, in *Emission Computed Tomography,* Esser, P. D., Ed., Society of Nuclear Medicine, New York, 1983, 163.
7. NEMA, A Guide to Revise Standards for Performance Measurements of Scintillation Cameras, Assoc. Stand. Publ. NU1-1986, National Electrical Manufacturers, Washington, D.C., 1986.
8. **Graham, L. S.,** Quality assurance of Anger cameras, in *Physics of Nuclear Medicine,* Recent Advances Medical Physics Monogr. No 10, Rao D. V., Chandra, R., and Graham, M. D., Eds., American Institute of Physics, Chicago, 1984, 68.
9. **Croft, B.,** *Single Photon Emission Computed Tomography,* Year Book Medical Publishers, Chicago, 1986, 177.
10. **Greer, K., Jaszezak, R., Harris, B., et al.,** Quality Control in SPECT, *J. Nucl. Med. Tech.,* 13, 76, 1985.
11. **Todd-Pokropek, A. E.,** Quality control in single photon emission computerized tomography, *J. Nucl. Med.,* 23, 52, 1982.

12. **Greer, K. L., Jaszezak, R. J., and Coleman, R. E.,** An overview of camera based SPECT system, *Med. Phys.*, 9, 455, 1982.
13. **Roger, W. L., Clinthorne, N. H., Harkness, B. A., et al.,** Field-flood requirements for emission computed tomography with an Anger camera, *J. Nucl. Med.*, 23, 162, 1982.
14. **Harkness, B. A., Rogers, W. L., Clinthorne, N. H., et al.,** SPECT: quality control procedures and artifact identification, *J. Nucl. Med. Tech.*, 11, 55, 1983.

Chapter 5

CLINICAL APPLICATIONS AND PROTOCOLS OF SINGLE PHOTON EMISSION COMPUTED TOMOGRAPHY

U. Raff and W. R. Hendee

TABLE OF CONTENTS

I. INTRODUCTION

Tomographic radionuclide imaging began in 1963 with the pioneering work of Kuhl and Edwards[1] performing section-scanning of the brain. After Kuhl's MARK III and MARK IV multidetector brain scanners, considerable time elapsed before commercial tomographic systems became available.[2] Finally, the Cleon 710 transaxial brain scanner and the Cleon 711 transaxial whole-body scanner were released. With the advent of a general-purpose SPECT system developed by Larsson,[3] tomographic imaging began to employ a rotating large-field-of-view scintillation camera. All major manufacturers now offer single- or dual-headed rotating tomographic systems that can be interfaced to any standard nuclear medicine computer.

Interest in single-photon emission computed tomography (SPECT) has grown considerably since the 10th Annual Symposium on the Sharing of Computer Programs and Technology in Nuclear Medicine in 1980.[4] At that time, attention was focused on limited-angle tomography with emphasis on rotating-quadrant-slant-hole collimators, seven-pinhole tomography, and coded apertures. While some interest in these techniques has remained,[5-6] attention has been focused principally on the rotating scintillation cameras. In the past few years, improved technology has enhanced the clinical relevance of SPECT in nuclear medicine. Nevertheless, SPECT still stands at the threshold of acceptance as a routine procedure in clinical medicine.

As pointed out by Ell,[7] emission-computed tomography preceded Hounsfield's development of X-ray transmission tomography (CT) by 6 years. Although this later modality was a quantum leap for diagnostic imaging, SPECT remained in the shadows for the next decade, with no practical impact on the medical field. Kuhl's[1] innovative ideas were somewhat ahead of their time, partly because instrumentation was still confined to experimental applications levels in laboratories and was not yet available clinically, and computer facilities were too limited to fulfill the requirements imposed by clinical applications of SPECT in hospitals.

With the advent of more cost effective hardware to support rotating scintillation cameras and dedicated nuclear medicine minicomputers, clinical SPECT has lately experienced a rapid growth and has become more attractive to clinical nuclear medicine services. Still, SPECT is far from achieving the same popularity as transmission X-ray tomography. The reasons are multiple: considerably fewer patients can be examined daily with SPECT than with CT; while CT is dedicated only to tomographic studies, SPECT units usually must be used for projection as well as for tomographic imaging; long acquisition times (in general, around 20 to 30 minutes per patient) and complicated, rather demanding quality assurance protocols are required for SPECT and mitigate against the use of this technology in smaller, service-oriented clinical programs. The two major advantages of SPECT over projection scintigraphy are the considerable improvement in contrast (since under- and overlying tissues do not interfere with the image plane of interest) and a full three-dimensional display capability. Difficulties in handling the noise characteristics of SPECT systems present problems, however. Artifacts, also, in reconstructed sections cannot be overlooked.[8] The overall increase in sensitivity of SPECT, compared to standard planar imaging, has been less than spectacular (10 to 15%). Problems associated with complex attenuation compensation[9-11] for correct visual identification of tomographic scintigrams and absolute quantification of radiotracer uptake have tempered the optimism generated by the SPECT methodology. Recent results, however, from several sites show some promise of overcoming these difficulties. In addition, the recent development of new radiopharmaceuticals has enhanced the clinical potential of SPECT, whether it is performed with special purpose instrumentation or rotating cameras. Decreasing costs, reliable hardware, software support and adequate documentation ultimately may promote SPECT into a clinical modality from the research tool that it has been over the past few years.

Special designs of detector heads (cut-off gamma camera[12]) and improved design of instrumentation ("long-hole" collimators[13] and slant-hole collimators[14]) have reduced the difficult task of choosing a general versus special purpose imaging device. Technological improvements in rotating cameras that permit the detector head to follow the body contour[15] will improve image quality to some extent. Contour-tracing is achieved by computer control of the camera's head or by combining horizontal and vertical motions of the imaging table.

II. BRAIN IMAGING

A. Introduction

The brain is a difficult candidate for SPECT imaging; the small fraction of radiotracer uptake in the brain and the resulting small number of photons available for imaging have necessitated for nearly two decades the use of high sensitivity, special purpose instruments for performance of tomographic brain studies.[16-18] With the development of radiopharmaceuticals which cross the normal blood-brain-barrier (BBB), investigation of the brain's metabolism no longer is restricted to the small number of positron-emitting isotopes used in positron emission tomography (PET) scanning. Labeled amphetamines that penetrate the BBB and remain long enough in the brain parenchyma to permit imaging can now be used with general purpose ECT equipment. These substances offer an alternative to the expense associated with the use of shortlived positron-emitting radiopharmaceuticals produced in on-site cyclotrons.

Until the appearance of labeled amphetamines to investigate the brain, nonlipophilic radiopharmaceuticals such as technetium pertechnetate or technetium glucoheptonate were used. According to Holman et al.,[19] "conventional brain scanning has always been misnamed" because it does not reflect normal brain function. ^{99m}Tc-based radiotracers concentrate only in pathological regions where the BBB has been damaged.

It is well known that the BBB is very selective. Substances that cross the BBB must have a transport system available; nonmetabolizable and non-diffusible substances are not transported. Lipid-soluble materials such as oxygen, carbon dioxide, and inert gasses massively penetrate the barrier.[20] A variety of drugs (analgesics and stimulants) such as nicotine, ethanol, imipramine, caffeine, heroin, cocaine, procaine, antipyrine and amphetamines, as well as common tranquilizers such as diazepam (valium), flunitrazepam, lorazepan and chlorpromazine, are known to reach rapid equilibrium with metabolites in the brain parenchyma. When these materials are labeled with radioactivity, the concentration of radiotracer in the brain depends primarily on the permeability of the BBB to the labeled drug, the degree of binding of the drug to the brain cells, the biological half-life, and the amount of radioactivity extracted by other organs (e.g., the liver, spleen, and kidneys).

The use of SPECT to study cerebral function in man has been summarized in several teaching editorials.[21-23] The slow development of adequate single-photon radiopharmaceuticals has prevented tomographic studies of the brain from becoming routine protocols in the clinical environment. Recent rather spectacular results of PET have stimulated additional efforts to investigate cerebral function with SPECT. In 1980, Hill[21] summarized the major advantages of transaxial systems over limited angle tomography for SPECT imaging of the brain. In 1981, Budinger[22] heralded the "revival of clinical nuclear medicine brain imaging", and 1 year later Coleman et al.[23] provided an overview of state of the art SPECT imaging of the brain.

Measurement of regional cerebral blood flow (rCBF) with SPECT appears promising, even though it is restricted to special purpose instrumentation since most SPECT systems are too insensitive for this application. Invasive intracarotid injection of ^{133}Xe[24] and ^{15}O-labeled water[25] were the early approaches to rCBF studies. High sensitivity is required to perform ^{133}Xe tomographic studies because of the fast washout of the radionuclide. Special instrumentation such as a bar-camera array system was developed to overcome this problem;[26,27] this approach failed, however, because of poor spatial resolution. Fazio et al.[28] studied rCBF using intracarotid infusion of ^{81m}Kr and a rotating SPECT camera; however, this approach is somewhat impractical because of its invasiveness. With the introduction of N-isopropyl-^{123}I-iodoamphetamine (^{123}I-IMP)[29-31] and, lately, other ^{123}I-labeled compounds such as hydroxyiodopropyldiamine (HIPDM)[32-35] and iodobenzene (IBZ),[36] some of the sensitivity problems can be overcome. Since ^{123}I-IMP remains a long time ($\simeq$2 days) in the brain parenchyma,[29] the sensitivity of the imaging device becomes less problematic compared to the use of ^{133}Xe with its fast washout.

In an overview of rotating camera systems for brain tomography, Coleman et al.[23] provide a comparison with scanner-based systems in terms of single-slice sensitivity and total-volume sensitivities. The total-volume sensitivity obtained by adding the single-slice-volume sensitivities together can be used as a parameter for the comparison of imaging systems; however, Coleman points out that the organ-volume sensitivity may be more appropriate for comparison purposes. The use of dual head rotating cameras, and even three scintillation cameras together with specially designed collimators, may be used to improve the total-volume sensitivity significantly. Some degree of optimism pervades Coleman's editorial in terms of imaging advances related to neurological metabolism. The future of brain imaging appears to depend largely on an improved relationship between radiopharmaceuticals and instrumentation design.

B. Study of Regional Cerebral Blood Flow

The measurement of brain perfusion is based on the assumption of local radiotracer distribution. Transaxial slices obtained by rapid tomographic scanning are, therefore, the only reliable approach since they eliminate nondesired activity outside the reconstructed section. For many years studies of blood flow and cerebral metabolism seemed to be approachable only by PET and costly single-photon-detection techniques. More recently, the single-photon approach using ^{133}Xe for the detection of focal hyperemia has become an attractive approach as it is cost effective, atraumatic, and expedient.

C. Use of ^{133}XE for rCBF Measurements

SPECT using inhalation and washout of ^{133}Xe was developed by Stokely et al.[26] Four groups of NaI(Tl) multicrystal detectors, each with 16 individual crystals, rotate around the patient and simultaneously acquire data for three tomographic slices. The sections are approximately 2 cm thick and their respective centers are about 4 cm apart. A 360° rotation is accomplished in 10 s. The images are recorded in a 64×64 matrix format. The very short acquisition time is required because of the fast arrival and washout of ^{133}Xe. The patient inhales a mixture of xenon-oxygen-air with 10 mCi/l ^{133}Xe for 1 min, followed by air over a 3-min washout period. Four 1-min measurements are obtained while the ^{133}Xe input function is determined by positioning a scintillation probe over an upper portion of the lung. Tomographic slices are computed by a filtered backprojection using arithmetic means of opposite-ray sums corrected for attenuation. Examples of ^{133}Xe rCBF in normal volunteers and patients who suffered stroke are shown in Figures 1 and 2.

When vascular disease has produced anatomical changes, concurrence between SPECT and CAT scans usually is observed. Changes in rCBF may be detected, however, early by SPECT before CT findings become apparent. Celsis et al.[37] present essentially the same technique as Bonte and Stokely:[27] rCBF is assessed by means of emission computed tomography of the inert gas concentration. Four tomograms, each collected for 1 min, are obtained with a fast rotating-single-photon tomograph. Two methods developed by Kanno and Lassen[38] are combined for data analysis. The first method, called "the sequence of picture method", analyzes the dynamics of buildup and clearance of activity in a given pixel over 4 min. The second method, labeled "the early picture method", analyzes differences

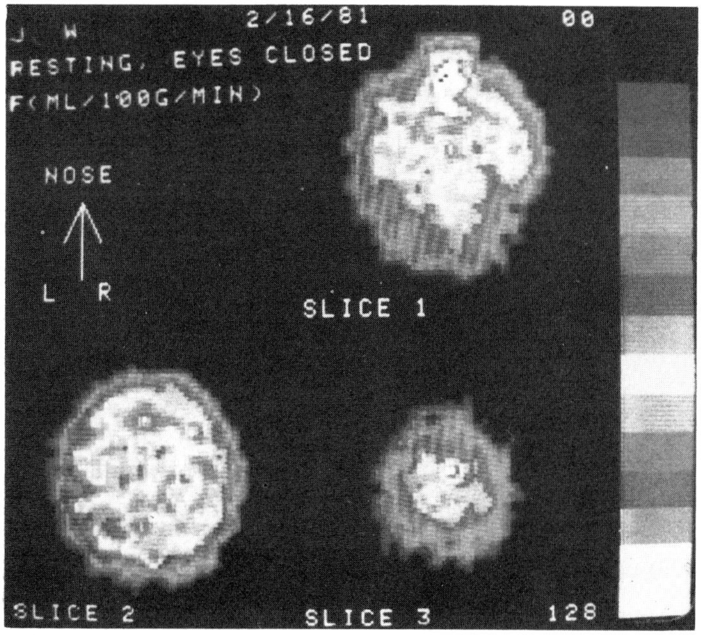

FIGURE 1. ^{133}Xe study of rCBF in a ''normal'' volunteer in resting state with eyes closed. Three tomographic sections (Slices 1-3) are displayed in a 16-color scale representing flow values from 0 (dark blue) to a maximum of 128 ml/100 g/min (white). In upper left-hand corner are subjects's data and an orientation symbol. Flow patterns of the three slices are within normal limits. (Subject 1). (From Bonte, F. J. and Stokely, E. M., *J. Nucl. Med.*, 22, 1049, 1981. With permission.)

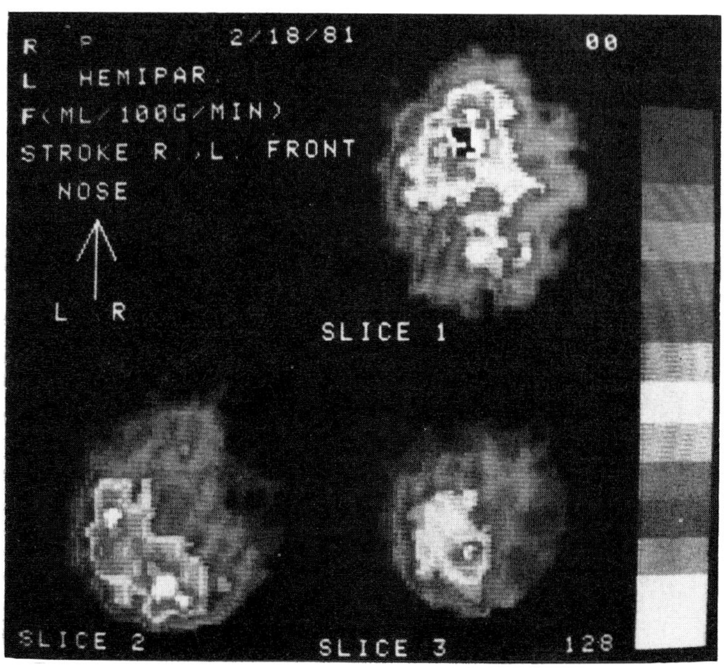

FIGURE 2. Tomographic rCBF study of 58-year-old hospitalized patient (Subject 2) with history of past left frontal and recent right strokes. Patterns of rCBF are abnormal. (From Bonte, F. J. and Stokely, E. M., *J. Nucl. Med.*, 22, 1049, 1981. With permission.)

in count rates between pixels in the early stages of ^{133}Xe appearance in the brain (0 to 2 min). In this latter approach, a low initial count rate in a given area is associated with no blood flow. Since the decay energy of ^{133}Xe is rather low (81 keV), difficulties in discriminating between primary and scatter radiation, with the corresponding loss in spatial resolution, must be expected. Therefore, the count rate in ischemic areas and the flow rate are overestimated. As a consequence, true flow rate is even lower than that recorded. The use of ^{127}Xe (half-life of 36.4 d and photon energies of 375 and 202.8 keV) may overcome this problem because of more efficient energy discrimination. The assumption of monoexponential clearance from each pixel is another source of error. Finally, spatial resolution is rather coarse with this technique and the resulting "partial volume effect" becomes important at high blood flows.

Activation of the visual cortex as recorded by dynamic ECT with ^{133}Xe has been described by Henriksen et al.[39] The technique is based on an increase in CBF in the visual cortex during visual stimulation, as shown in Figure 3. A 35% increase in CBF in primary and associated visual cortices has been measured. This technique illustrates the use of an interesting atraumatic method to quantify a well-known physiological process. A two-dimensional conventional method using inhalation of ^{133}Xe with static detectors over both occipital regions yielded only a 15% increase in CBF observed during visual activity.[40] Better localization and higher amplitude of response are obtained with tomographic techniques.

D. Radiolabeled Amines in rCBF Measurements

The idea of using radiolabeled amines for study of brain metabolism is not new. Kuhl et al.[52-53] mentioned several years ago that radiotracers other than Xenon-133 could be used. IMP is a lipophilic tracer capable of crossing the intact BBB and remaining in the brain parenchyma for a reasonable time (approximately 48 h) after intravenous injection. Pioneering work with brain tomography using ^{123}I-IMP[41,42] has been done by Hill et al.[30] The multidetector brain system developed at Harvard[17,43-48] was used to study 46 patients with IMP. Perfusion abnormalities were observed in nearly all patients. Results can be summarized as follows: white and gray matter of the cerebral cortex can be differentiated well in normal patients. The regional uptake of IMP is influenced by external stimulation. Examples of normal ^{123}I-IMP transaxial images are shown in Figures 4 and 5. The use of IMP to study patients with acute cerebral infarction is superior to transmission-computerized tomography. Hyperperfusion corresponding to EEG seizure focus was registered for one patient during seizure activity (Figure 6). An IMP study obtained after acute onset of right hemiparesis and aphasia is shown in Figure 7. An absence of activity was observed in patients with brain tumors, in correlation with CT results. Initial experience using IMP as a brain-imaging agent shows promise for future work on neurologic diseases, including those classified as functional disorders which may be accompanied by altered amine kinetics and function. Magistretti et al.[49] reported results similar to Hill et al. concerning the delineation of elliptic foci during seizure activity.

Hill et al.[50] have summarized the properties of radiolabeled amines, their possible mechanism of localization in the brain, and their metabolism, once they have crossed the BBB. These investigators employed the Harvard multidetector brain system in their studies, using a dual-channel mode to eliminate the effects of ^{124}I contamination (2.1 to 4.6%). From these studies, the following clinical indications are recommended for the use of IMP:

1. Acute cerebral infarction where a CT scan may be normal over a week or more until anatomic abnormalities are detectable.
2. Before and after endarterectomy to assess the success of surgical intervention.
3. Epilepsy in cases where the extent and localization of hypermetabolic foci are important for treatment and follow-up.

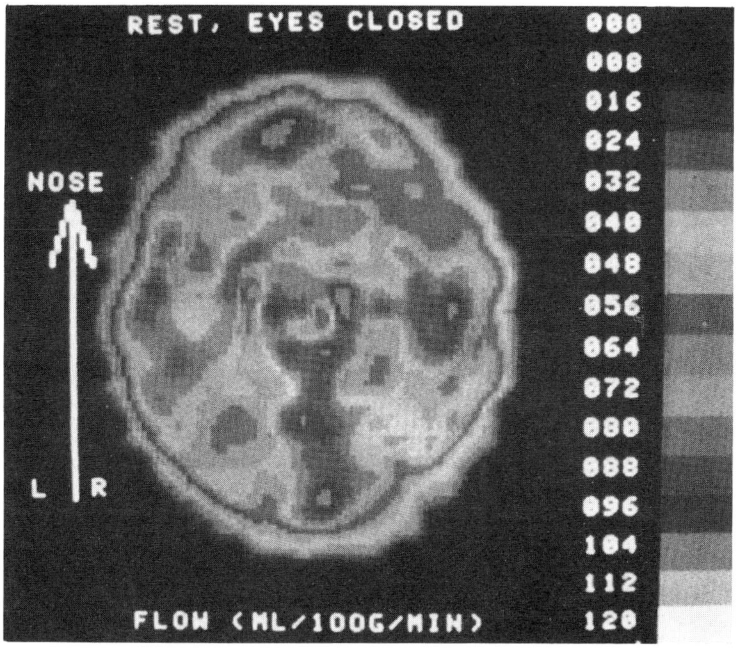

A

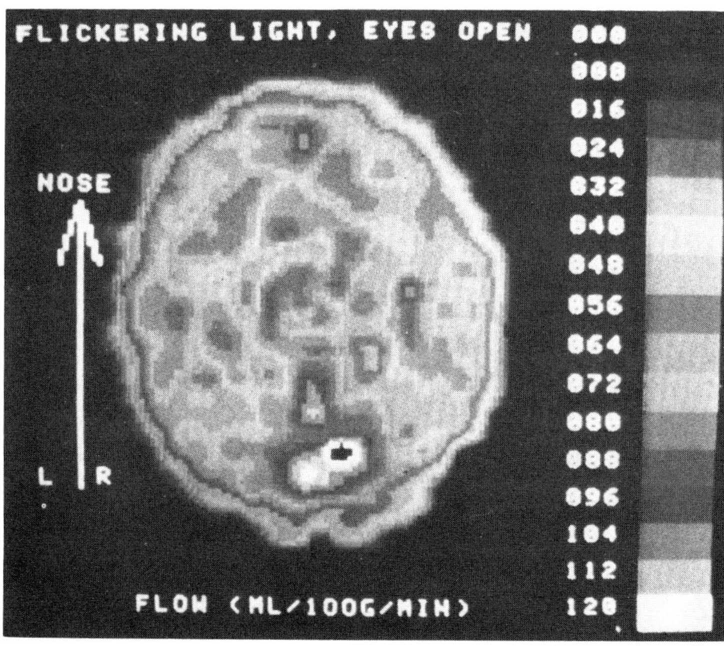

B

FIGURE 3. (A) The rCBF in a normal man during resting state with eyes closed (in a slice 5 cm above the orbito-meatal line). (B) The flow in the same man during stimulation of the visual cortex with flickering light when the eyes are open. (From Henriksen, I. et al., *Eur. J. Nucl. Med.*, 6, 487, 1981. With permission.)

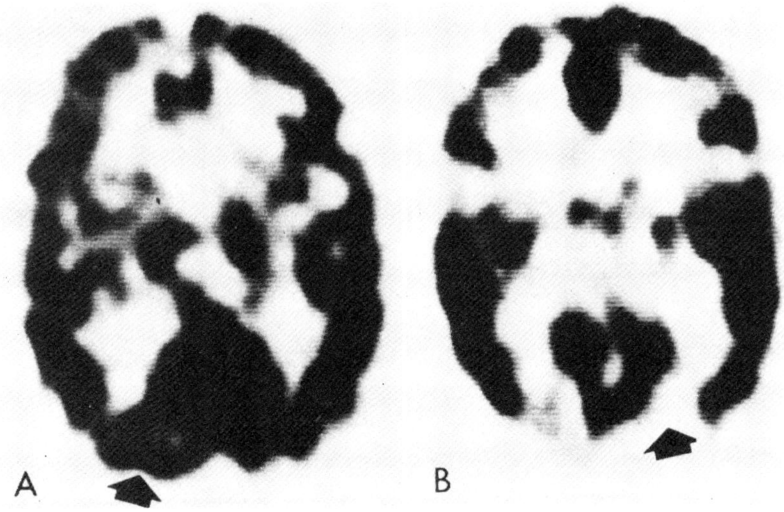

FIGURE 4. (A) Normal ^{123}I-iodoamphetamine scan obtained in a patient during visual and auditory stimulation. Note the relative increased blood flow to the occipital visual perceptive areas (arrow). (B) ^{123}I-iodoamphetamine image obtained in a patient with eyes closed during and immediately following injection. Note the markedly decreased perfusion to the occipital visual perceptual areas (arrow). (From Holman, B. L., *Invest. Radiol.*, 17, 206, 1985. With permission.)

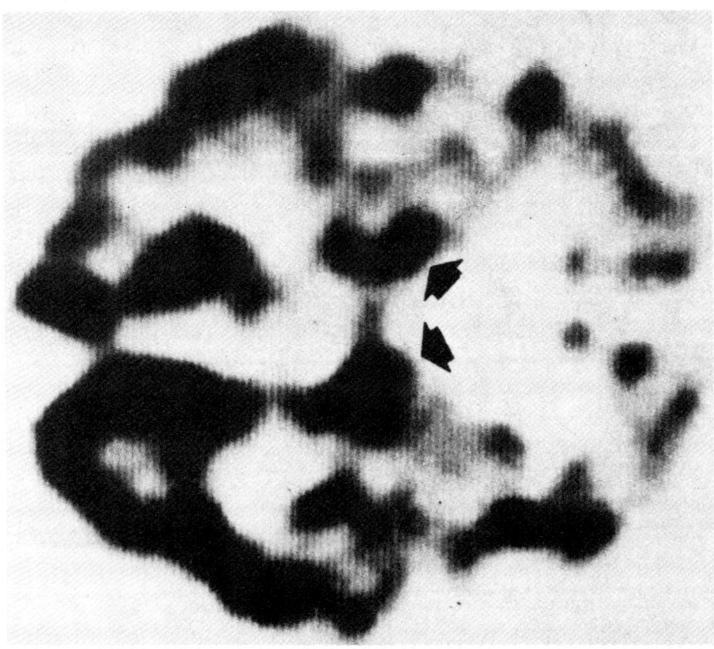

FIGURE 5. Normal ^{123}I-iodoamphetamine transaxial image. The cortical uptake appears to be related to gray matter blood flow with good demarcation of the interlobar fissure. In this tomographic slice, taken 2 cm above the orbitomeatal line, the basal ganglia are clearly defined (arrows). (From Holman, B. L., *Invest. Radiol.*, 17, 206, 1985. With permission.)

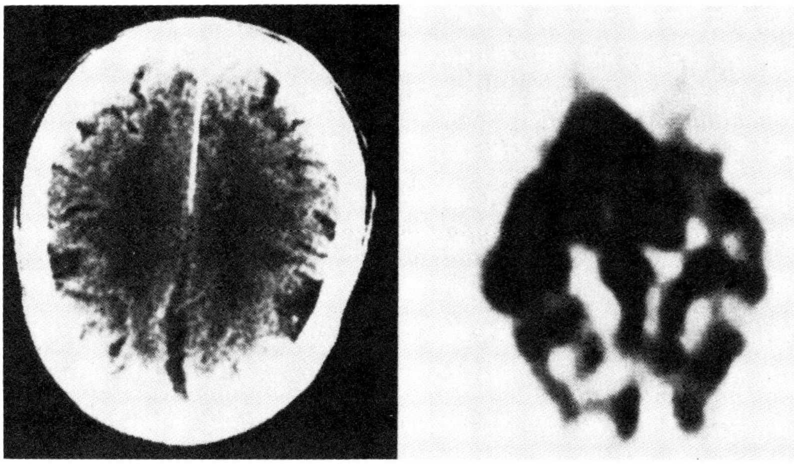

FIGURE 6. Study from a patient with hemiballism (left). During study, patient had uncontrollable flaying on entire right side of body. Tomographic image demonstrates hyperfused seizure focus in left parietal region. TCT study is normal (right). (From Hill, T. C. et al., *J. Nucl. Med.*, 23, 191, 1982. With permission.)

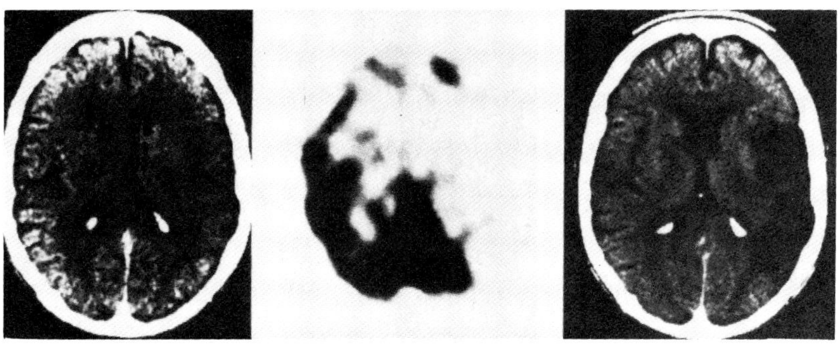

FIGURE 7. Initial TCT, obtained on day of an acute onset of right hemiparesis and aphasia, is normal (left). IMP study shows absent perfusion in territory of left middle cerebral artery (center). Follow-up TCT study 6 after acute event shows a low-density area in left parietal lobe (right). Note that resultant infarct appears smaller than ischemic tissue demonstrated on IMP study. (From Hill, T. C. et al., *J. Nucl. Med.*, 23, 191, 1982. With permission.)

4. When an ambiguous clinical pattern is observed with no evidence of structural lesions by CT scan examination.

Kuhl and co-workers[29] quantified local CBF using IMP tomography. Their model was validated for CBF quantitation with a modification of a method for arterial input sampling. Initial experiments included autoradiograms of rat brains showing the distribution of IMP activity in the local CBF pattern. The extraction rate was 92% (CBF = 33 ml/100 g/min and arterial blood pH = 7.33) for intracarotid first-pass injection in monkeys and the washout rate yielded a half-life of 1.8 min for 8% of trapped activity and 63 min for the remainder. Good contrast between gray and white matter is observed at 5 min but tends to disappear within 1 h. IMP, which is almost completely extracted in the first-pass phase through the brain, is bound in proportion to local CBF. This distribution map is maintained for at least 1 h, during which the activity diminishes slowly because of its replenishment by new IMP

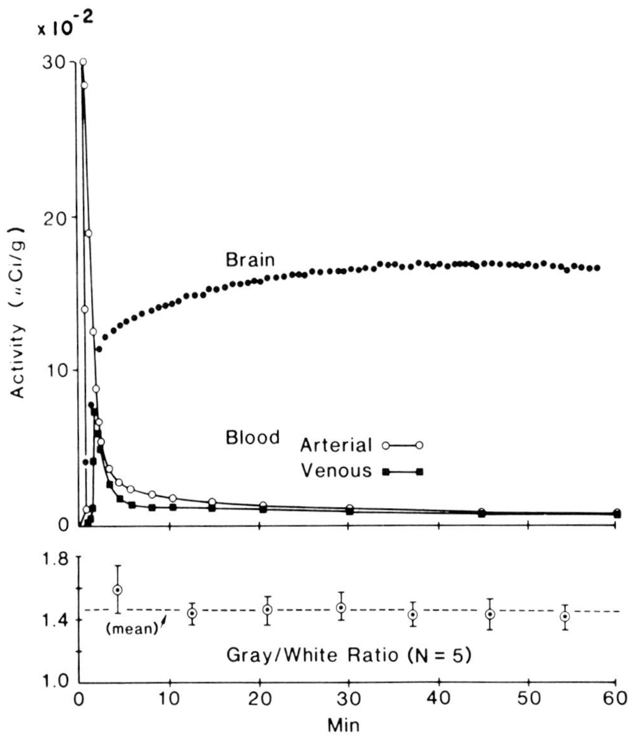

FIGURE 8. (Top) Time course of brain and blood activity during first hour after i.v. injection of IMP in normal human subject. Brain activity was measured from continuous sequence of ECT scans. (Bottom) ECT-determined ration of gray- to white-matter LCBF was relatively stable over 1 h in five human subjects. (From Kuhl, D. E. et al., *J. Nucl. Med.*, 23, 196, 1982. With permission.)

from the pulmonary reservoir. As revealed by time-activity curves, IMP experiences rapid metabolism. Time-activity curves measured from arterial and venous blood sampling reveal a rapid increase in blood activity immediately after injection, followed by a decrease within 5 min. Over the same time interval, the IMP activity measured in the brain reaches approximately 75% of its maximum value (Figure 8). The organ distribution of activity in humans after intravenous injection of IMP is shown in Figure 9. The rCBF ratio of gray to white matter was stable over 1 h. The IMP-SPECT approach to brain-flow imaging also has the advantage of demonstrating blood-flow patterns in smaller structures. While regional IMP activity in brain tissue reflects rCBF in patients with cerebral disorders, large deficits of IMP uptake reveal important structural alterations, as shown for a stroke patient in Figure 10.

Several questions related to the lipophilicity and trapping of IMP in nonspecific binding sites in the brain and capillary endothelium remain unanswered.[41] Difficulties arise since cerebral IMP uptake depends not only on cerebral perfusion but also on cerebral metabolism. Kuhl and co-workers have concluded that alterations in local CBF cause a proportional alteration in local IMP activity. Trapping and release mechanisms, however, for IMP are probably also dependent on other metabolic conditions for different brain diseases. Kuhl et al. observed no trapping in gliomas, in spite of their characterization as hypervascularized tissue. It seems that discrepancies between local CBF and IMP trapping in diseased brain parenchyma result in a decreased localized accumulation of IMP. This locally decreased activity may indicate a limitation for CBF quantitation with IMP.

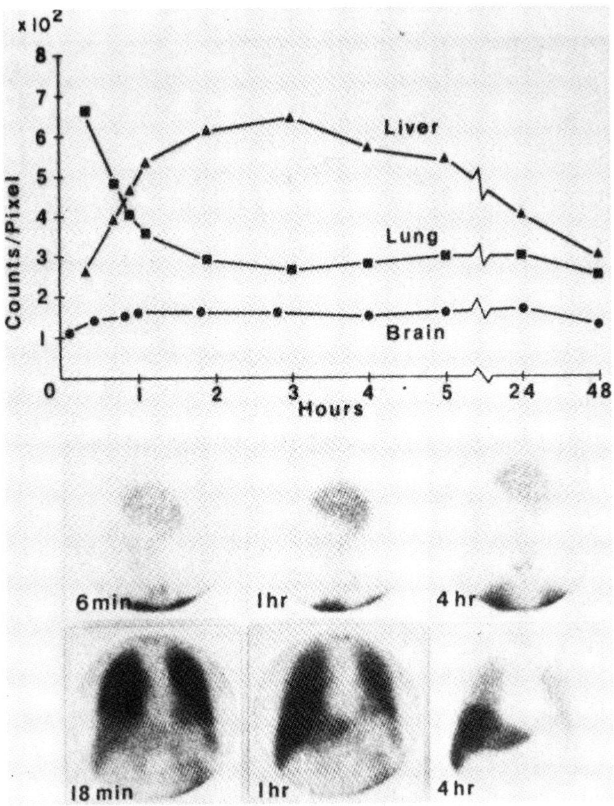

FIGURE 9. Organ distribution of activity in a human after i.v. injection of IMP. Uptake is immediate in the brain and lungs but progressive to 3 h in liver. There is rapid washout of much of lung activity, but the brain activity remains constant during first 24 h. All data are corrected for physical decay. Scintiphotos of head trunk are shown for different times. Note faint image of thyroid iodide uptake (no K1 was given to this subject) and no evidence of eye uptake. (From Kuhl, D. E. et al., *J. Nucl. Med.*, 23, 196, 1982. With permission.)

A technique using ^{123}I-isopropyl-amphetamine for rCBF was compared recently to the ^{133}Xe inhalation method by Lassen et al.[51] With IMP the input curve was not recorded since it would require arterial sampling and would fall, therefore, into the category of invasive techniques. The ^{123}I was obtained by a (p, 5n) reaction, which avoids the contamination of ^{124}I inherent to the standard (p, 2n) reaction. An area to area difference of CBF was used as a reference for normal tomograms. This is correct whenever the extraction fraction and the fractional washout are the same for all areas examined. Lassen et al.[51] found excellent agreement in all cases between ^{123}Xe CBF tomograms and IMP tomograms taken over the first 10 min. IMP scans were continued in series of 10 min over 1 h. Initial asymmetry between diseased area and normal contralateral area decreases with time. This results in a loss of contrast with time since a washout of the initial asymmetry is observed over a 1-h delay. Unfortunately, a true quantitation cannot be obtained due to the many imperfections of the SPECT technique (scatter, attenuation, reconstruction, low resolution). A tendency to outline the brain tissue better was observed with IMP relative to ^{133}Xe. The high first-pass extraction efficiency, the slow washout rate, the high brain-blood ratios, and the physical properties of ^{123}I (half-life: 13 h, energy: 159 keV) favor SPECT IMP for local CBF mapping over ^{133}Xe.

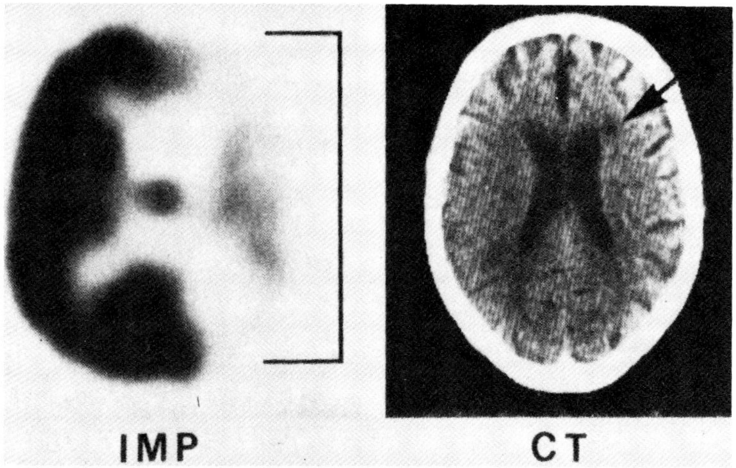

FIGURE 10. IMP tomography in stroke. These brain scans of a 57-year-old hypertensive man were made 3 months after he experienced sudden onset of left hemiparesis. Permanent reduction (21%) in CBF of entire right hemisphere (bracket) is clearly demonstrated by IMP tomography. The only abnormalities seen in CT scan were bilateral diffuse atrophy and a small lacunar infarct (arrow). (From Kuhl, D. E. et al., *J. Nucl. Med.*, 23, 196, 1982. With permission.)

From the viewpoint of clinical utility, ^{133}Xe seems to offer more than ^{123}I: longer half-life, lower cost, shorter study time, lower radiation dose, and no traumatic techniques required. Studies with ^{133}Xe can be repeated within 15 min, while a 2-d delay must be considered with IMP. However, inhaled ^{133}Xe does have some practical drawbacks, including: low solubility in tissue, with a small fraction of inhaled activity passing from the lungs to the blood pool; low X-ray energy (81 keV), making scatter discrimination difficult; a nonconstant partition coefficient in abnormal brain regions. Interest in IMP has increased considerably over the past 2 years because it permits rCBF mapping with general purpose rotating scintillation cameras.

Tomographic assessment of cerebral perfusion using a continuous carotid infusion of ^{81m}Kr and a rotating scintillation camera has been reported by Fazio et al.[28] Several advantages of this approach are listed: blood-flow distribution within brain structures (white and gray matter, basal ganglions) can be visualized accurately; alterations in perfusion can be well-located; patterns of collateral circulation are well-defined and can be evaluated accurately; high sensitivity and specificity in detecting blood-flow changes are observed during physiological activation studies. An example of a patient with reversible ischemic attack from occlusion of the right internal cerebral artery is shown in Figure 11. Administration of ^{81m}Kr under steady state conditions allows the accumulation of high count rate images at a relatively low radiation dose (^{81m}Kr half-life: 13 s). Rapid sequential changes of brain function can be assessed well by this method. Some disadvantages may prevent the method from becoming a routine clinical procedure: hemispheric images rather than global cerebral perfusion are produced; the technique is relatively invasive; and absolute measurements of blood flow are difficult to obtain.

E. The Role of SPECT in Space Occupying Disease

Emission CT started with brain-scanning when Kuhl and Edwards published their first results in 1963.[1] In the following years, scintigraphic investigation of the brain was restricted to space-occupying disease and ^{99m}Tc became the only conventional radiotracer able to penetrate the damaged BBB. It is not surprising that, with the advent of X-ray transmission

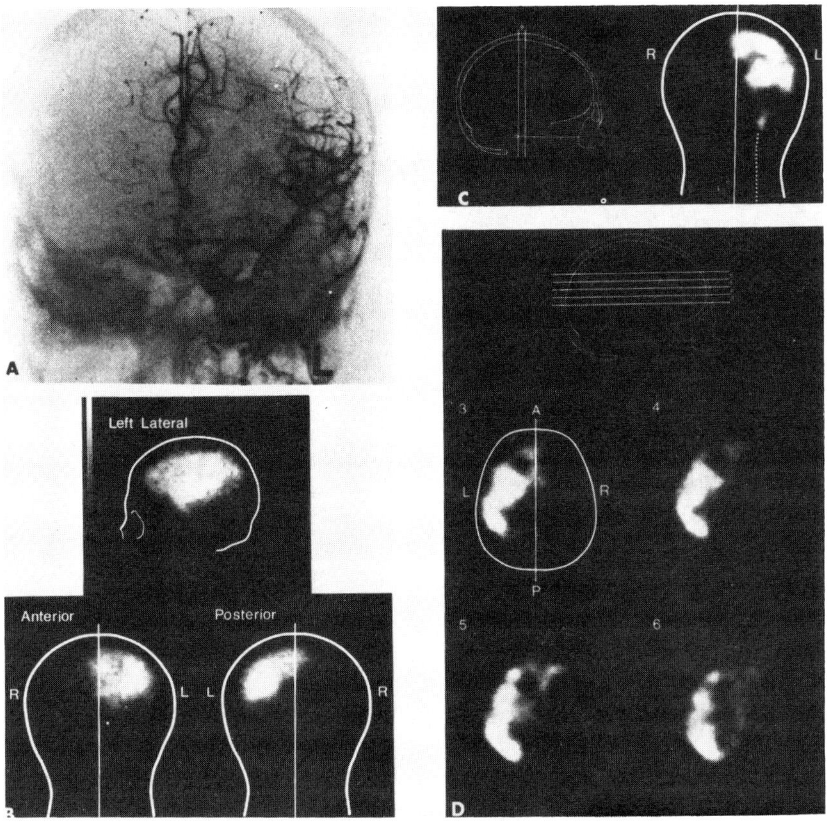

FIGURE 11. Occlusion of right internal carotid artery. (A) Left carotid angiogram. (B) Conventional ^{81m}Kr two-dimensional projections (infusion in left carotid artery). (C) Perfusion in a coronal tomographic section, passing $\simeq$12 cm behind the glabella. (D) Perfusion in set of horizontal sections. (From Fazio, F. et al., *J. Nucl. Med.*, 21, 1139, 1980. With permission.)

CT scanners, the number of brain scans decreased substantially and tomographic radiosotopic explorations were discontinued due to the unavailability of commonly used instrumentation and the absence of suitable radiopharmaceuticals. In the early 1980s rotating Anger cameras revived interest in tomographic scanning of the brain. With the appearance of improved software and the pioneering work of many investigators, radionuclide-computed tomography reappeared, and results of brain scanning with ^{99m}Tc appeared in the literature.[54-57] Early approaches included the detector used by Jaszczak et al.[58] and Keye's "Humongotron".[59] Revolving around the patient's head at a constant angular velocity, Jaszczak's device yielded a total scan time of approximately 20 min.

In subsequent years, the brain's morphology has been investigated using mainly ^{99m}Tc pertechnetate, glucoheptonate, and DTPA. Research has been oriented toward detection of primary tumors, metastatic disease, basal lesions, separation of skull and intracranial abnormalities, and better definition of the medial extent of cranial abnormalities.[60] Comparison of ECT results with transmission scans yielded comparable accuracy between the emission tomographic approach and the transmission technique for selected groups of patients. Separation of superficial and deep intracranial abnormalities has improved the detectability of lesions located near the midline in the cerebellum or near the base of the skull. ECT is also promising for distinguishing brain from skull metastases and for resulting ambiguous diagnoses in planar-delayed imaging. The overall increase in sensitivity of SPECT over conventional planar imaging (approximately 10%) is deceivingly low. Improvement was reported

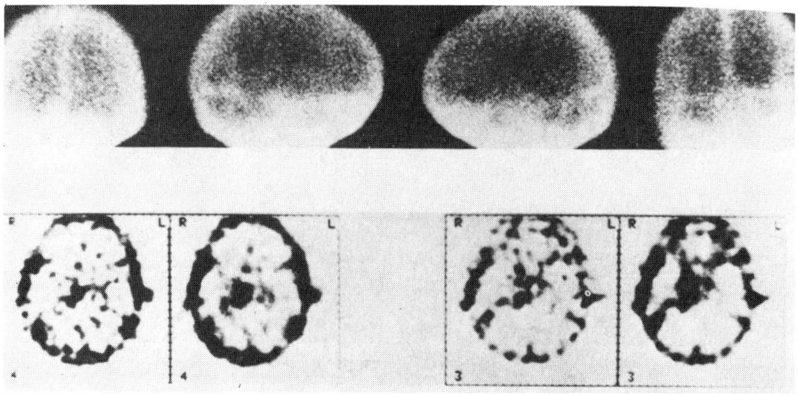

FIGURE 12. This 45-year-old female had a long history of right-sided facial pain. Five years ago, bilateral carotid angiography was performed with negative outcome. She was readmitted for investigation, with more intense right sided facial pain. Standard 4-view gamma camera scan of the brain appears normal. A dynamic perfusion sequence was entirely normal. In the SPECT scan, tomograms of this patient show an area of increased uptake, round in shape, near to the mid-line, and in the proximity of the right petrous apex. At operation, a right-sided syncitial petrous apex meningioma was found. (From Ell, P. J. and Khan, O., *Sem. Nucl. Med.*, 11, 50, 1981. With permission.)

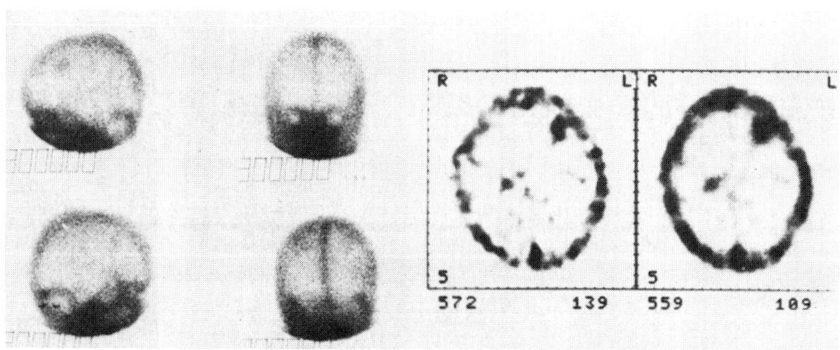

FIGURE 13. This female patient, aged 50 years, with a 4-year history of carcinoma of the left breast, presented with a recent episode of focal epilepsy. Gamma-camera brain scan showed a single abnormality in the static 4-view study (left frontal area). In the SPECT scan, two lesions are shown: one in the left frontal lobe and another in the right parietal lobe deep in the substance of the brain, close to the mid-line. (From Ell, P. J. and Khan, O., *Sem. Nucl. Med.* 11, 50, 1981. With permission.)

by Carril et al.[61] for the detection of tumors and infarcts (10% for detection of neoplasms) when the ECT approach was used in addition to planar scintigraphy. Watson et al.[62] seem to be the only group who found no improvement in SPECT compared to planar imaging. The rationale for use of SPECT in brain imaging has been described by Ell,[7] who gives a diagnostic flow chart for examination of cerebrovascular disease and for detection of neoplasms. The merits of SPECT brain studies for space-occupying disease are summarized in Figures 12 and 13. Oyameda et al.[63] concluded their analysis with the statement that transmission tomography is superior to ECT for intracranial detection of lesions. This situation seemed to be reversed for the detection of skull metastases.

As a result of these studies, the need for new radiopharmaceuticals to explore metabolic function and to detect physiopathologic conditions has become obvious. Hence, traditional ^{99m}Tc based radiotracers have essentially been abandoned for this purpose as the need for new brain imaging agents has become apparent.

III. MYOCARDIAL IMAGING

A. Introduction

Since the first correct description of acute myocardial infarction (MI) by Herrick in 1912,[64] numerous methods have been developed to identify and treat patients with cardiovascular disease. Risk factors identified in the patient's anamnesis, abnormalities found in the EKG (segmental ST changes), or increases of the serum creatinekinase isoenzyme level are detected in patients with cardiovascular disease. These findings, however, are neither sensitive nor specific enough to facilitate triaging of the patient within the healthcare system. Over the past decade, myocardial perfusion imaging[65-67] and radionuclide angiography[66,67] have become established as useful screening methods for the detection of coronary artery disease (CAD). The clinical utility of these new techniques has not yet been fully determined; nevertheless, they are providing clinicians with a sensitive tool to assess cardiac physiology and pathophysiology. Lately, regional myocardial metabolism has become a rapidly evolving field of research using PET.[68,69] PET techniques, however, are restricted to only a few selected sites because of their high implementation and operational costs. Conventional procedures in nuclear cardiology utilize gamma-emitting radiotracers such as ^{99m}Tc, ^{131}I, and ^{201}Tl. These tracers are neither metabolites nor physiologic substrates, and their behavior with respect to myocardial tissue determines their role in the diagnosis of myocardial disease.

With the appearance of commercially available low cost rotating scintillation cameras,[70] myocardial perfusion tomography became a routine procedure in many nuclear medicine departments. In earlier limited-angle tomographic approaches[71,72] that use coded apertures such as seven-pinhole and rotating slant-hole collimators, multiple images of the heart are projected simultaneously on the detector's face by means of special collimators. In the rotating detector approach,[70] full-angular sampling of the data is achieved, as opposed to the limited-angle tomographic method. At this time, rotational SPECT is indeed slowly replacing other tomographic techniques.

Tomographic studies to study regional perfusion with agents such as ^{201}Tl help to improve the localization and quantification of acute and chronic myocardial disease. ^{201}Tl is currently the best isotope for investigation of CAD, even though its specificity in stress studies is not fully understood.[73] The use of ^{201}Tl in detection of CAD and its indication for stress and redistribution imaging are reviewed in articles by McKillop[65] and Smalling.[75] The clinical usefulness of ^{201}Tl for screening patients for CAD is discussed by Hamilton.[76]

^{99m}Tc stannous pyrophosphate (^{99m}Tc PyP)[77-81] acts in the opposite fashion to ^{201}Tl: only damaged tissue shows an affinity for the radiotracer, permitting relatively good infarct sizing.[82-86] Uptake of ^{99m}Tc PyP depends on regional blood flow, calcification, and infarcted tissue. The greatest sensitivity for the detection of acute MI is observed within 48 to 72 h after occlusion of the coronary artery. As a consequence, imaging with ^{99m}Tc PyP has only limited value in an intensive care unit because of the delay time for uptake of the tracer. Although SPECT imaging with ^{99m}Tc PPI has not drawn as much attention as ^{201}Tl perfusion studies, several investigators have published results with this agent over the past few years.[87-90]

B. Myocardial SPECT Imaging, Planar Imaging, and Angiography

In some cardiovascular nuclear medicine programs, myocardial SPECT with rotating Anger cameras is slowly becoming as a noninvasive technique to assess CAD in symptomatic patients. There is, however, reluctance in many hospitals to discard planar ^{201}Tl imaging (three or four views for stress and redistribution) in favor of the tomograhic approach, in part because of the slow acceptance of SPECT technology in the nuclear medicine community. Improved quantitation of myocardial perfusion based on planar ^{201}Tl images remains a serious competitor for SPECT imaging of the heart.[91,92] A continuous but slow improvement in SPECT quantification is in progress and will ultimately determine if SPECT of the myocardium will become a viable routine protocol. In all likelihood, invasive ventriculography and arteriography will survive as the "gold standard" whenever identification of stenosed vessels and quantification of luminal flows are required. As a counterpart, myocardial SPECT (rotating camera,[70] seven-pinhole collimators,[93] rotating slant-hole collimators[94]) may evolve toward an "ideal" noninvasive technique for screening patients for myocardial disease.

Since the rotating camera offers full-angular sampling and is therefore not subject to the artifacts inherent in limited-angle tomography, some improvement in perfusion deficiency and infarct sizing should be expected. Compared to planar imaging, the sensitivity of SPECT is 10% higher with no change in specificity.[75] This improvement in sensitivity for detection of CAD has been achieved for the anterior and posterior wall sections, apical sections, and septum of the myocardium.[75] The role of SPECT in idiopathic cardiomyopathies, including those not of CAD origin, has not been established. The real benefit of perfusion SPECT studies may be for ICU admissions, since more than half of the suspected acute MI yield negative angiographic results.

Qualitatively, myocardial SPECT images may yield more accurate information than planar scintigraphy because of the considerable increase in image contrast. The measurement of activity distributions from tomographic images may lead ultimately to quantification of total and regional radiotracer uptake in the myocardium and hence quantification of the extent of perfusion changes over time for myocardial disease.

For many years, ^{201}Tl myocardial perfusion imaging has been widely accepted as a routine procedure for the evaluation of CAD, even though its usefulness, indications, and limitations are still debated. Clinical indications for ^{201}Tl imaging have been discussed in several articles[63,74,75,95-100] and its clinical usefulness in terms of sensitivity and specificity for analysis of myocardial perfusion has been analyzed critically.[76]

From coronary angiography, it is generally accepted that a critical CAD state has been reached when the degree of stenosis is equal to or exceeds 70% in one or more major coronary vessels or proximal and distal branches. A subcritical state of arterial occlusion is considered as in the range of 50 to 70% stenosis. When a 50% degree of stenosis is diagnosed angiographically, the patient's symptoms may be difficult to assess, especially when they are atypical or when collateral flow is present. Improvements obtained with SPECT imaging could increase the clinical usefulness of ^{201}Tl in the assessment of myocardial perfusion. The major benefit might be expected for patients with atypical angina symptoms (probability of CAD: 50%), angiographically documented borderline cases (50% occlusion of one or more coronary arteries), and following myocardial revascularization after coronary artery bypass grafting. In patients with remote MI, tomographic sections may provide the crucial quantitative assessment of viable myocardial tissue. In patients with acute MI, tomography may improve the quantitation of possible residual ischemia after onset of the acute symptoms. For this application, angiographically documented upper and lower normal limits for myocardial perfusion in tomographic planes must be established.

The strategy to assess CAD and to determine the amount of viable myocardial tissue with ^{201}Tl in ECT studies is similar to the procedure used in planar imaging. Stress imaging is followed by redistribution imaging 2 to 4 h later. Stress imaging reflects perfusion, while the redistribution images show functional myocardial cell mass. If the stress tomograms show abnormalities and the redistribution images show normal perfusion, myocardial ischemia is present. If no changes can be observed between stress and redistribution patterns, abnormal tomograms and quantitation of relative perfusion may indicate regional MI, and rest imaging may be considered 24 h later. With rest imaging, scars can be diagnosed if the perfusion pattern of the tomographic sections does not change. Severe CAD (above the critical limit of 70% luminal stenosis) is indicated if reversible regional perfusion is observed.

In cases where partial reperfusion is seen in the redistribution tomograms, myocardial ischemia can be diagnosed; rest imaging may be considered if more precise information is desired.

Unless fibrosis of myocardial tissue is present, underperfusion is typical for stress sections through the left ventricle of patients with stenosed coronary vessels. The redistribution process is more complex and not fully understood. The gradual uptake of radiotracer may indicate a critical degree of stenosis in some major vessels; however, collateral flow supplying the ischemic zone during the time delay following exercise cannot be excluded. Rest imaging yields valuable information in cases of acute or remote MI, possibly during coronary artery spasm conditions, and in patients with persistent chest pain. For patients who can be stressed, rest imaging should always be performed in combination with exercise and redistribution. For patients unable to withstand stress conditions, pharmacologic coronary vasodilation can be induced before injection of ^{201}Tl.[101-104] The sensitivity and specificity of this approach have been reported equal to the results obtained with physical exercise.

Analysis of ^{201}Tl tomograms is performed visually and by applying some semi-quantitative criterion based on a circumferential profile analysis around the annular region of the left ventricle. Any type of quantitative analysis and display format used in other tomographic methods[105] (e.g., seven-pinhole tomography) can be applied to rotating-camera tomograms. Until recently, most quantitation could be performed only by comparing results obtained from a small group of normal volunteers (i.e., considered free of CAD, but not documented by arteriography) to results obtained for abnormal patients with documented MI or CAD. At this time, it is difficult to make a definitive statement concerning the improvement in sensitivity and specificity of rotational tomography compared to planar imaging and to other tomographic techniques. It is not surprising that a slight increase in sensitivity, compared to planar imaging, has been reported for myocardial disease assessed with stress and redistribution perfusion tomograms.

C. Use of ^{201}Tl in SPECT Studies with Rotating Cameras

Since the first reported myocardial perfusion studies with ^{201}Tl,[106-113] improvements in instrumentation and software have contributed to a better understanding of ^{201}Tl perfusion to assess CAD. Thallium (from the Greek "*thallos:* blossoming twig") injected intravenously as thallium chloride is stable in solution as monovalent Tl^+ cation. The ^{201}Tl isotope (half-life: 73 h) decays by electron capture (EC) to ^{201}Hg; 58% of the ^{201}Tl decay goes to the ground state of ^{201}Hg and 34% to an excited state of mercury with energy 167.4 keV; the remaining 8% of ^{201}Tl decays into a 32.19-keV level of ^{201}Hg. Imaging is performed with the lower energy X-rays of mercury ranging from 69 to 83 keV and with the 167.4 keV (magnetic dipole) transition to the mercury ground state.[114] In general, the pulse-height window is set to 40% over the first peak and to 20% over the second peak.

Stress imaging is started after injection of approximately 2 to 3 mCi of ^{201}TlCl. Approximately 4% of the injected ^{201}Tl is extracted from the blood. The uptake of ^{201}Tl by the myocardium reflects mainly the blood supply to the heart. Data acquisition postinjection with a single-head large-field-of-view camera is generally performed over 180° from a right anterior oblique (RAO) to a left posterior oblique (LPO) position. A total acquisition time of approximately 20 min is considered adequate to scan most patients. It has also been observed that the patient's discomfort is reasonably low for these scan times. On the other hand, problems associated with ^{201}Tl redistribution, washout, and uptake arise with an increase in scan time.

Problems associated with SPECT imaging of the heart are multiple. In normal myocardial tissue, ^{201}Tl uptake reflects regional perfusion through the sodium-potassium pump.[65] Idiopathic abnormalities impair myocardial uptake of ^{201}Tl, hence ^{201}Tl abnormalities are not entirely specific for CAD. Patients under medication may also not yield the correct distribution pattern for ^{201}Tl. Drugs such as Digoxin and Propranolol decrease the extraction of ^{201}Tl uptake, while Dipyridamole increases the uptake considerably.[103]

No final consensus has been achieved for the optimal data acquisition protocol in a clinical setting.[115] Multiple phantom studies have been performed by various groups[116-120] to establish a protocol for ^{201}Tl perfusion tomography with single-headed rotating cameras. One major difficulty arises with the desire to included adequate attenuation compensation into the reconstruction algorithm.[121] The complexity of the human chest and the myocardium's anatomical location complicate the correction process. Information from the anterior wall is obliterated through the lung tissue and overlying ribs. Radioactivity originating from the posterior and inferior wall is attenuated by the presence of other organs with a density different from the lung parenchyma. Myocardial SPECT does not provide quantitative information about absolute radiotracer concentrations; hence, recent efforts have been oriented toward attenuation problems[121] and scatter corrections[122,123] to obtain the best possible relative quantitation. New approaches to correction for Compton scatter have yielded some improvement in contrast and spatial resolution in phantom studies by decreasing the slightly overestimated activity in the organ.[122-123] Blurring at the organ edges may also be reduced to some extent. Application of this approach to clinical myocardial perfusion studies has yet to be made.

Resolution of tomographic slices is affected by the low-energy photons of ^{201}Tl (poor discrimination of scatter components) and by the motion of the heart which inevitably blurs the edges of the organ. With the recent possibility of acquiring data from noncircular orbits or rotating cameras[125] or from the motion of the patient relative to circular rotating cameras, some improvement in spatial resolution can be expected.

A clinical ^{201}Tl SPECT protocol can be described by the following steps:

1. A 32-million-count flood image is acquired either without a collimator using a point source of 200 to 300 μCi of ^{201}Tl located at a distance of approximately 5 useful field-of-view diameters or with a collimator using a ^{201}Tl extended flood source. This image is obtained preferably at the beginning of the day, together with a check of the center of rotation as part of the daily routine quality control protocol for the SPECT camera. A 40% pulse-height window is used over the 78-keV photopeak, and a 20% window is used over the second 167-keV photopeak if multiple-window capability is available. The use of a high resolution collimator is recommended.
2. The patient is stressed next to the SPECT camera until onset of typical symptoms: chest pain, exhaustion, maximum heart rate, hypertension, ST segmental changes in ECG, and/or serious arrhythmia. After injection of 2 to 3 mCi of $^{201}TlCl$, imaging is started immediately after exercise.
3. The stressed patient, holding both arms behind his head, lies supine on the scan table. The CRT scope is used to correctly position the patient's myocardium within the field of view of the camera while moving the camera's head over 180° from a 45° LPO to a 45° RAO position. For circular motion, the camera's head is generally brought as close as possible to the lateral side of the patient's chest. In cases where noncircular motion is available, the patient remains as close as possible to the collimator's face either by following the camera's circular motion or by moving the camera in a noncircular orbit around the patient.
4. Planar views in 64 × 64 matrices are collected for 32 views (32 s per view) or for 16 views (1 min per view) from an LPO to RAO position. Total data collection time is approximately 16 min. A typical patient SPECT acquisition file (16 views over 180°) is shown in Figure 14. The entire procedure involves no longer than 20 min. In case a doubleheaded tomographic unit is used to acquire the data, the opposite camera head moves from an RAO position to an LPO (counterclockwise) orientation

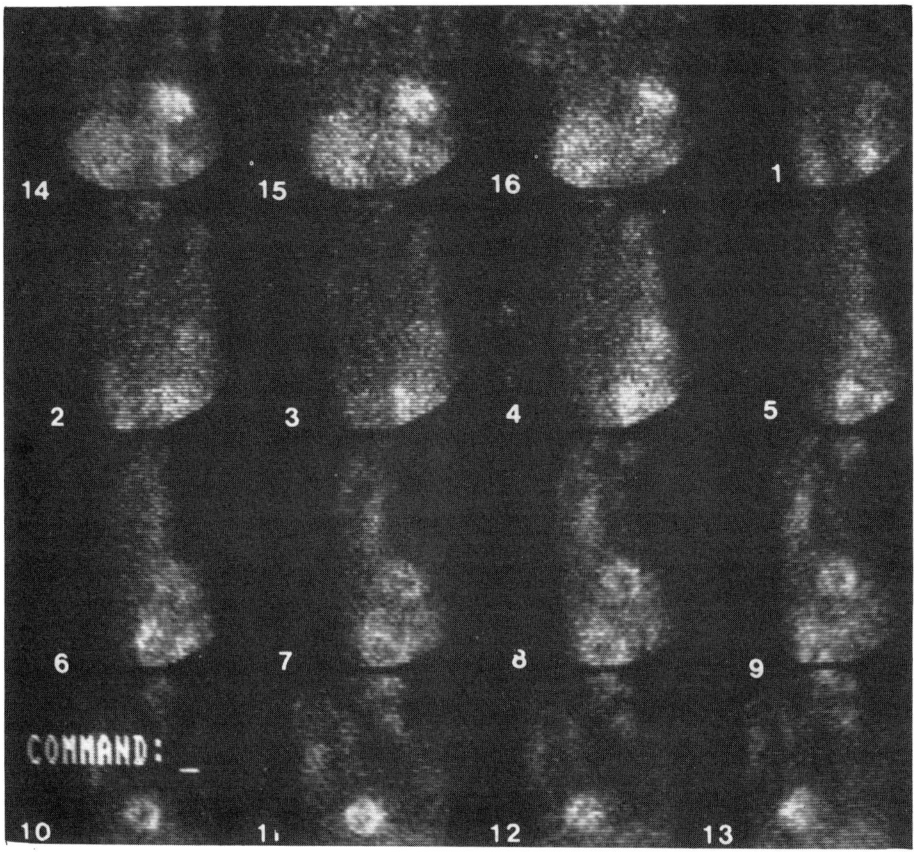

FIGURE 14. ^{201}Tl redistribution data for myocardial perfusion study. The SPECT acquisition file has a total of 16 planar views (64 × 64 matrices) collected over 180° from an LPO position (starting at frame 1) to an RAO position (ending at frame 16; frames 14 to 16 are mirrored). Myocardium-to-surrounding-lung activity was approximately 3:1.

to collect the opposite views which with a single-head device could be obtained only by full 360° rotation. The extremely low count-rate densities observed in cardiac ^{201}Tl SPECT images (20 to 90 counts maximum per planar view) yield very poor information on the opposite side of the heart because of its asymmetrical location in the chest.

5. Planar views usually are flood-corrected, although this seems not to be mandatory because of the very low count densities observed in the thallium acquisition data (target to background ratio of about 2:1). These low count densities mask most artifacts resulting from nonuniformities or from small offsets of the center of rotation (on the order of 3 mm or 1 pixel in a 128 × 128 matrix for a 15-in. LFOV camera). Reconstruction can be performed simultaneously during data collection or in batch mode at the end of the day. In most commercially available systems, reconstruction of tomographic slices is based on a standard filtered backprojection (FBP) algorithm using a linear interpolation scheme for the profiles to account for the mismatch of the projected filtered profiles at an angle with a pixel of the square matrix. Using a standard 16-bit minicomputer with floating-point hardware capabilities, reconstruction time per tomographic slice is approximately 10 s for a 16 view data collection cycle over 180° and approximately 20 s for a 32 view collection process over the same angular range. Transaxial tomographic myocardial sections obtained from the collected planar views displayed in Figure 14 are shown in Figure 15. Array processors make it possible to

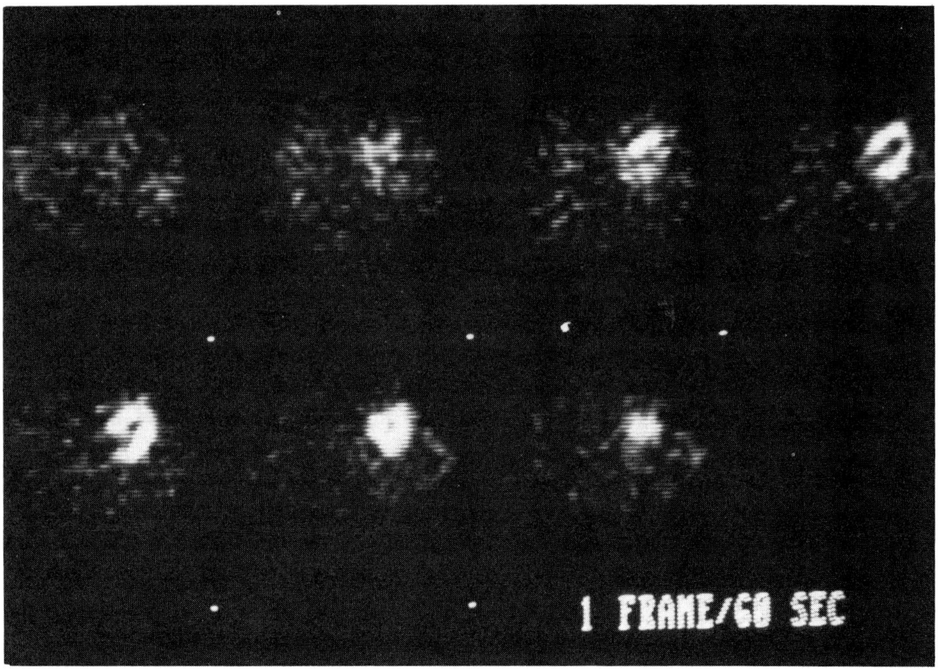

FIGURE 15. Tomographic transaxial views of the myocardium obtained with the data displayed in Figure 14. Tomographic slices (each 1.3 cm thick) are perpendicular to the long axis of the patient's body. The orientation is given by an observer viewing from the feet toward the head.

obtain results as soon as data collection is complete or within a short time after completion ranging from seconds to several minutes, depending largely on the type of computer and hardware used if the reconstruction is performed postacquisition. Photon attenuation compensation can be included during the reconstruction if data collection is performed over 360°.

6. From the set of slices transaxial to the longitudinal axis of the body, tomographic slices perpendicular to the longitudinal axis of the left ventricle are obtained by defining interactively the caudal and cephalad angulation of the myocardium on a video screen (Figure 16). Tomographic sections orthogonal to the left ventricle's long axis are then obtained after applying three-dimensional linear interpolation to the original set of transaxial sections.[126] Tomograms in this oblique orientation have the advantage of improved visualization of the myocardial structure and allow a more adequate relative quantitation of regional perfusion.[127]
7. Tomographic slices from apex to base, as shown in Figure 17 are displayed with the observer looking along the left ventricle's axis toward the base of the myocardium. An outline of the right ventricle can be observed on the left side of the left ventricle. Slice thickness can vary between 1.2 and 2 cm.
8. Depending on the myocardium's size, four to seven tomographic sections are usually used to quantify regional perfusion. In general, circumferential analysis is performed and the relative radiotracer activity around the myocardium is preserved.
9. Redistribution tomography is performed 2 to 4 h later by repeating steps 4 to 8; results obtained are compared to the exercise patterns.
10. If planar imaging is discarded in favor of SPECT imaging, stress and redistribution tomograms as well as relative activity curves must be compared to upper and lower normal limits. If the ^{201}Tl perfusion protocol is based on planar stress and redistribution

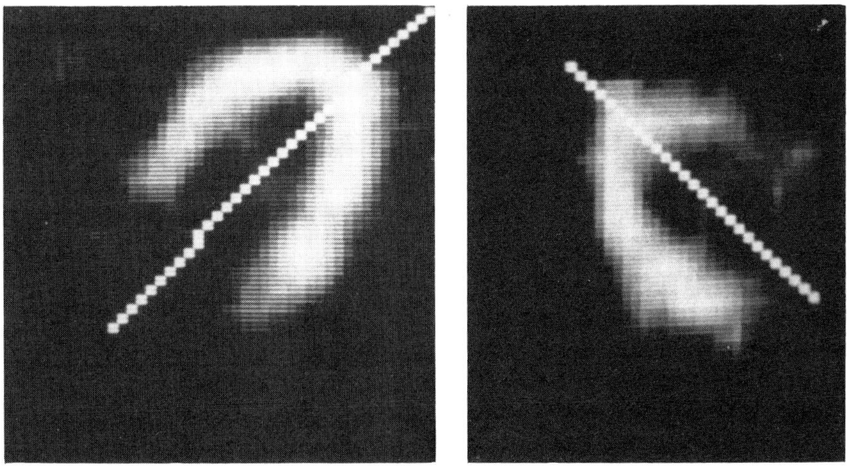

A B

FIGURE 16. Interactive selection of cephalad and caudal angulation of the left-ventricular long axis. A three-dimensional linear interpolation is applied to the tomographic transaxial data set. Caudal (A) and cephalad (B) angles of the myocardium's left-ventricular long axis are determined interactively with a joystick.

imaging, SPECT can be used as an add-on modality. Redistribution and rest imaging is performed only for comparative purposes.

11. If considered necessary, rest imaging is performed 24 h later.

D. Clinical Results of ^{201}Tl Imaging

Early myocardial perfusion tomography with rotating cameras was applied to a small population of "normal" patients (volunteers) with no known myocardial history and to larger groups of patients with clinically documented transmural myocardial necrosis based on electrocardiographic or enzymatic evidence. An overall 10 to 15% increase in sensitivity over planar imaging was reported for the tomographic technique with no change in specificity. A decrease in sensitivity with infarct age was observed. Tomographic imaging improved the visual detection and delineation of transmural inferior subendocardial MI and transmural anterior MI.

Kirsch et al.[131] studied 95 patients with ^{201}Tl SPECT and compared the results to angiography and planar scintigraphy; 23 patients had a normal coronary angiogram. Patients who underwent ^{201}Tl perfusion were studied only at rest. The results of Kirsch et al. showed a considerably higher sensitivity for SPECT (93%) compared to planar imaging (68%), especially for the detection of perfusion defects in the posterior wall of the myocardium. Small myocardia and hearts with high left ventricular ejection fractions resulting in a washout of the myocardial sections seem to be poorly suited for SPECT studies. Small hypertrophic heart yielded higher false negative results, and large hypertrophic hearts (with or without cardiomyopathies) led to an increase in the number of false positives. In the latter case, specificity decreased slightly because of an increase in the number of false positives (decrease in true normals). The increase in false positive rate was attributed to attenuation effects on data collected over 360°. Redistribution effects during data acquisition seemed to be less severe than anticipated, in concordance with preliminary results by McIntyre et al.[132]

Much effort has been directed to comparison of results obtained for 180° versus 360° rotation.[116-120] No definite consensus seems to be available at this time. In institutions where routine SPECT ^{201}Tl is performed, this controversy seems to be resolved from a practical

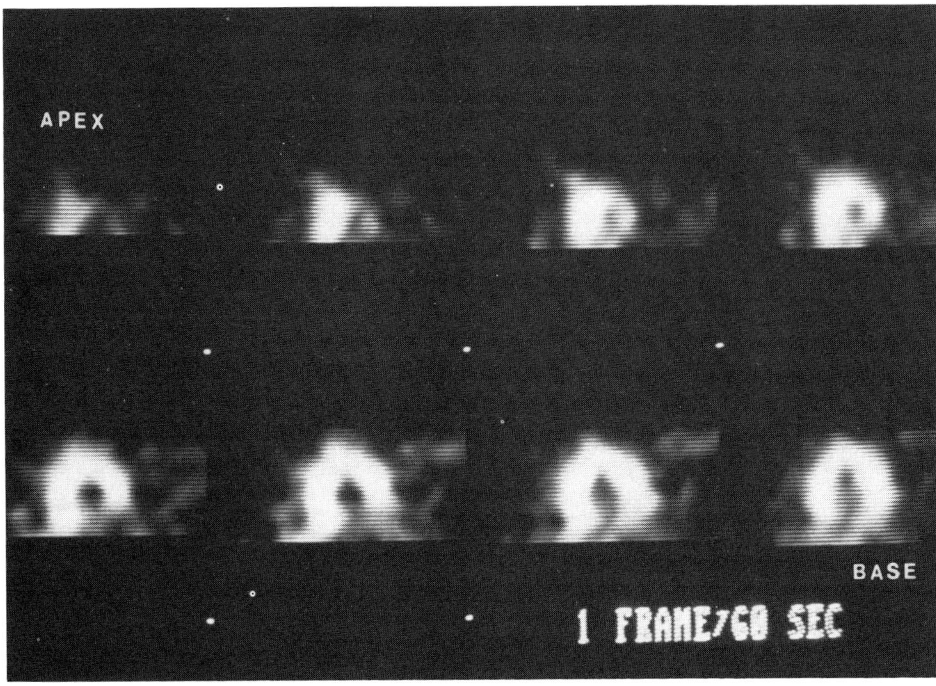

FIGURE 17. Transaxial slices perpendicular to the myocardium's left-ventricular long axis. Tomographic sections start at the apex and end near the base. Each slice is approximately 1.3 cm thick. Exercise and redistribution perfusion patterns show photopenic defect in inferolateral left-ventricular myocardium. Postinferolateral myocardial infarction was diagnosed. A gated blood-pool study showed akinesis in left ventricular inferolateral and inferoapical regions. The right ventricular apex was akinetic.

point of view. Because of the myocardium's asymmetric location in the chest, a 180° scan from a 45° LPO to a 45° RAO seems to be the only logical approach for a single-headed tomographic camera. The energy discrimination of scattered photons is rather poor for ^{201}Tl so that views collected on the distal side of the heart are of inferior quality; these data substantially degrade the good information collected with the 180° scan on the proximal side of the myocardium. That is, the higher image contrast obtained from a 180° scan contributes to better image quality. Coleman's[120] double-headed camera, which allows data collection over 360° in the same amount of time and with the same count density as over 180°, is an interesting approach; it is doubtful, however, that this approach will become part of standard ECT equipment in community hospitals.

Studies with a modified Iowa heart phantom (Figure 18) loaded with ^{201}Tl (myocardial to background activity ratio of 2:1) have been performed at the University of Colorado, yielding the following results:[133]

1. The LPO starting position for a 180° scan is relatively critical. The lesion size and depth simulating a lack of perfusion is dependent on the starting angle. Best results were obtained for a symmetric 180° scan around the myocardium.
2. With single-headed large-field-of-view cameras, the 180° scan yields better results than the 360° approach in terms of organ shape and resolution.
3. Angular undersampling (16 views over 180°) seems not to affect the quality of the tomograms. Decreasing the number of views therefore provides a proportional increase in count densities in the raw data. Lesion sizes and organ geometry improve visually more with increased photons than with an increased number of data acquisition stations

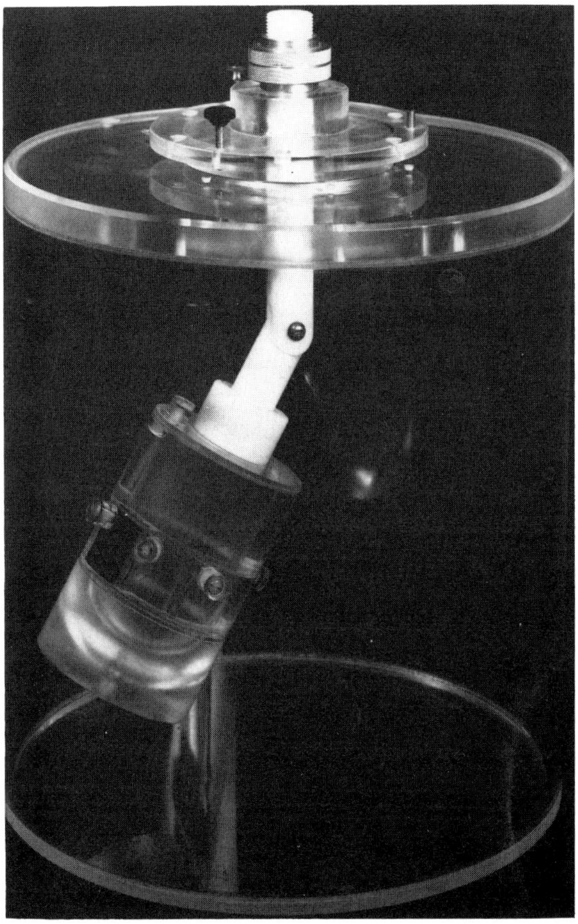

FIGURE 18. Iowa heart phantom used at the University of Colorado Medical School to assess acquisition parameters for myocardial SPECT studies. Angulation of the heart's long axis determines caudal angle (approximately 45°). Cephalad angulation is obtained by rotating the cylindrical phantom around the long axis (approximately 30°).

4. The extremely low count densities encountered in SPECT ^{201}Tl perfusion studies (20 to 90 counts max/planar view) suggest that clinically acceptable reconstructions can be obtained with matrices no larger than 64 $\times$ 64.

Recently, Caldwell et al.[134] used an animal model to study the problem of accurate quantitation of regional blood flow to determine viable and infarcted myocardial mass. Regions with perfusion defects showed an overestimation of flow. Good correlation between calculated values and measured weights of infarcted myocardial mass was obtained by Keyes et al.;[135] these investigators showed that ^{201}Tl perfusion studies had a high promise for quantification of acute myocardial injuries.

Quantification of ^{201}Tl uptake by the myocardium has shown little progress. Recently Garcia et al.[136] described a method for quantification of the relative three-dimensional uptake of ^{201}Tl in the myocardium. The basic idea is not new and the strategy used by these authors is essentially that applied to tomograms obtained by other tomographic techniques such as seven-pinhole. The technique uses the maximal count circumferential profiles of short-axis (oblique) and long-axis (sagittal) tomograms of the heart, with the three-dimensional dis-

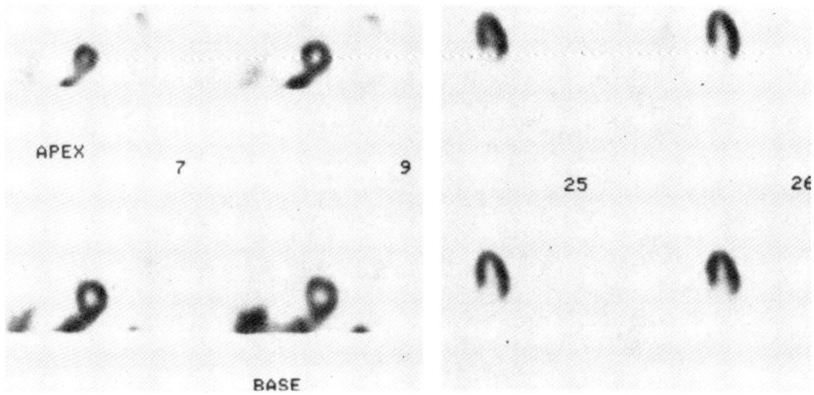

FIGURE 19. Tomograms obtained in cucumber (short axis) projection (left) and horizontal long-axis projection (right) in normal subject. Uptake of ^{99m}Tc TBI [hexakis (*t*-butyl-isonitrile)] is uniform thorughout left ventricle. Left lobe of liver is separated from inferoposterior wall of left ventricle on short-axis images. On horizontal long-axis images, apex of left ventricle is at the top of the horseshoe, septum to left, and lateral wall at right. (From Holman, B. L. et al., *J. Nucl. Med.*, 25, 1350, 1984. With permission.)

tribution mapped onto a two-dimensional polar representation. No corrections for scattering and attenuation were included. An abnormal ^{201}Tl perfusion map or washout was obtained by automatic comparison with lower limits of normal profiles. Normal limits were obtained as curves defined by 2.5 standard deviations below the mean value of the circumferential activity. These normal limits were taken from a group of 25 patients having less than 5% likelihood of CAD based on Bayesian analysis. Analysis by Garcia et al. of ^{201}Tl washout seemed not to improve detection and localization of CAD. The accuracy in percentage of abnormal myocardium is influenced by many factors that can contribute to considerable error in measuring the size of perfusion defects or remote MI. The object size (small transmural perfusion defects may be masked, while large defects may be overestimated), the motion of the heart and chest, as well as myocardial thickness, have to be considered during analysis. Acquisition, preprocessing, reconstruction, and the method of relative quantification all substantially affect the evaluation of lower limits of normal profiles. Nevertheless, this computerized method yields a reproducible quantitative assessment of myocardial ^{201}Tl uptake.

Presently, myocardial perfusion scintigraphy with ^{201}Tl seems to be the most well-established method for routine assessment of CAD in humans. However, ^{201}Tl does not have optimal physical properties, and a ^{99m}Tc-based radiotracer that could replace ^{201}Tl has been sought for over 4 years. Preliminary results obtained with a new ^{99m}Tc labeled myocardial imaging agent, hexakis (*t*-butylisonitrile) Tc (I)(^{99m}Tc TBI) have been reported recently by Holman et al.[137] The biodistribution of ^{99m}Tc TBI was studied in four normal patients and in two subjects with CAD. Preliminary results from animal studies indicate that ^{99m}Tc TBI is promptly extracted from the blood pool by the myocardium. The radiotracer remains in the myocardium for several hours with approximately constant concentration. Planar, tomographic, and gated myocardial images were obtained for 3 patients at rest between 1 and 4 h after injection. The ratio of heart to lung activity was found to be 1.5:1 in these 3 subjects after 1 h, while the liver uptake was increasing steadily over the same period of time to yield a liver to heart activity ratio of 3.4:1. Tomographic sections of the heart are shown in Figure 19. Perfusion defects due to remote MI and transient ischemia could be well visualized with ^{99m}Tc TBI.

A ^{99m}Tc based radiotracer has two major advantages over ^{201}Tl: high photon yield and higher energy, permitting better energy discrimination and, therefore, better resolution. Since ^{99m}Tc TBI seems to remain fixed in the myocardium, reversible ischemia may be imaged as late as 4 h after injection. This also indicates, however, that two injections may be necessary to distinguish properly between stress-induced ischemia and irreversible myocardial injury.

A teaching editorial by Mullani et al.[138] gives an overview of the basic principles dictating the choice of a satisfactory myocardial perfusion imaging agent. After the characteristics of an optimal imaging agent are defined, the properties of ^{99m}Tc TBI are reviewed in terms of the four fundamental characteristics of a perfusion tracer for *in vivo* imaging: the energy of the emitted photons, the physical half-life of the isotope, the myocardial extraction and retention of the radiotracer, and, finally, the clinical safety, radiation dose and toxicity. It appears that the lack of redistribution observed with ^{99m}Tc TBI will prevent this radiotracer from becoming widely accepted in clinical practice. Since a clinically useful redistribution seems not to occur, the half-life of a potential substitute for ^{201}Tl becomes critical. Compared to ^{201}Tl, the extraction efficiency for ^{99m}Tc TBI appears to be suboptimal, resulting in a relatively poor myocardium to background ratio and, therefore, relatively poor image quality. This fact may not be compensated by the higher emission energy of ^{99m}Tc. At the present time, myocardial SPECT imaging with rotating cameras may not play an important role with this type of ^{99m}Tc based imaging agent, because SPECT yields only a marginal increase in sensitivity and specificity with regard to myocardial injuries, even though the development and use of a new perfusion imaging agent by Holman and colleagues[137] provides an important step forward toward an improved myocardial perfusion imaging.

E. Gated Cardiac SPECT Studies

Gated-blood-pool emission-computed tomography (GSPECT) has been used recently by different groups of investigators[139-141] as a noninvasive technique to assess ventricular wall motion. Tamaki et al.[142] selected 3 normal volunteers and a small group of 15 patients with angiographically documented myocardial injuries to study planar and ECT gated-blood-pool imaging. A LFOV general-purpose rotating camera collected 16 images over 180° from an LPO (45° left posterior oblique) to an RAO (45° right anterior oblique) position with 1 min/view. Data were acquired in the R-wave synchronized frame mode from each station. Transaxial tomographic sections were used to reconstruct oblique transaxial, frontal, oblique frontal, and sagittal sections through the myocardium. The principal advantage of GSPECT is the visualization of all four cardiac chambers and the possibility of quantifying their function. Systolic contraction and diastolic expansion of the ventricles, together with the corresponding volume changes in right and left atria, were well-presented in a cine-mode display. The LV wall motion could be displayed especially well in the frontal oblique view perpendicular to the long axis of the LV. GSPECT may permit more precise quantification of regional and global myocardial function compared to planar gated-blood-pool imaging.

A segmental motion of the LV has been measured by Barat and co-workers[143] using the GSPECT technique. The validity of their method was assessed in terms of contrast angiocardiography. ECG data were collected during 20 min over 360° using a LFOV camera. The framing rate at each of the 64 stations was 8 per cardiac cycle. After reconstruction, sagittal slices containing the LV chamber were selected to quantify the wall motion, with the results compared to contrast ventriculography. Patients (66) with chest pain were referred to cardiac catheterization and were examined with the GSPECT technique. Analysis of regional wall motion was performed with both techniques. Coordinates of ED and ES outlines of apical dimple and LV aortic junction were used to define the center of the ventricular contraction, as shown in Figure 20. The LV outline in ED and ES for the GSPECT slice was assessed by Fourier analysis (amplitude and phase). Regional segmentation of the LV wall was then performed using the approach outlined for angiographic images. The regional

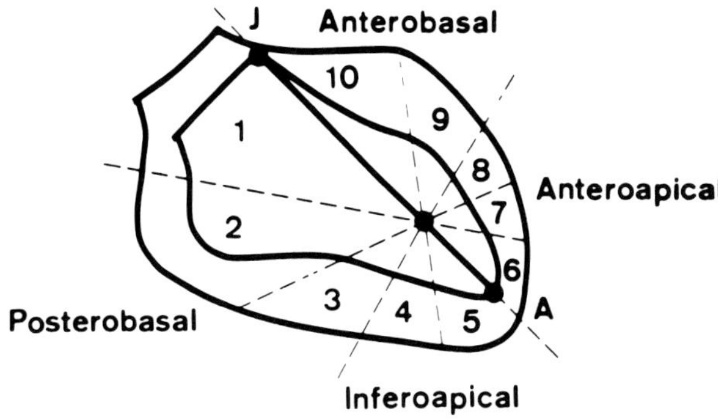

FIGURE 20. Cardiac outlines at ED and ES. Center of contraction is on line joining LV-aortic junction (J) to apex (A), as described in text; it forms center of ten 36° radial sectors. These are grouped into four conventional anatomic regions whose adjacent names include sectors as follows: posterobasal (2,3), inferoapical (4,5), anteroapical (6-8), and anterobasal (9,10). (From Barat, J. L. et al., *J. Nucl. Med.*, 25, 1167, 1984. With permission.)

wall motion for these latter images was measured as a percentage shortening of the mean radius of each individual sector. Figure 21 shows a normal and an akinetic heart documented with ventriculography and GSPECT. Because of suppression of background and overlying myocardial activities in the GSPECT approach, quantification of regional wall motion is not restricted to an approximate evaluation. The method of describing wall motion radially toward a center of contraction[144] was applied to both contrast ventriculography and GSPECT. Inter- and intraobserver variations in results were attributed to variable operator interventions in the two approaches. Although only one plane through the major axis of the heart was used for the dynamic study, Barat's method can be applied to any plane containing this axis. Regional myocardial wall motion seems to be approachable with the GSPECT technique, with results correlating well with contrast angiography. The noninvasive nature of GSPECT may promote this innovative technique to a routine procedure for evaluation of cardiac dynamic function.

F. Infarct Avid SPECT Imaging

Some isolated attempts to perform tomographic studies with ^{99m}Tc PyP in humans are described in the literature.[87-90] After acquisition of tomographic raw data, the patients are injected with approximately 20 mCi of ^{99m}Tc pertechnetate to provide red blood cell labeling resulting from the presence of the stannous ion in the pyrophosphate complex. Leaving the patient in the same position, tomographic blood-pool imaging is then restarted. According to Holman et al.,[145] this method, called "double-tracer tomography", has improved specificity. By superimposing the blood-pool image onto the ^{99m}Tc PyP image, the focal uptake in infarcted areas can be discerned. This focal activity is restricted to the walls of the ventricle. The use of the ^{99m}Tc red blood cell technique is necessary for accurate localization of pyrophosphate uptake in the tomographic plane.

The potential of ^{99m}Tc PyP tomography is limited, primarily because a time delay of 24 h is needed after the onset of acute MI. Portable small-field-of-view cameras with SPECT capabilities would be useful for this study, but they are not available at this time. These limitations explain in part why myocardial SPECT procedures using infarct avid agents have had no major impact on the diagnosis of myocardial injuries.

G. Role of SPECT in Myocardial Imaging

Several issues concerning the use of SPECT with rotating cameras in nuclear cardiology

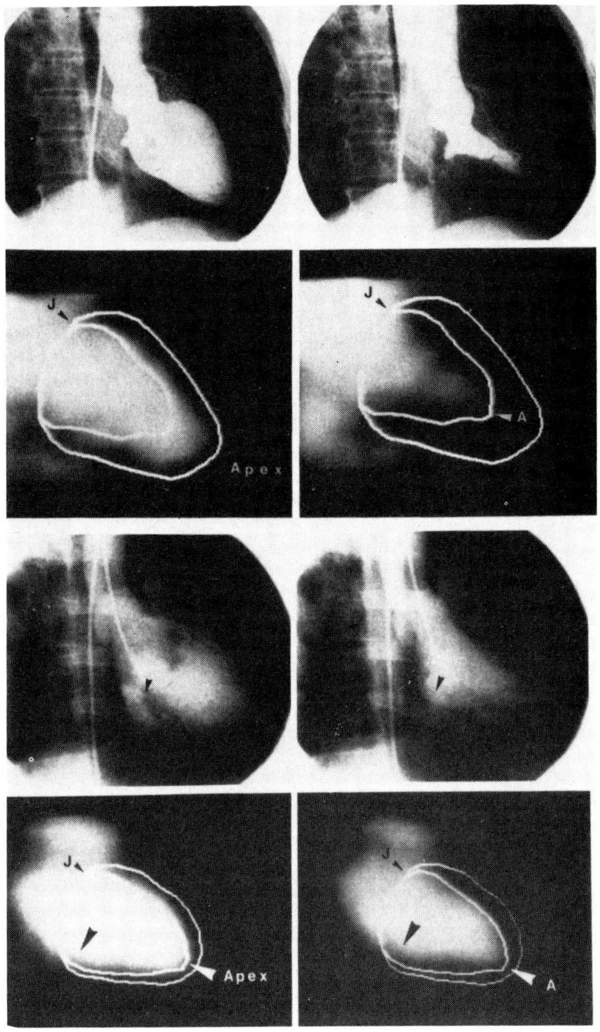

FIGURE 21. Images from two patients: upper 4 normal, lower 4 showing inferobasal akinetic region due to infarct (arrow). Left column diastolic, right systolic. Lines 1 and 3 from contrast ventriculography, 30° RAO; lines 2 and 4 from GSPECT, sagittal slice containing long LV axis. (From Barat, J. L. et al., *J. Nucl. Med.*, 25, 1167, 1984. With permission.)

remain to be answered. Early SPECT results with rotating cameras reflect essentially the same enthusiasm that was observed earlier with the seven-pinhole tomographic technique. There is little doubt but that high-contrast tomograms free from underlying and overlying activities are qualitatively superior to planar scintigraphic ^{201}Tl images. If there is any clinically relevant superiority of the rotating-camera approach over the seven-pinhole technique,[146] it has to be attributed to the full-angular sample of rotational tomography; rotational tomograms are relatively free from the artifacts observed with limited-angle tomographic techniques.

At the present time the planar ^{201}Tl imaging protocol seems to remain the practical clinical approach to myocardial perfusion. In addition, most dedicated minicomputers are offering a quantitative planar ^{201}Tl evaluation. With the improved quantitative analysis of planar thallium images by Goris et al.[92] the borderline superiority of SPECT over planar imaging may diminish even more and could eventually vanish. So far, SPECT with rotating cameras has proven to be attractive for myocardial perfusion studies since it yields high quality images. This fact alone does not justify the exclusive use of this relatively complicated and sophisticated technique to gain more insight into the extent of myocardial injuries. A marginal diagnostic superiority of SPECT with rotating cameras may yet be demonstrated; at this time, continued investigations about the clinical usefulness and practicality of SPECT should continue to determine its future role in nuclear cardiology.[75]

IV. LIVER AND SPLEEN IMAGING

A. Introduction

Radiographic exploration of the liver/spleen system is a complex issue. Standard X-ray examinations of liver and spleen do not depict the subtle changes in tissue density that are indicative of pathologic processes. Radiography and angiography are moderately helpful in studies of these organs because of their low sensitivity for detecting specific diseases. Over the past decade, attention has increasingly focused on X-ray transmission tomography, ultrasound, and nuclear medicine planar imaging for delineation of the liver/spleen system. Since normal and abnormal liver tissue have approximately the same density, the contrast of CT scans is generally poor. Ultrasound examinations are competitive with nuclear medicine for studies of the liver and spleen, and the choice of examination or examination sequence varies from one institution to another and with the particular pathologic condition suspected of being present.

Today, nuclear medicine imaging of the liver and spleen with a large-field-of-view camera is one of the more practical, noninvasive examinations of this organ system. Nuclear medicine imaging of the liver and spleen has the advantage of detecting physiologic changes before morphologic alterations can be detected with other imaging modalities. Tomographic (SPECT) imaging of the liver and spleen is easy to accomplish for various reasons: the data collection is straightforward, the technique is relatively operator-independent once the data acquisition is started, the cost is moderate, the method noninvasive, and the time per study is comparable to planar imaging (approximately 30 min total).[147] SPECT imaging of liver and spleen is more appealing than conventional planar scintigraphy since it yields high contrast images free from under- and overlying activity and may therefore permit better detection and quantification of lesions.[148]

B. Tomography of Liver and Spleen

Like planar imaging, the SPECT approach to liver disease yields insight into physiological and/or functional changes that cannot be detected by X-ray transmission CT scans. The liver is a common site of metastases from primary malignancies in organs; these metastases appear as "cold" spots in scintigraphic images. Primary cancers that frequently metastasize to the liver include lymphoma, Hodgkin's disease, breast cancer, melanoma, bronchus cancer, osteosarcoma, and hypernephroma.

SPECT liver/spleen studies yield high-count-density images (200 to 500 counts per pixel in a 64×64 image; 50 to 125 counts per pixel in a 128×128 image). Typical SPECT artifacts, such as those resulting from small nonuniformities in camera sensitivity, can yield disturbing artifacts that may easily be interpreted as a decrease in radiotracer uptake. Consequently, flood-correction of data before processing is very important in liver/spleen studies. If the data collection is performed in a 64×64 matrix, a 32- to 40-million-count flood image (acquisition time approximately 20 min) is required to correct the raw images before processing. If data acquisition is performed in a 128×128 matrix, a flood image of approximately 130 million counts is required (acquisition time approximately $1^1/_2$ h). The offset of the camera's center of rotation can be expressed as a fractional number of pixels

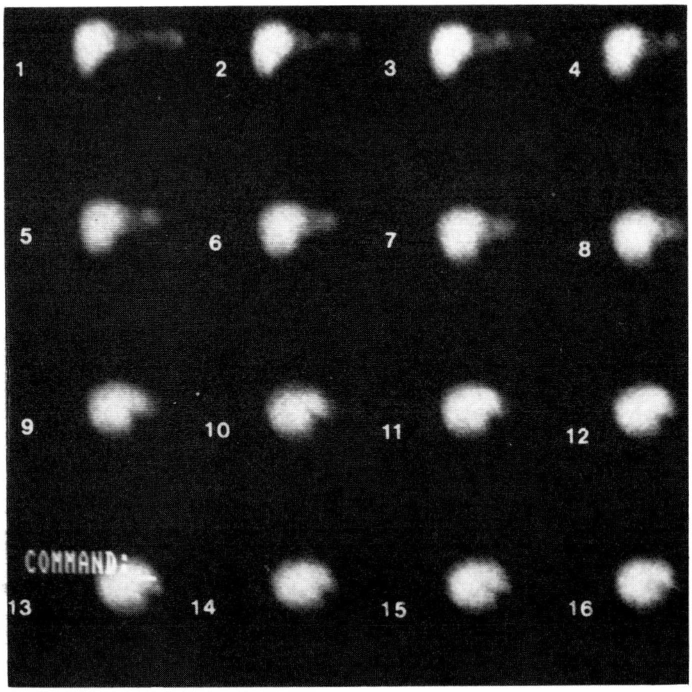

FIGURE 22. SPECT acquisition file for liver/spleen sulfur colloid study. A total of 64 views was collected into 64 × 64 matrices over 360°. The first 16 views of the study are displayed starting in the upper left in an anterior position.

and can be applied to the raw data during reconstruction. The offset of the camera's center of rotation can also be corrected, for example, to be less than 0.5 pixel in a 256 × 256 matrix of a LFOV camera. These procedures shall be part of the routine protocol of a department performing SPECT routine liver/spleen studies.

A standard protocol for liver/spleen tomography includes the following steps:

1. Injection of 5 to 8 mCi of ^{99m}Tc sulfur or albumin colloid.
2. Registration of specific points approximating the patient's outline for attenuation correction of data. If the ECT systems provide noncircular motion to improve resolution by following the body contour, the outline of the patient's cross section is automatically determined.
3. Acquisition of 64 views (30 s/station) over 360° around the patient. Data collection may be done either into 64 × 64 matrices or 128 × 128 matrices for a LFOV camera, since liver/spleen studies yield high count densities. The first 16 views of a patient SPECT acquisition file are shown in Figure 22.
4. Reconstruction can be started during acquisition once data collection over 180° has been accomplished. This is necessary with some attenuation correction schemes. As an alternative, data may be stored on some form of mass storage for later batch processing.
5. Display in formats that include transaxial, coronal, and sagittal slices. Transaxial slices obtained from the raw data shown in Figure 22 are displayed in Figure 23A. Coronal and sagittal sections are shown for the same patient in Figures 23B and 23C, respectively.

For routine clinical liver/spleen SPECT studies, the number of scheduled patients must be adapted to the facilities that are available in each individual institution. A complete liver/

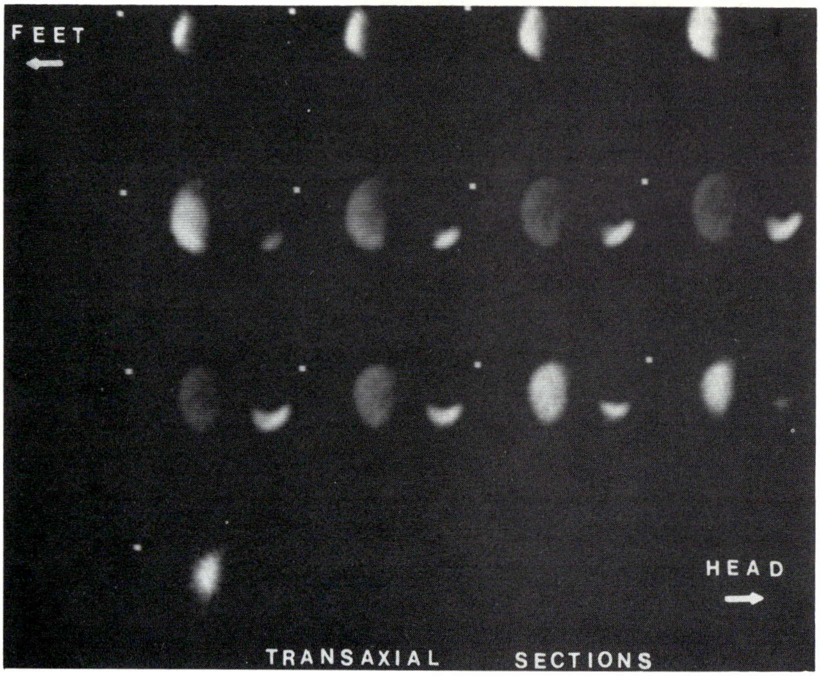

FIGURE 23A. Transaxial slices obtained from liver data shown in Figure 22. The observer is viewing the tomographic sections from the patient's feet toward the head.

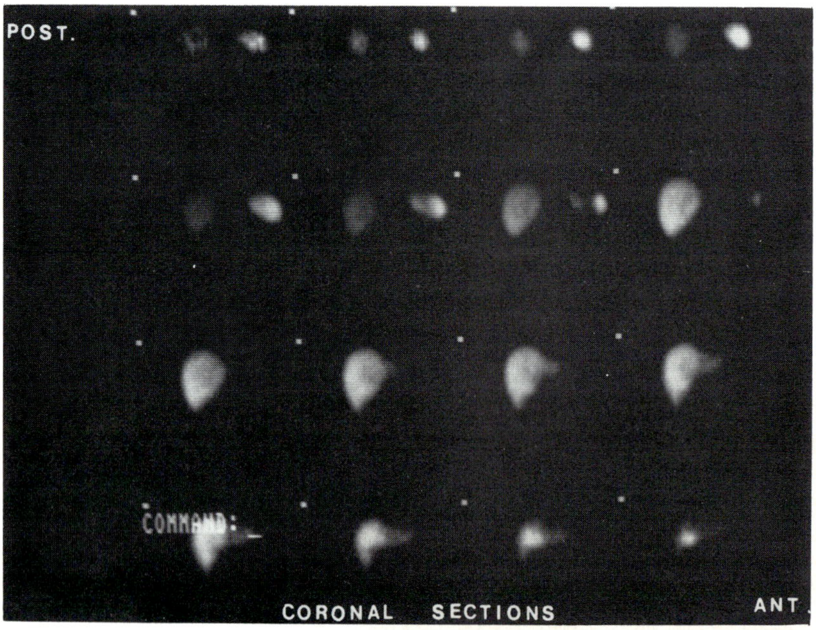

FIGURE 23B. Coronal slices obtained from the set of transaxial slices shown in Figure 23A. Sections are displayed from a posterior-to-anterior position starting at the top image row from left to right.

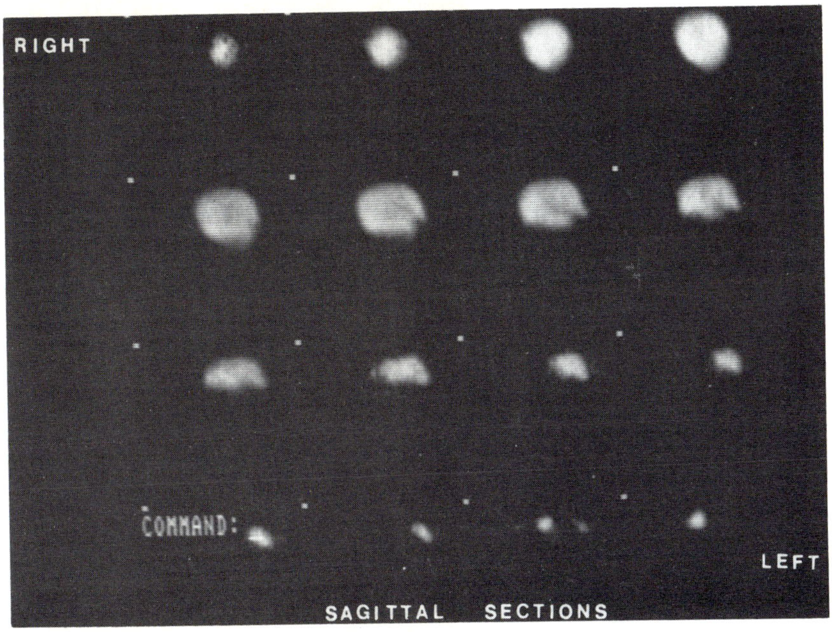

FIGURE 23C. Sagittal sections obtained from the set of transaxial slices shown in Figure 23A. Sections are displayed from the patient's right side to his left side. The displayed liver/spleen scan did not show any abnormalities.

spleen SPECT study (data collection and reconstruction) may take as long as 1 h, since as many as 20 transaxial sections may be required. In addition, a similar number of coronal and sagittal slices may be requested. Depending on the work load of the institution, a dedicated SPECT unit may alleviate the time problem.

C. Clinical Results

The study of hepatic function is a very complicated task; hence, most SPECT studies of the liver have been limited to space-occupying diseases where transmission tomography is unable to provide a reliable diagnosis. Accuracy in the localization and extent of lesions has increased with SPECT techniques, thereby reducing the misstaging of tumors. When the liver is involved with metastases, the localization of regions of reduced activity in the liver can be improved with the ECT approach of rotating LFOV cameras. Today, lesions from 2 to 10 cm can be detected relatively well using the tomographic approach. The potential of the SPECT approach to lesion detection is illustrated in Figure 24.

With the availability of emission-computed tomography, a new imaging strategy for liver/spleen disease now needs to be defined. CT scans excel in speed and resolution and yield significant anatomical detail; however, the technique lacks contrast resolution. When anatomy is not of primary concern, ECT could be considered a first choice for patient examinations. However, complete studies (acquisition, reconstruction, and interpretation) are very time consuming. Due to inherent limitations in the spatial resolution provided by radionuclide section-scanning, liver and spleen volume measurements are difficult.[149] When they are available, however, they yield good correlation with CT data.

Many patients have undergone SPECT studies as a prospective trial to assess the clinical usefulness of emission tomography of the liver. Dendy et al.[150] analyzed a group of 373 patients. Their results did not demonstrate a significant increase in the accuracy of diagnosing liver disease, probably because only one transaxial section was used for comparison with

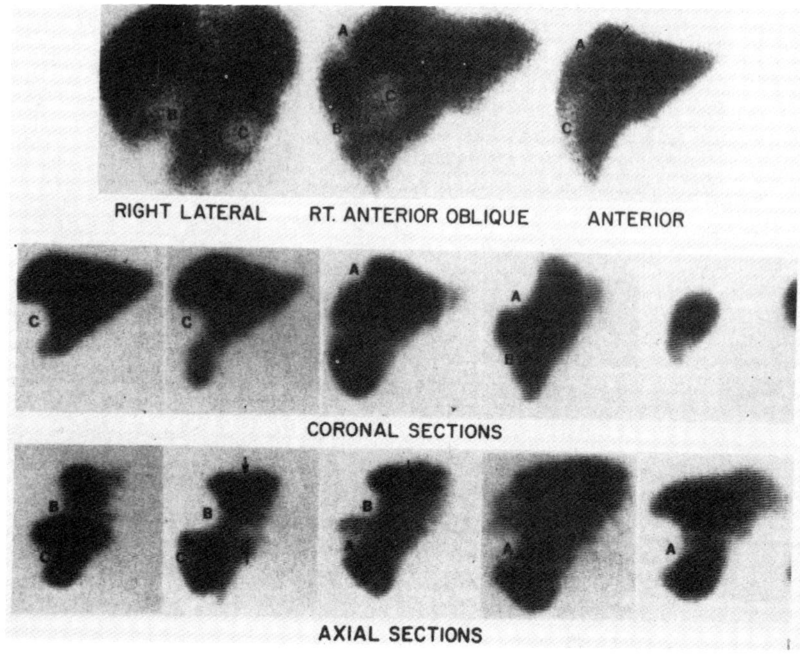

FIGURE 24. Multiple mass lesions in liver are shown by ^{99m}Tc sulfur colloid study in patient with colon carcinoma. In anterior, right lateral, and right anterior oblique projections, corresponding photopenic foci are identified with letters and same lesions are noted in tomographic views (axial and coronal). Additional defects found only by tomography are identified with arrows. (From DeLand, F. H. et al., *J. Nucl. Med.*, 25, 1375, 1984. With permission.)

planar images. Another group of investigators[151] analyzed results obtained from 53 patients with documented primary gastrointestinal cancer and possible hepatic metastases. Berche et al.[151] compared their findings with various techniques: surgery, echography, planar scintigraphy, laboratory hepatic tests, and carcinoembryonic antigens. Their conclusion was that ECT is a very sensitive approach for detection of metastases in the liver, equivalent to surgery and superior to all other techniques. In a more recent study involving 130 examined patients, Strauss et al.[152] used Bayesian analysis to assess the reliability of SPECT and conventional planar scintigraphy at different prevalences of metastatic disease. The final diagnosis was a higher sensitivity, specificity, and accuracy for ECT than for planar imaging, with superiority of SPECT at low disease prevalence. Despite the conflicting results reported on the sensitivity and specificity of planar scintigraphy, the true positive rate of SPECT seems to be higher by approximately 10%. In the Strauss et al.[152] study, 65 patients with 156 metastases documented by CT were used to assess sensitivity of the SPECT approach. Figure 25 shows the true positive percentages of SPECT results in these 65 patients for various lesion diameters. The sensitivity of SPECT was found to be 35% for metastases having a diameter of 1.0 to 1.5 cm, 52% for lesions of 1.5 to 2.0 cm, 68% for lesions with a diameter of 2.0 to 2.5 cm, and over 90% for metastases exceeding a diameter of 3.5 cm. Figure 26 shows a 4.2-cm metastasis in the right lateral part of the liver that could be detected by CT, planar and SPECT imaging. Figure 27 shows an example of 1.9-cm lesion detected by CT and SPECT only. Strauss et al.,[152] applying Bayesian analysis to their data, found that at 20% disease prevalence, the posterior probability of false negative with SPECT was lower than 2% and at 80% prevalence it was 21%. Bayesian analysis applied to planar imaging yielded a posterior probability of false negative of 5% at 20% disease prevalence and of 47% at 80% prevalence. The true positive posterior probability with SPECT was

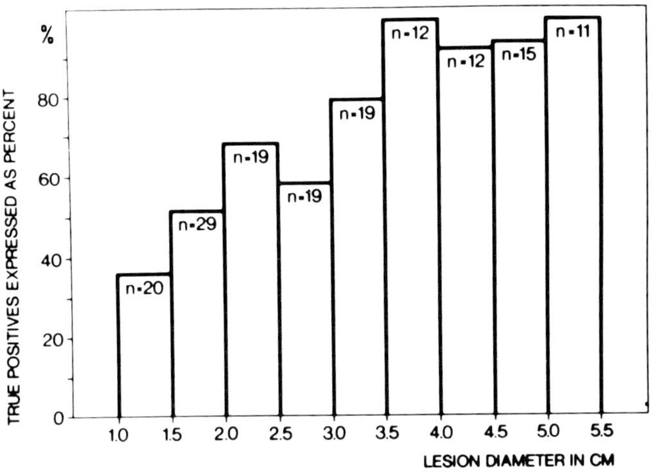

FIGURE 25. True-positive results of SPECT examination in 65 patients who had 156 hepatic lesions. TCT served as reference method and was used to determine diameters of lesions. (From Strauss, L. et al., *J. Nucl. Med.*, 23, 1059, 1982. With permission.)

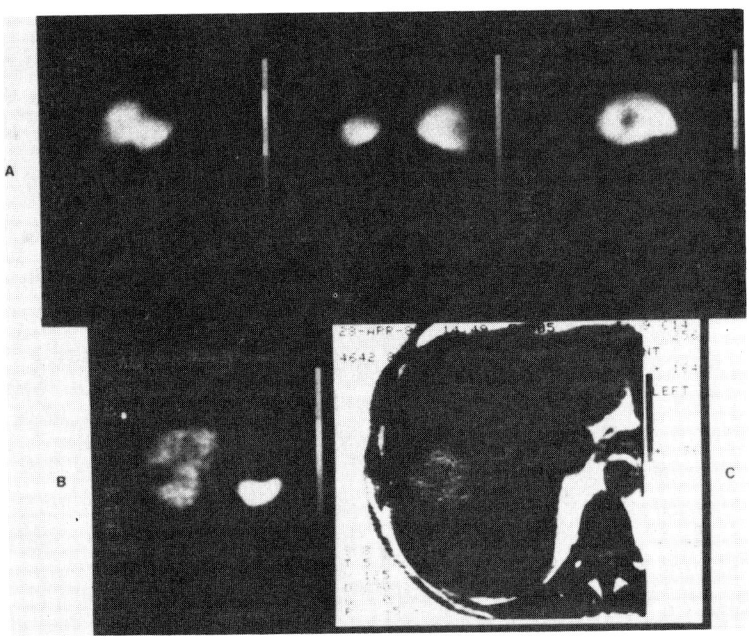

FIGURE 26. (A) Top row: conventional scintigrams in anterior, posterior, and right lateral view. (B) Bottom row, left: single-photon emission computed tomography, transverse slice. (C) Bottom row, right: portion of TCT slice showing the 4.2-cm metastasis. All imaging procedures demonstrated defect in right lateral part of liver. (From Strauss, L., et al., *J. Nucl. Med.*, 23, 1059, 1982. With permission.)

68% at 20% disease prevalence and 97% at 80% prevalence. Planar imaging yielded a true positive posterior probability of 57% at 20% prevalence and 96% at 80% prevalence. Dividing the liver into three sections (right, middle, and left), Strauss et al.[152] found that the rate of true positives was lowest in the middle section of the liver; a lesion of 2 to 3 cm in diameter yielded a true positive rate of 56%, while lesions over 3 cm in diameter were needed for a

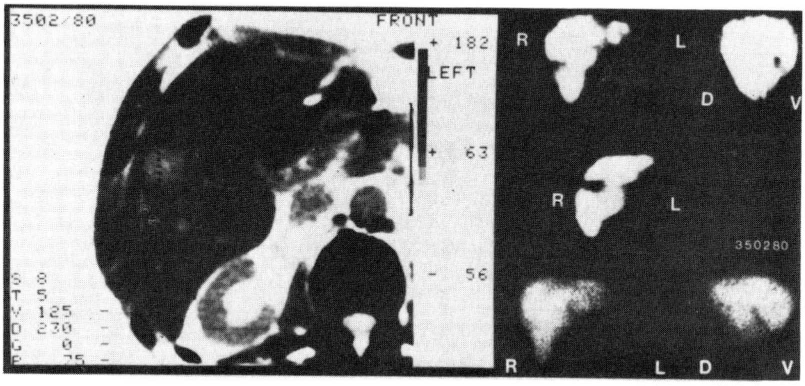

FIGURE 27. Left: TCT slice showing 1.9-cm metastasis. This mass was seen clearly only in TCT and SPECT images. Bottom row, right: conventional anterior and right lateral scintigrams. Middle row, right: single-photon emission computed tomography, transverse slice. Top row, right: reconstructed frontal and sagittal SPECT views. (From Strauss, L. et al., *J. Nucl. Med.*, 23, 1059, 1982. With permission.)

true positive rate of 80%. Only 52% of all hepatic lesions with a diameter of 1.5 to 2 cm could be visualized with SPECT. However, SPECT seems to be preferable to conventional scintigraphy at low disease prevalence.

A recent extensive study by Croft and Teates[153] reports results of liver/spleen tomography obtained with 110 patients. Patients were injected with 8 mCi of ^{99m}Tc sulfur or albumin colloid. Data were collected in 64 views over 360° into 64 × 64 matrices, and tomograms were reconstructed into the same matrix size. Sensitivity and specificity of SPECT data were then compared to those from other institutions. Sensitivity and specificity did not improve substantially, however, compared to the numbers obtained with conventional planar scintigraphy.

Efforts to find new applications of SPECT in detecting and characterizing hepatic tumors have been described recently by Gyves et al.[154] Hepatic tumor microcirculation was investigated with SPECT by combining the results of transaxial tomography with ^{99m}Tc sulfur colloid with those obtained after hepatic-arterial injection of ^{99m}Tc macroaggregated human serum albumin (MAA). ^{99m}Tc MAA perfusion was used to assess hypo- and hypervascularization of colorectal and carcinoid tumors relative to normal liver. Figure 28 shows transaxial tomographic sections taken 48 h apart using ^{99m}Tc sulfur colloid uptake and ^{99m}Tc hepatic artery infusion of ^{99m}Tc MAA. A rim of increased activity around the tumor area is easily identified. Important differences in blood distribution can be quantified better with the SPECT approach than with contrast angiography. Tumors greater than 8 to 9 cm showed a hypovascularized cave surrounded by a rim of increased activity. The maximum radius of solid nodules was 4.2 cm, probably indicating a maximum depth of tumor hypervascularity of about 4 cm. The potential of designing a therapeutic protocol based on microspheres directed against hypervascularized tumors is presently being investigated.

Space occupying disease occurs less frequently in the spleen than in the liver. SPECT may assume a special role in evaluating splenic volumes when enlargement and infiltration of the spleen precede noticeable changes in the liver. Phantom studies[155] have shown that the volume of liver and spleen may be evaluated within 90 to 95% accuracy with the SPECT approach. Detection of hematomas in spleen trauma is approached best by SPECT because of the low sensitivity of other imaging approaches such as sonography and computed tomography.

Several questions must be answered in future investigations:

1. Whereas SPECT permits detection of lesions as small as 1 cm, its sensitivity is poor

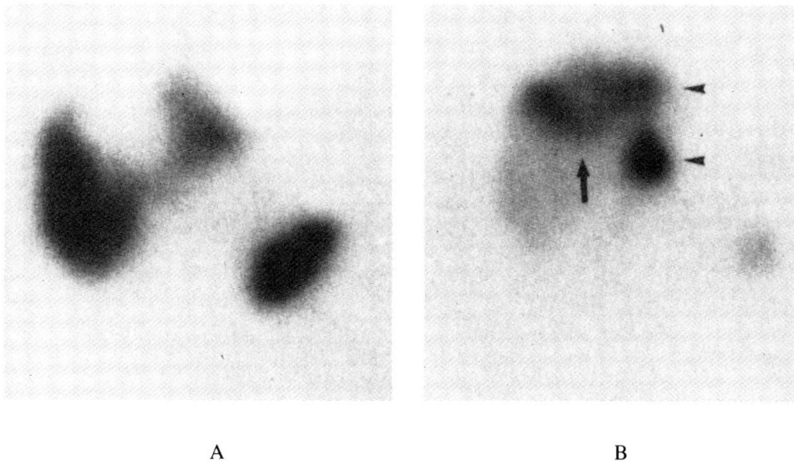

FIGURE 28. (A) Transaxial tomographic section through ^{99m}Tc SC liver-spleen scintigram, showing large focal defect in patient with proven metastatic colon cancer. (B) Comparable transaxial tomographic slice after hepatic-arterial infusion of ^{99m}Tc MAA, showing rim of increased activity at periphery of metastatic nodule (←). There is also extrahepatic perfusion to stomach (←). (From Gyves, J. W. et al., *J. Nucl. Med.*, 25, 972, 1984. With permission.)

for small lesions in the middle third of the liver. Small defects simulating metastases may be merely localized impressions of the kidney and gallbladder. Small defects beneath the hilus may be easily missed, and some large lesions in the left third of the liver may not be identified correctly.[152]

2. Liver motion degrades spatial resolution. Motion over 1 to 2 cm caused by respiration is observed for patients in the supine position. The liver's deformability is difficult to control, and its shape varies to a large extent from patient to patient.
3. The liver is a relatively large organ, and the attenuation and scatter of radiation are serious problems.
4. The volume of liver and spleen is important to the characterization of some specific diseases. Detection of changes in volume is, important, therefore, as long as a relatively accurate estimate can be obtained through increased resolution. This increase in resolution may be expected from rotating cameras following the patient's body contour.
5. Although the potential of SPECT for characterizing space-occupying liver/spleen disease has been recognized, practical time limits can significantly restrict the number of patients examined, unless the workload of a department allows ECT units to be dedicated exclusively to tomographic studies. The use of array processors and an increase in instrumentation sophistication may help reduce these time limitations; these additions, however, increase the cost of acquisition and maintenance of the equipment.

There is still no consensus on the magnitude of the improvement of SPECT over planar scintigraphy for routine liver/spleen studies. A marginal improvement of 5% to 10% relative to planar imaging for the use of SPECT in space occupying diseases is rather discouraging. Even with state of the art equipment, SPECT seems to be confined to the role of an add-on imaging modality for liver/spleen studies. More studies are needed to establish the exact role of SPECT in liver/spleen studies.

V. LUNG IMAGING

A. Introduction

Radioisotope techniques for evaluation of pulmonary functions began with the pioneering work of Taplin et al.[156] in 1963. Radioisotope scanning of the lung using ^{131}I- and ^{51}Cr-labeled MAA as radiotracers for the detection of pulmonary emboli was first described by Wagner et al.[157] in 1964. One year later, Taplin and Poe[158] described a dual-lung scanning technique for evaluation of regional pulmonary arterial blood flow and bronchial patency. Preliminary ventilation studies were performed by inhalation of aerosols containing ^{131}I-labeled MAA, ^{197}Hg chlormerodrin and colloidal ^{198}Au. Intravenous scans were obtained after injection of ^{131}I MAA. Colloidal ^{198}Au was preferred to the other radiotracers because of its rapid clearance with no absorption from the gastrointestinal tract. The low energy of ^{125}I, ^{197}Hg, and ^{99m}Tc isotopes, however, was more desirable because studies could be obtained on the same day.

Lung ventilation and perfusion scans (V/Q) are now among the more common procedures of every nuclear medicine department.[159] The conventional planar posterior, anterior, lateral and oblique perfusion views are obtained with ^{99m}Tc-labeled MAA, while the ventilation portion of the study traditionally uses ^{133}Xe.[160] V/Q scans are the most sensitive approach for detection of pulmonary embolism and should always be performed before pulmonary angiography. The role of ^{133}Xe and radiolabeled aerosols in chronic obstructive pulmonary disease was discussed by Taplin et al.[161]

Perfusion images are difficult to interpret because of the complex anatomy and physiology of the lungs and because they present a two-dimensional representation of a very large organ. Additional difficulties generated in V/Q scans are created by the different energies of ^{133}Xe (80 keV) and ^{99m}Tc (140 keV) used for imaging. The low energy ventilation images are characterized by relatively poor spatial resolution (approximately 5 cm).

With the availability of LFOV rotating cameras that offer routine emission-computed tomography, it seems reasonable to consider the lung as a good candidate for SPECT tomographic imaging. The reasons are multiple:

1. The SPECT approach using rotating cameras over a range of 360° is adapted well to the anatomy. Other nonrotating SPECT techniques have specific advantages for smaller organs but are not applicable to the large size of the pulmonary system.
2. The count density of ^{99m}Tc-labeled MAA perfusion imaging is high enough to produce quality tomographic images.
3. The lungs present a relatively uniform source of activity because they are composed of a fairly homogeneous tissue of low density so that attenuation compensation is less critical than for other organs. The degree of attenuation (μ is approximately equal to $0.06\ cm^{-1}$ for ^{99m}Tc) is fairly independent of the viewing angle around the chest.
4. Because of a complex blood supply system, the localization of perfusion and/or ventilation defects, and their respective sizes and shapes, are enhanced by the SPECT approach; this advantage may alleviate the difficult interpretation of multiple overlapping segmental lung divisions.

Some difficulties, however, which are specific to the pulmonary system can complicate the diagnostic process based on tomographic sections. The spine and ribs are localized, undesirable structures of high density that are superimposed on the organ to be imaged. The myocardium also interferes with interpretation because of its higher density and motion. The most disturbing problem is natural respiration motion, which degrades spatial resolution.

B. Tomography of the Lung

Very little work has been done in the field of lung tomography. Perfusion tomographic sections can be obtained with ^{99m}Tc MAA, while ventilation images use the ^{81m}Kr isotope ($T_{1/2}$ = 13 s). ^{133}Xe used for ventilation imaging after a single breath cannot be used in tomographic imaging because it cannot be administered continuously to the patient, as can

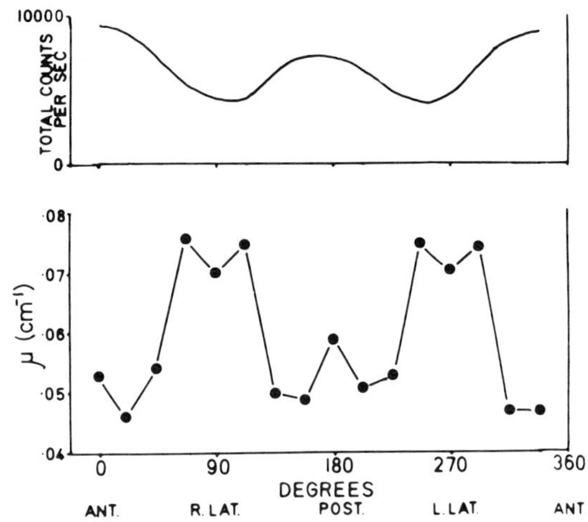

FIGURE 29. Variation of μ measured with the transmission source rotated round a normal subject (lower curve) and the relationship between total counts and angle-of-view for the same subject during a perfusion scan with ^{99m}Tc macroaggregates (upper curve). (From Ell, P. J. and Holman, B. L., Eds., *Computed Emission Tomography*, Oxford University Press, New York 1982. With permission.)

the short half-life isotope ^{81m}Kr. With ^{133}Xe, the equilibrium state is reached within 5 to 10 s. ^{81m}Kr also has the advantage of a satisfactory imaging energy (190 keV).

Phantom studies using paraffin wax and sawdust to simulate lung tissue have been performed by Macey and Marshall.[162] Rectangular boxes of sizes from 1 to 5 cm were introduced into the "lung" tissue to simulate a lack of perfusion. A 1-cm^2 defect was found to be the borderline defect size. Various thresholding levels were used to determine the areas obtained from cross-sectional images and for comparison to the true area of the phantom. A lower threshold of 20% gave the correct result, while 10% overestimated the respective lung areas by 12%. The total number of counts detected in all tomographic sections showed excellent linearity with the measured activity in mCi/ml of injected ^{99m}Tc. This result implies the potential of a good relative quantitation of lung perfusion in different segments.

The transmission emission method[163] can be used to assess absolute quantitation of radiotracer uptake. Macey and Marshall[162] showed that the accuracy was better than 10% for routine perfusion lung scans. These investigators, therefore, used the same approach to quantify regional uptake in selected lung areas using SPECT imaging with a rotating camera. Accurate quantitation can be obtained only by use of some method for attenuation compensation. Although lung tissue has a fairly constant attenuation coefficient, the accuracy of the procedure is influenced by the presence of other soft tissue, bones, and myocardium. The variation of the linear attenuation coefficient μ as a function of the angle of view obtained with the transmission method is shown for a normal subject in Figure 29. Total counts per frame as a function of angle is shown in the upper part of the same figure. Macey and Marshall have established the following protocol for SPECT lung imaging:

1. A transmission flood source (10 mCi of ^{99m}Tc) mounted on a specially designed holder (Figure 30) rotates around the patient in the supine position. A 16-view (5 s/view) data file is generated with a 1-min AP view to be able to perform the transmission emission quantitation procedure. The count rate per unit area through the patient's chest is obtained for each angular view using a 20% lower threshold.
2. The count rate of the flood source per unit area recorded by the camera is measured

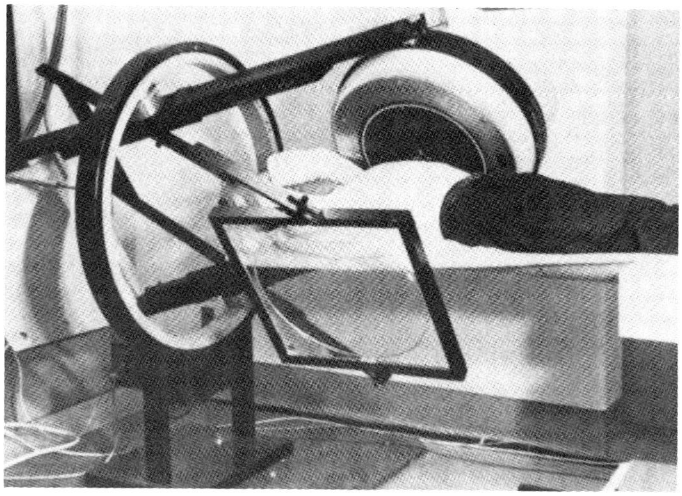

FIGURE 30. Arrangement for transmission imaging. Plane flood source (Plexiglas vessel) and camera are attached to the rotating ring. (From Maeda, H. et al., *J. Nucl. Med.*, 22, 815, 1981. With permission.)

while the patient is injected with 3 mCi of ^{99m}Tc, MAA for the perfusion study. The injected activity is measured accurately by determining the activity before administration and the activity remaining in the syringe.

3. The rotating camera collects 64 views over 360° with 5 s/view. A 1-min frame is collected in the anterior and posterior views. The SPECT data collection is then repeated using continuous inhalation of a ^{81m}Kr air mixture for the tomographic ventilation study.
4. Tomographic reconstruction with perfusion and ventilation data is performed with a standard filtered backprojection algorithm. Attenuation correction is performed using an average value of 0.06/cm for the attenuation coefficient. Opposing views are averaged before backprojection.
5. Coronal and sagittal slices are reconstructed from the set of transaxial sections. Slices are approximately 1.2 cm thick.
6. Coronal, sagittal, and transaxial slices are combined to obtain depth independent images of anterior and posterior views, lateral views, and transaxial sections of any desired thickness.

Normal perfusion and ventilation tomograms are shown in Figures 31 and 32. Tomographic sections are shown in Figure 33 for a case of angiographically documented pulmonary embolism. The extent of lack of perfusion is apparent in various lung segments. Figure 34 shows normal conventional planar perfusion images obtained with ^{99m}Tc MAA. Perfusion can be observed in the transaxial basal sections. The ventilation scan is normal.

C. Clinical Results

Despite the lack of experience in SPECT imaging of the lungs in a clinical setting, the future looks promising. Osborne et al.[164] have compared the SPECT approach to planar scintigraphy and selective angiography in animals. The lower lobe segmental pulmonary arteries of six dogs were embolized, and pulmonary perfusion using ^{99m}Tc-labeled microspheres was studied with rotating camera tomography, planar scintigraphy, and angiography. The selective angiography was the most sensitive approach for the detection of emboli. The SPECT technique yielded higher sensitivity than did conventional two-dimensional imaging.

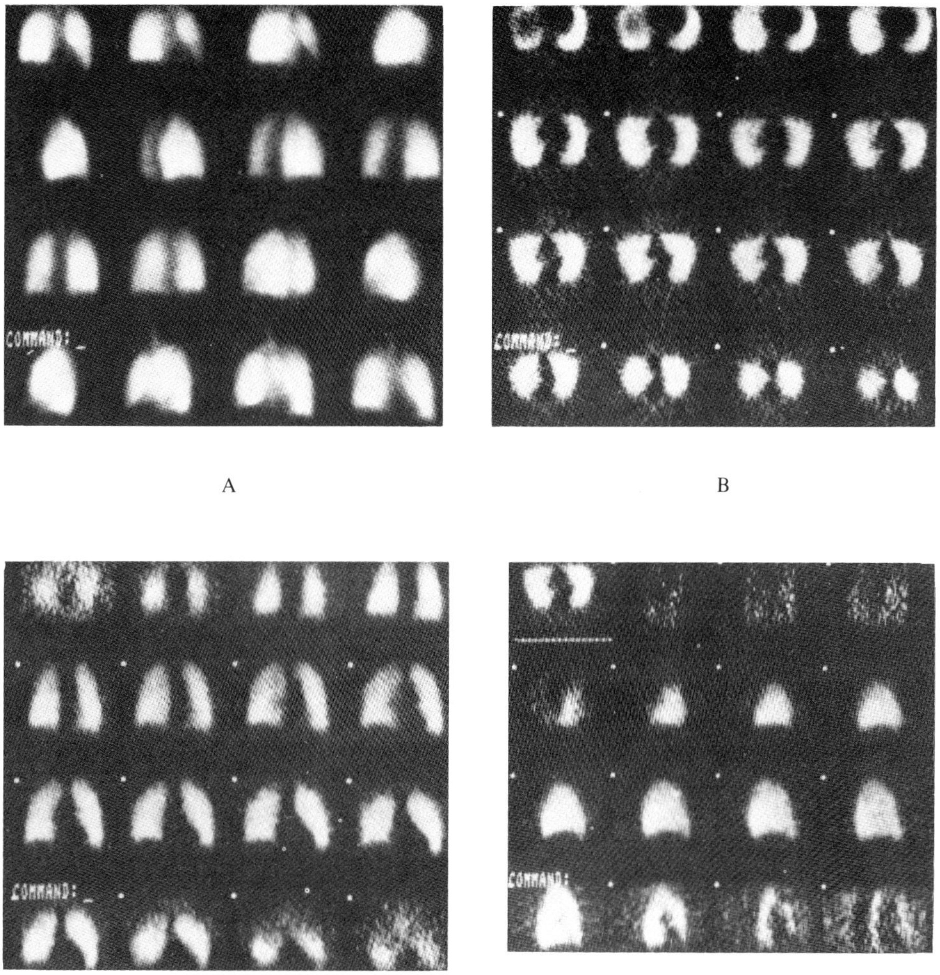

A B

C D

FIGURE 31. Perfusion scan of normal subject with ^{99m}Tc macroaggregates. (A) Acquisition file. Each image is the sum of four consecutive views (B) Transverse slices. (C) Coronal slices. (D) Sagittal slices. (From Maeda, H. et al, *J. Nucl. Med.*, 22, 815, 1981. With permission.)

At 4 and 8 weeks the perfusion defects were found to be smaller than in the acute case. Altered perfusion pattern was observed over a period of 8 weeks, partially due to the fragmentation of the emboli and to blood supply from adjacent lung areas maintaining the distal segments to the emboli functional. In these experiments, the autopsied animals showed a significant reduction of perfusion defects with the proximal segmented emboli unchanged from their initial location. The suggestion of perfusion defects at the periphery of the lung may be enhanced with a combination of emission and transmission images obtained from a planar ^{99m}Tc source. The nonspecificity of a perfusion defect, however, seems to limit the diagnosis of pulmonary emboli in clinical environments.[165] A combination of conventional V/Q scans with the SPECT technique might improve the specificity.

Tomographic ventilation exploration of the lungs with ^{99m}Tc-labeled aerosols[166-169] has been suggested. SPECT ventilation studies with radioactive gases are limited by the duration of the study (approximately 30 min) and by the relatively high cost compared to, for example, a ^{81m}Kr generator.

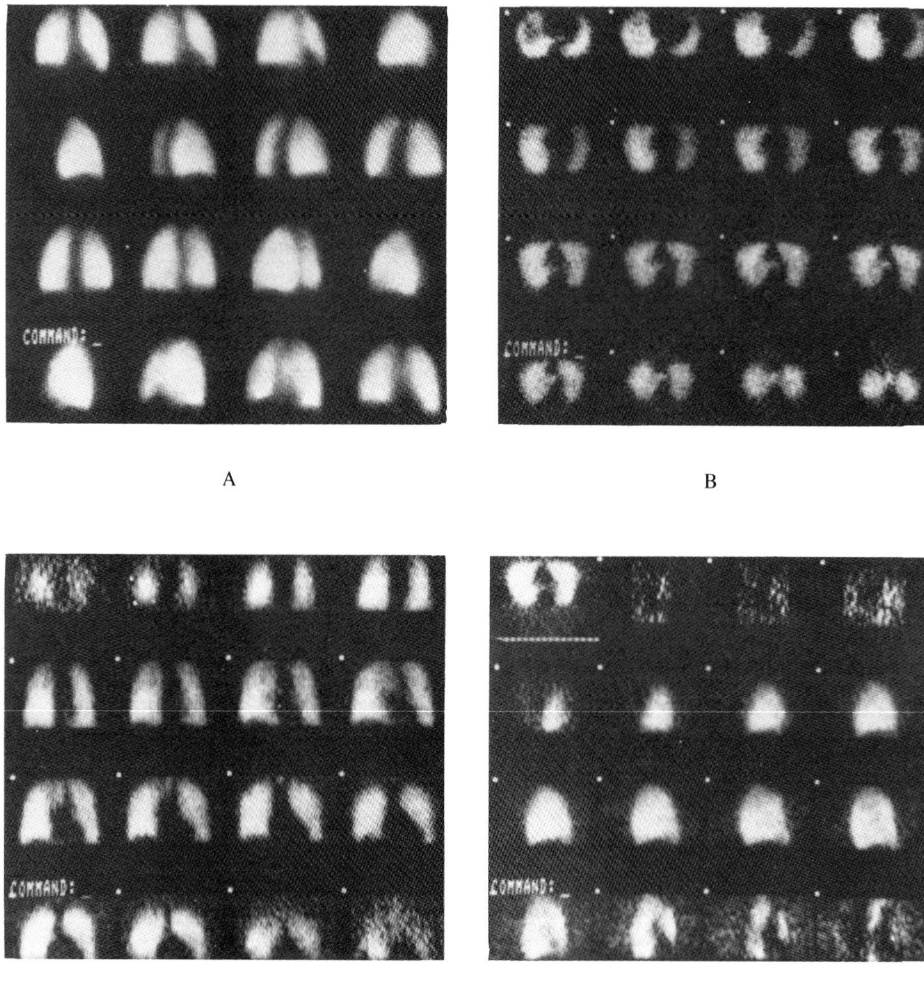

FIGURE 32. Ventilation scan of normal subject with ^{81m}Kr. (A) Acquisition file. Each image is the sum of four consecutive views. (B) Transverse slices. (C) Coronal slices. (D) Sagittal slices. (From Maeda, H. et al., *J. Nucl. Med.*, 22, 815, 1981. With permission.)

Only a few patient studies have been published. A study by Donaldson et al. consisted of 84 patients with suspected pulmonary emboli.[170] Tomography using ^{99m}Tc MAA was compared to planar scintigraphy. Data of angiographically documented pulmonary emboli obtained with cardiac catheterization were available in 12 cases. Excellent correlation was observed between tomograms and angiography. Section scanning yielded higher sensitivity than the two-dimensional planar projections of the lung scans. In eight patients, SPECT revealed the presence of perfusion defects, while planar images were normal. Coronal planes obtained from the transaxial sections offer the best approach to detection of segmental perfusion defects. It appears that the noninvasive SPECT approach may be a good alternative to cardiac catheterization. The SPECT approach also offers the relatively small advantage of increasing the sensitivity for detection of pulmonary emboli by approximately 10%. Similar results were reported by LeJeune's group.[171] According to these investigators, however, a small group of 30 patients did not confirm the superiority of tomography over conventional planar imaging. Nevertheless, the extent and localization of perfusion defects are enhanced

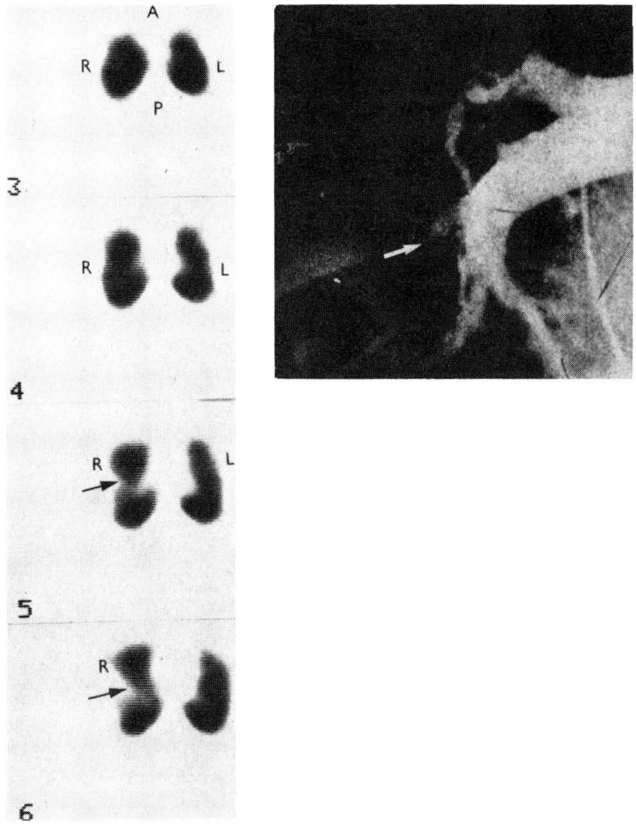

FIGURE 33. (a), (b) Angiographic/section scan correlation. The occluded lateral right middle lobe branch (arrow) is clearly visualized as a segmental defect seen in transverse sections 5 and 6 (R = right; L = left; A = anterior; P = posterior). (From Donaldson, R. M. et al., *Clin. Radiol.*, 33, 389, 1982. With permission.)

due to increased contrast. Applications to cases of cardiomegaly are presently under investigation.

Recently, the feasibility of lung tomography for interstitial lung disease (ILD) has been studied with ^{67}Ga citrate. Preliminary results showed the feasibility of localizing the extension of ^{67}Ga uptake in lungs. Quantitation of radiotrace uptake, and comparison to planar ^{67}Ga lung scintigraphy, is presently under study, in which the regional uptake in tomograms will be compared to the semiquantitative Line Index introduced by Line et al.[172,173] Tomography appears to provide the clinician with better contrast images in lung diseases without yielding an increase in sensitivity sufficient to justify a routine clinical protocol. The role of SPECT in lung imaging with ^{67}Ga has yet to be defined.

VI. OTHER ORGAN IMAGING

A. Introduction

For many reasons, SPECT is close to being accepted as a clinical tool for selected studies in community hospitals. A marginal increase in diagnostic sensitivity has prevented a rapid proliferation of SPECT imaging and explains, therefore, why very few results have been reported concerning SPECT studies of organs other than the myocardium, the brain, and

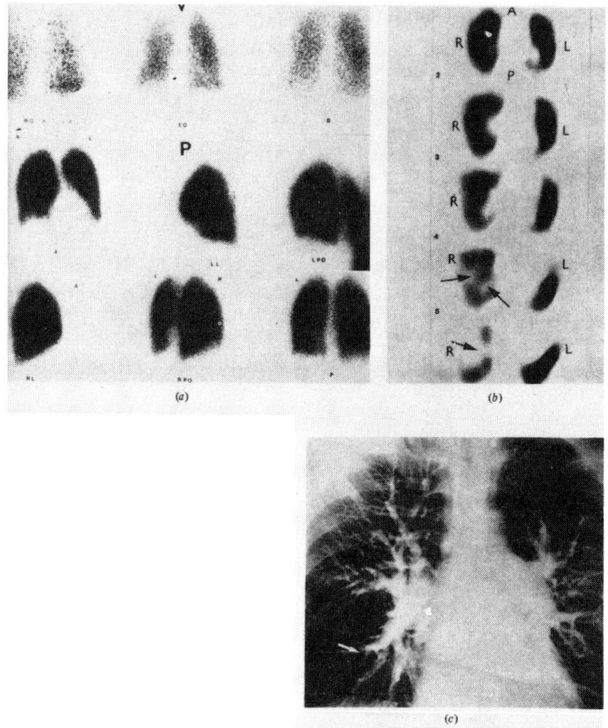

FIGURE 34. (a) Normal planar ventilation (V) and perfusion (P) scans. (b) Transverse section scan (selected frames) demonstrated a perfusion defect in basal sections of the right lung (arrows). (c) Arterial cut-off visualized in the pulmonary angiogram (arrow). (From Donaldson, R. M. et al., *Clin. Radiol.*, 33, 389, 1982. With permission.)

the liver/spleen system. Some isolated research and preliminary results have been reported, however, in the literature for kidneys, bones, thyroid, pituitary, and adrenals.

B. Kidneys

Volume measurements of smaller organs such as the kidneys[174] appear to be a possible application of the SPECT method.[175] Kidney volumes of both normal patients and those with renal disease have been estimated using the rotating-camera approach. SPECT measurements of kidney volume agree well with ultrasound results. In all likelihood, the SPECT technique will ultimately be useful in certain renal diseases and in transplant rejections when kidney volume increases. An algorithm developed by Tauxe et al.[175] to determine organ volume by SPECT has been published recently. The method has been applied to kidney studies of nine patients and appears to be a productive first step toward the absolute quantitation of radioactivity in the kidneys.

C. Adrenal Gland

Intimately related to renal scintigraphy is the potential of adrenal imaging.[176] Radiotracers such as ^{75}Se selenomethylcholesterol have been used to image adrenal adenomas which produce excess aldosterone and to distinguish the adenoma from the adrenal cortex that normally produces this hormone. SPECT may be used to identify the depth of the adrenals

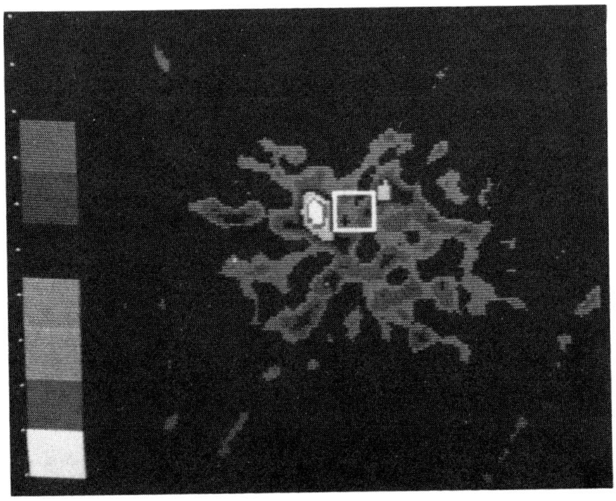

FIGURE 35. SPECT of adrenal hyperplasia, 14 d [^{75}Se]-selenomethylcholesterol image: one of four sections encompassing the two adrenals, showing the tip of the left and middle of the right adrenal with an interadrenal region of interest. (From Macey, D. J. and Marshall, R., in *Computed Emission Tomography*, Ell, P. J. and Holman, B. L., Eds., Oxford University Press, New York, chap. 19, 1982. With permission.)

required for adrenal quantitation.[177] An example of an adrenal hyperplasia case studied with SPECT is shown in Figure 35. Using a phantom at different depths of tissue equivalent material, Hawkins et al.[178] developed a calibration curve that relates adrenal depth to activity. Good results were obtained in a clinical trial involving a group of 10 patients with adrenal disorders when the uptake of the administered dose (approximately 200 μCi) was measured with SPECT.

D. Thyroid

Shapiro et al.[179] have approached the measurement of thyroid volume with SPECT. This measurement is of particular value when determining the appropriate dosage for a radioiodine treatment,[180] as the dosage is varied according to the thyroid's weight and, therefore, volume. While the uptake of radioiodine is known accurately, the thyroid volume is difficult to estimate and large errors (up to 100%) are often made.[181] Only ultrasound with three-dimensional measurements[182] has previously shown some success in the evaluation of thyroid volume.

Shapiro's group studied two thyroid phantoms:

1. The standard Picker phantom with a volume of 40 cm^3
2. A three-dimensional thyroid phantom with a volume of 29 cc placed in water so that the anterior face of the phantom was 1 cm below the surface

High accuracy for volume measurements by SPECT was obtained in both cases (101.8% of the true volume for the Picker phantom and 98.9% of the true volume for the second phantom).

E. Bones

The diagnostic value of SPECT in bone scanning is presently being investigated. Few results have been published. In some images at the levels of the thyroid and pelvis, multiple

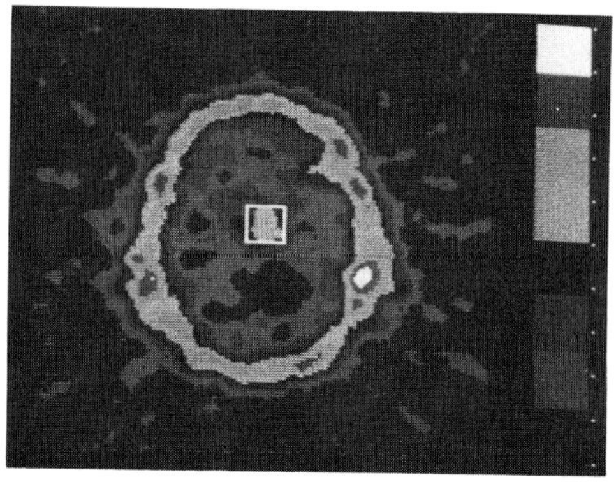

A

FIGURE 36. SPECT of pituitary microadenoma causing hyperprolactinemia and secondary amenorrhea. (A) Region of interest over the active pituitary area, C_1 counts, A pixels. (B) Region of interest extended over the pituitary environment, C_2 counts, B pixels. The target activity per pixel T is equal to C_1/A. The background activity per pixel B is equal to $(C_2 - C_1)/(B - A)$. The pituitary target-to-background ratio T/B is normal for $0.7 < T/B < 1.25$. The ratio is abnormal for $T/B > 1.27$, leaving a borderline range between normal and abnormal. (From Macey, D. J. and Marshall, R., in *Computed Emission Tomography,* Ell, P. J. and Holman, B. L., Eds., Oxford University Press, New York, chap. 19, 1982. With permission.)

overlying structures of different densities interfere in a two-dimensional projection image. Use of tomography may help to reduce this interference. The first results of SPECT using a rotating slant-hole collimator were published by Pavel et al.[183] for sectional tomography of the hip. In certain cases, the lower neck uptake in bone scans is difficult to interpret and some benefit from SPECT may be obtained[184] in terms of a three-dimensional visualization and localization of certain tumors and abnormal tissue configurations.

F. Pituitary Gland

Pituitary adenomal structures are very small (microadenomas) and difficult to discern in transmission tomography. Their density is close to the density of normal glandular tissue and the skull creates artifacts that interfere with visualization of the adenomas. Tomoscanners II and IIS (J&P Engineering) have been used by Shapiro et al. to study the application of emission tomography to the endocrine system.[185] A total of 15 mCi of ^{99m}Tc pertechnetate was injected into the patient and ECT imaging was performed 40 min later; conventional brain scintigraphy was started 20 min after injection. SPECT was able to show tumors not visible with standard planar imaging. An example of a pituitary microadenoma studied with SPECT is shown in Figure 36.

SPECT has also been useful in therapy situations. Labeled radiotracers binding to the pituitary therapy drug bromocriptine allow the monitoring of the state of hyperactive adenomas. A decrease in activity which could not be observed by other radiological techniques was identified by SPECT and used to assess the effectiveness of therapy.

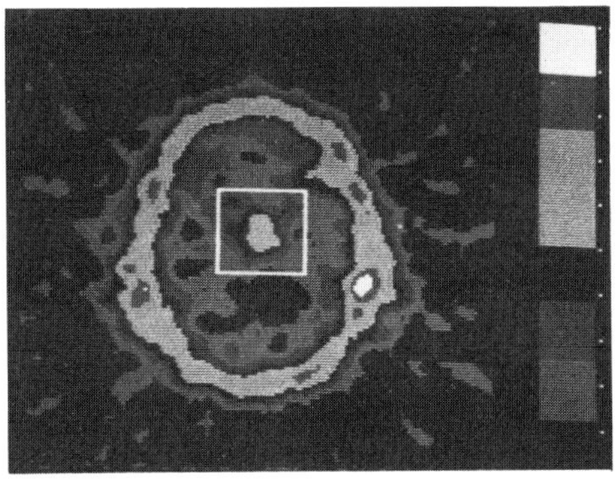

FIGURE 36B.

REFERENCES

1. **Kuhl, D. E. and Edwards, R. Q.,** Image separation radioisotope scanning, *Radiology,* 80, 653, 1963.
2. **Stoddart, H. F. and Stoddart, H. A.,** A new development in single gamma transaxial tomography. Union Carbide focussed collimator scanner, *IEEE Trans. Nucl. Sci.,* NS-26, 2710, 1979.
3. **Larsson, St. A.,** Gamma camera emission tomography. Development and properties of a multisectional emission computed tomography system, *Acta Radiol. (Suppl.),* 363, 1980.
4. **Sorenson, J. A. (Book Coordinator),** *Single Photon Emission Computed Tomography and Other Selected Computer Topics,* Society of Nuclear Medicine, New York, 1980.
5. **Paxman, R. G., Schmith, W. E., and Barrett, H. H.,** Two algorithms for use with an orthogonal-view coded aperture system, *J. Nucl. Med.,* 25, 700, 1984.
6. **Koral, K. F., Nolder, C., Ciliax, G., Rogers, W. L., and Keyes, J. W., Jr.,** Simulated ECT of the left ventricle using rotating slant-hole collimator and two camera positions, *J. Nucl. Med.,* 25, 343, 1984.
7. **Ell, P. J.,** The brain. The role of single-photon emission computed tomography (SPECT) in the diagnosis of space-occupying disease, in *Computed Emission Tomography,* Ell, P. J. and Holman, B. L., Eds., Oxford University Press, New York, 1982, chap. 14.
8. **Todd-Pokropek, A. E. and Jarritt, P. H.,** The noise characteristics of SPECT systems, in *Computed Emission Tomography,* Ell, P. J. and Holman, B. L., Eds., Oxford University Press, New York, 1982, chap. 12.
9. **Budinger, T. F.,** Physical attributes of single-photon tomography, *J. Nucl. Med.,* 21, 579, 1980.
10. **Gullberg, G. T., Malko, J. A., and Eisner, R. L.,** Boundary determination methods for attenuation correction in single photon emission computed tomography, in *Emission Computed Tomography: Current Trends,* Esser, P. D., Ed., 13th Annu. Symp. Sharing Comput. Programs Tech. Nucl. Med., Society of Nuclear Medicine, New York, 1983.
11. **Moore, S. C.,** Attenuation compensation, in *Computed Emission Tomography,* Ell, P. J. and Holman, B. L., Eds., Oxford University Press, New York, 1982, chap. 11.
12. **Larsson, S. A., Bergstrand, G., Bergstedt, H., Berg, J., Flygare, O., Per-Olof, S., Anderson, N., and Lagergren, C.,** A special cut-off gamma camera for high resolution SPECT of the head, *J. Nucl. Med.,* 25, 1023, 1984.
13. **Esser, P. D., Alderson, P. O., Mitnick, R. J., and Arliss, J. J.,** Angled-collimator SPECT (A-SPECT): An improved approach to cranial single photon emission tomography, *J. Nucl. Med.,* 25, 805, 1984.
14. **Polak, J. F., Holman, B. L., Moretti, J. L., Eisner, R. L., Lister-James, J., and English, R. J.,** I-123 HIPDM brain imaging with a rotating gamma camera and slant-hole collimator, *J. Nucl. Med.,* 25, 495, 1984.
15. **Gottschalk, S. C., Salem, D., Lim, C. B., Binhim, D., and Wake, R. H.,** SPECT resolution and uniformity improvements by noncircular orbit, *J. Nucl. Med.,* 24, 822, 1983.
16. **Kuhl, D. E., Edwards, R. Q., Ricci, A. R., Yacob, R. J., Mich, T. J., and Alavi, A.,** The Mark-IV system for radionuclide computed tomography of the brain, *Radiology,* 121, 405, 1976.
17. **Zimmerman, R. E., Kirsch, C-M., Lovett, R. D., and Hill, T. C.,** Single photon emission computed tomography with short focal length detectors, in *Single Photon Emission Computed Tomography and Other Selected Topics,* Sorenson, J. A., Ed., Society of Nuclear Medicine, New York, 1980, 147.

18. **Bonte, F. and Stokely, E. M.,** Single-photon tomographic study of regional cerebral blood flow after stroke: concise communication, *J. Nucl. Med.,* 22, 1049, 1981.
19. **Holman, B. L., Hill, T. C., and Magistretti, P. L.,** Brain imaging with emission computed tomography and radiolabeled amines, *Invest. Radiol.,* 17, 206, 1982.
20. **Oldendorf, W. H.,** *The Quest For An Image of Brain,* Raven Press, New York, 1980, chap. 5.
21. **Hill, T. C.,** Single-photon emission computed tomography to study cerebral function in man, *J. Nucl. Med.,* 21, 1197, 1980.
22. **Budinger, T. F.,** Revival of clinical nuclear medicine brain imaging, *J. Nucl. Med.,* 22, 1094, 1981.
23. **Coleman, R. E., Drayer, B. P., and Jaszczak, R. J.,** Studying regional brain function: a challenge for SPECT, *J. Nucl. Med.,* 23, 266, 1982.
24. **Lassen, N. A. and Ingvar, D. H.,** Radioisotope assessment of regional cerebral flow, in *Progress In Nuclear Medicine,* Vol. I., Potchen, E. J. and McCready, V. R., Eds., S. Karger, Basel, 1972, 376.
25. **Ter-Pogossian, M. M., Eichling, J. O., Davis, D. O., Welch, M. J., and Metzger, J. M.,** The determination of regional cerebral blood flow by means of water labeled with radioactive oxygen-15, *Radiology,* 93, 31, 1969.
26. **Stokely, E. M., Sveinsdottir, E., Lassen, N. A., and Rommer, P.,** A single photon dynamic computer assisted tomograph (DCTA) for imaging brain function in multiple cross sections, *J. Assist. Tomogr.,* 4, 230, 1980.
27. **Bonte, F. J. and Stokely, E. M.,** Single-photon tomographic study of regional cerebral blood flow after stroke: concise communication, *J. Nucl. Med.,* 22, 1049, 1981.
28. **Fazio, F., Fieschi, C., Collice, M., Nardini, M., Banfi, F., Possa, M., and Spinelli, F.,** Tomographic assessment of cerebral perfusion using a single-photon emitter (krypton-81m) and a rotating gamma camera, *J. Nucl. Med.,* 21, 1139, 1980.
29. **Kuhl, D. E., Barrio, J. R., Huang, S. C., Selin, C., Ackermann, R. F., Lear, J. L., Wu, J. L., Lin, T. H., and Phelps, M. E.,** Quantifying local cerebral blood flow by N-isopropyl-p-[^{123}I]iodoamphetamine (IMP) tomography, *J. Nucl. Med.,* 23, 196, 1982.
30. **Hill, T. C., Holman, B. L., Lovett, R., O'Leary, D. H., Front, D., Magistretti, P., Zimmerman, R. E., Moore, S., Clouse, M. E., Wu, J. L., Lin, T. H., and Baldwin, R. M.,** Initial experience with SPECT (single-photon computerized tomography) of the brain using N-isopropyl I-123 p-iodoamphetamine: concise communication, *J. Nucl. Med.,* 23, 191, 1982.
31. **Lear, J. L., Ackermann, R. F., Kameyama, M., and Kuhl, D. E.,** Evaluation of (I-123)-N-isopropyl-p-iodoamphetamine as a tracer for local cerebral blood flow using direct autoradiographic comparison, *J. Cereb. Blood Flow Metab.,* 2, 179, 1982.
32. **Fazio, F., Gerundini, P., Gillardi, M. C., Lenzi, G. L., Taddei, G., Piancentini, M., Colombo, F., Colombo, R., Kung, H. F., and Blau, M.,** Single photon emission computerized tomography (SPECT) evaluation of the brain imaging agent, (I-123)HIPDM in man with rotating gamma camera, *J. Nucl. Med.,* 24 (Abstr.), 5, 1983.
33. **Fazio, F., Gerundini, P., Lenzi, G. L., Collice, M., Gilardi, M. C., Taddei, G., Piacentini, M., Colombo, F., Colombo, R., Kung, H. F., and Blau, M.,** Evaluation of cerebrovascular disorders using the brain imaging agent, (I-123)HIPDM, and single photon emission computerized tomography (SPECT), *J. Nucl. Med.,* 24 (Abstr.), 5, 1983.
34. **Kung, H., Tramposch, K., Wicks, R., and Blau, M.,** Synthesis and biodistribution of I-123 HIPDM: A new brain perfusion imaging agent, *J. Nucl. Med.,* 23 (Abstr.), 22, 1982.
35. **Holman, B. L., Lee, R. G. L., Hill, T. C., Lovett, R. D., and Lister-James, J.,** A comparison of two cerebral perfusion tracers, N-isopropyl I-123 p-iodoamphetamine and I-123 HIPDM, in the human, *J. Nucl. Med.,* 25, 25, 1984.
36. **Frey, K. A., Wieland, D. M., Brown, L. E., Rogers, W. L., and Agranoff, B. W.,** Development of a tomographic myelin scan, *Ann. Neurol.,* 10, 214, 1981.
37. **Celsis, P., Goldman, T., Henriksen, L., and Lassen, N. A.,** A method for calculating regional cerebral blood flow from emission computed tomography of inert gas concentrations, *J. Comput. Assist. Tomog.,* 5, 641, 1981.
38. **Kanno, I. and Lassen, N. A.,** Two methods for calculating cerebral blood flow from emission computed tomography of inert gas concentrations, *J. Comput. Assist. Tomogr.,* 3, 71, 1979.
39. **Henriksen, I., Paulson, O. B., and Lassen, N. A.,** Visual cortex activation recorded by dynamic emission computed tomography of inhaled xenon-133, *Eur. J. Nucl. Med.,* 6, 487, 1981.
40. **Maximilian, V. A., Prohovnik, I., and Risberg, J.,** Cerebral hemodynamic response to mental activation in normo- and hypercapnia, *Stroke,* 11, 342, 1980.
41. **Winchell, H. S., Baldwin, R. M., and Lin, T. H.,** Development of I-123-labeled amines for brain studies: localization of I-123 iodophenylalkyl amines in rat brain, *J. Nucl. Med.,* 21, 940, 1980.
42. **Winchell, H. S., Horst, W. D., Braun, L., Oldendorf, W. H., Hattner, R., and Parker, H.,** N-isopropyl [^{123}I]p-iodoamphetamine: Single-pass brain uptake and washout; binding to brain synaptosomes; and localization in dog and monkey brain, *J. Nucl. Med.,* 21, 947, 1980.

43. **Zimmerman, R. E., Judy, P. F., and Hill, T. C.,** Performance measurements of an emission tomographic brain scanner, *J. Nucl. Med.*, 20 (Abstr.), 628, 1979.
44. **Zimmerman, R. E., Judy, P. F., and Hill, T. C.,** Evaluation of the performance of an emission computed tomography scanner, *Med. Phys.*, 5 (Abstr.), 314, 1978.
45. **Flower, M. A., Parker, R. P., Coles, I. P., Fox, R. A., and Trott, N. G.,** Feasibility of absolute activity measurements using the Cleon emission tomography system, *Radiology*, 133, 497, 1979.
46. **Jarritt, P. H., Ell, P. J., Myers, M. J., Brown, N. J. G., and Deacon, J. M.,** A new transverse-section brain imager for single-gamma emitters, *J. Nucl. Med.*, 20, 319, 1979.
47. **Kirsch, C-M., Moore, S. C., Zimmerman, R. E., English, R. J., and Holman, B. L.,** Characteristics of a scanning, multidetector, single-photon ECT body imager, *J. Nucl. Med.*, 22, 726, 1981.
48. **Zimmerman, R. E., Kirsch, C.-M., and Lane, H. R.,** Single photon emission computed tomography with short focal length determination, in *Single Photon Emission Computed Tomography and Other Selected Computer Topics.* Proc. of the 10th Annu. Symp. Soc. Nucl. Med. Comput. Counc., Miami Beach, FL, 1980, 147.
49. **Magistretti, P., Uren, R., Blume, H., Schomer, D., and Royal, H.,** Delineation of epileptic focus by single photon emission tomography, *Eur. J. Nucl. Med.*, 7, 484, 1982.
50. **Hill, T. C., Holman, B. L., and Magistretti, P. L.,** Emission-computed tomography of the brain with radiolabelled amines, in *Computed Emission Tomography*, Ell, P. J. and Holman, B. L., Eds., Oxford University Press, New York, 1982, chap. 15.
51. **Lassen, N. A., Henriksen, L., Holm, S., Barry, D. I., Paulson, O. B., Vorstrup, S., Rapin, J., le Poncin-Lafitte, M., Moretti, J. L., Askienazy, S., and Raynaud, C.,** Cerebral blood-flow tomography: Xenon-133 compared with isopropyl-amphetamine-iodine-123: concise communication, *J. Nucl. Med.*, 24, 17, 1983.
52. **Kuhl, D. E., Wu, J. L., Lin, T. H., Selin, C., and Phelps, M.,** Mapping local cerebral blood flow by means of emission computed tomography of N-isopropyl-p(123-I)-iodoamphetamine (IMP), *J. Cerebral Blood Flow Metab. (Suppl. 1)*, I, 25, 1981.
53. **Kuhl, D. E., Wu, J. L., Lin, T. H., Selin, C., and Phelps, M.,** Mapping local cerebral blood flow by means of emission computed tomography of N-isopropyl-p (123-I)-Iodoamphetamine (IMP), *J. Nucl. Med.*, 22, 16, 1981.
54. **Ell, P. J. and Khan, O.,** Emission computerized tomography: clinical applications, *Sem. Nucl. Med.*, XI, 50, 1981.
55. **Dendy, P. P., McNab, J. W., MacDonald, A. F., Keyes, W. J., and Cannill, J. M.,** An evaluation of transverse axial emission tomography of the brain in the clinical situation, *Br. J. Radiol.*, 50, 555, 1977.
56. **Wooley, J. L., Williams, B., and Venkatesh, S.,** Cranial isotope section scanning, *Clin. Radiol.*, 28, 517, 1977.
57. **Cowan, R. J. and Watson, N. E.,** Special characteristics and potential of single photon emission computed tomography in the brain, *Sem. Nucl. Med.*, X, 335, 1980.
58. **Jaszczak, R. J., Murphy, P. H., Huard, D., and Burdine, J. A.,** Radionuclide emission computed tomography of the head with ^{99m}Tc and a scintillation camera, *J. Nucl. Med.*, 18, 373, 1977.
59. **Keyes, J. W., Jr., Orlandea, N., Heetderks, W. J., Leonard, P. F., and Rogers, W. L.,** The humongotron-a scintillation-camera transaxial tomograph, *J. Nucl. Med.*, 18, 381, 1977.
60. **Hill, T. C., Lovett, R. D., and McNeil, B. J.,** Observations on the clinical value of emission tomography, *J. Nucl. Med.*, 21, 613, 1980.
61. **Carril, J. M., MacDonald, A. F., Dendy, P. P., Keyes, W. I., Undrill, P. E., and Mallard, J. R.,** Cranial scintigraphy: value of adding emission computed tomographic sections to conventional pertechnetate images (512 cases), *J. Nucl. Med.*, 20, 1117, 1979.
62. **Watson, N. E., Jr., Cowan, R. J., Ball, M. R., Moody, D. M., Laster, D. W., and Maynard, C. D.,** A comparison of brain imaging with gamma camera, single-photon emission computed tomography, and transmission computed tomography: concise communication, *J. Nucl. Med.*, 21, 507, 1980.
63. **Oyamada, I., Terui, S., Fukukita, H., Kawai, H., and Nagaiwa, K.,** Clinical evaluation of single photon emission computed tomography of the brain, *Eur. J. Nucl. Med.*, 7, 439, 1982.
64. **Herrick, J. B.,** Clinical factors of sudden obstruction of the coronary arteries, *JAMA*, 58, 1971, 1912.
65. **McKillop, J. J.,** Is ^{201}thallium imaging clinically valuable in coronary artery disease?, *Crit. Rev. Diag. Imaging*, 18, 167, 1981.
66. **Ritchie, J. L.,** Exercise myocardial imaging and radionuclide angiography: uses, abuses, and limitations in the evaluation of coronary artery disease, in *Cardiovascular Medicine*, Vol. 1, Vogel, J. H. K., Ed., Raven Press, New York, 1982, 7.
67. **Borer, J. S., Bacharach, S. L., and Green, M. V.,** Radionuclide imaging in the evaluation of ventricular function — techniques and application in coronary, valvular, and cardiomyopathic diseases: selected topics, in *Cardiovascular Medicine*, Vol. 1, Vogel, J. H. K., Ed., Raven Press, New York, 1982, 15.
68. **Sobel, B. E. and Geltman, E. M.,** Localization and quantification of myocardial ischemia and infarction with positron emission tomography, in *Cardiovascular Medicine*, Vol. 1, Vogel, J. H. K., Ed., Raven Press, New York, 1982, 33.

69. **Schelbert, H. R.,** The heart, in *Computed Emission Tomography,* Ell, P. J. and Holman, B. L., Eds., Oxford University Press, New York, 1982, chap. 3.
70. **Larsson, St. A.,** Gamma camera emission tomography. Development and properties of a multisectional emission computed tomography system, *Acta Radiol. (Suppl.),* 363, 1980.
71. **Vogel, R. A., Kirch, D. L., LeFree, M. T., and Steele, P. P.,** A new method of multiplanar emission tomography using a seven pinhole collimator and an Anger scintillation camera, *J. Nucl. Med.,* 22, 48, 1981.
72. **Koral, K. F., Nolder, C., Ciliax, G., Rogers, W. L., and Keyes, J. W., Jr.,** Simulated ECT of the left ventricle using rotating slant-hole collimator and two camera positions, *J. Nucl. Med.,* 25, 343, 1984.
73. **Losse, B., Kuhn, H., Kronert, H., Rafflenbohel, D., Feinendegen, L. E., and Loogen, F.,** Exercise thallium-201 myocardial perfusion imaging in patients with normal coronary angiogram and ventriculogram, *Circulation (Suppl.),* 60 (Abstr.), 148, 1977.
74. **Holman, B. L. and Wynne, J.,** Thallium-201 — when should we use it?, *J. Nucl. Med.,* 20, 1206, 1979.
75. **Smalling, R. W.,** The SPECTrum of thallium-201 imaging in coronary artery disease, *J. Nucl. Med.,* 24, 854, 1983.
76. **Hamilton, G. W.,** Myocardial imaging with thallium-201: the controversy over its clinical usefulness in ischemic heart disease, *J. Nucl. Med.,* 20, 1201, 1979.
77. **Buja, L. M., Parkey, R. W., Stokely, E. M., Bonte, F. J., and Willerson, J. T.,** Pathophysiology of technetium-99m stannous pyrophosphate and thallium-201 scintigraphy of acute anterior myocardial infarcts in dogs, *J. Clin. Invest.,* 57, 1508, 1976.
78. **Buja, L. M., Tofe, A. J., Kulkarni, P. V., Mukherjee, A., Parkey, R. W., Francis, M. D., Bonte, F. J., and Willerson, J. T.,** Sites and mechanisms of localization of technetium-99m phosphorus radiopharmaceuticals in acute myocardial infarcts and other tissues, *J. Clin. Inv.,* 60, 724, 1977.
79. **Buja, L. M., Poliner, L. R., Parkey, R. W., Pulido, J. I., Hutcheson, D., and Platt, M. R., Mills, L. J., Bonte, F. J., and Willerson, J. T.,** Clinicopathologic study of persistently positive technetium-99m stannous pyrophosphate myocardial scintigrams and myocytolytic degeneration after acute myocardial infarction, *Circulation,* 56, 1016, 1977.
80. **Poliner, L. R., Buja, L. M., Parkey, R. W., Bonte, F. J., and Willerson, J. R.,** Clinico-pathologic findings in 52 patients studied by technetium-99m stannous pyrophosphate myocardial scintigraphy, *Circulation,* 59, 257, 1979.
81. **Parkey, R. W., Kulkarni, P. V., Lewis, S. E., Datz, F. L., Dehmer, G. J., Gutekunst, D. P., Buja, L. M., Bonte, F. J., and Willerson, J. T.,** Effect of coronary blood flow and site of injection of Tc-99m PPi detection of early canine myocardial infarcts, *J. Nucl. Med.,* 22, 133, 1981.
82. **Stokely, E. M., Buja, L. M., Lewis, S. E., Parkey, R. W., Bonte, J., Harris, R. A., Jr., and Willerson, J. T.,** Measurement of acute myocardial infarcts in dogs from 99m Tc-stannous pyrophosphate scintigrams, *J. Nucl. Med.,* 17, 1, 1976.
83. **Berger, H. J., Gottschalk, A., and Zaret, B. L.,** Dual radionuclide study of acute myocardial infarction. Comparison of thallium-201 and technetium-99m stannous pyrophosphate imaging in man, *Ann. Intern. Med.,* 88, 145, 1978.
84. **Willerson, J. T., Parkey, R. W., Stokely, E. M., Bonte, F. J., Lewis, S., Harris, R. A., Blomquist, G., Poliner, L. R., and Buja, L. M.,** Infarct sizing with technetium-99m stannous pyrophosphate scintigraphy in dogs and man; relationship between scintigraphic and precordial mapping estimates of infarct size in patients, *Cardiovasc. Res.,* 11, 291, 1977.
85. **Lewis, S. E., Stokely, E. M., Devons, M. D., Bonte, J. F., Buja, L. M., Parkey, R. W., and Willerson, J. T.,** Quantitation of experimental canine infarct size with multipinhole and rotating-slanthole tomography, *J. Nucl. Med.,* 22, 1000, 1981.
86. **Lewis, S. E.,** A letter to the editor, *J. Nucl. Med.,* 12, 939, 1981.
87. **Sing, H. M., Berggren, M. J., Gustafson, D. E., Dewanjee, M. K., Bahn, R. C., and Ritman, E. L.,** Emission-computed tomography and its application to imaging of acute myocardial infarction in intact dogs using Tc-99m pyrophosphate, *J. Nucl. Med.,* 20, 50, 1979.
88. **Stokely, E. M., Tipton, D. M., and Buja, L. M.,** Quantitation of experimental canine infarct size using multipinhole single-photon tomography, *J. Nucl. Med.,* 22, 5, 1981.
89. **Lewis, S. E., Corbett, J., Morgan, C., Izquierdo, C., Huxley, R., Nicod, P., Devous, M., Buja, L. M., and Willerson, J. T.,** Single photon emission tomographic sizing of experimental myocardial infarcts: comparison of infarct-avid and perfusion methods, *Clin. Res.,* 30, 201A, 1982.
90. **Abdullah, A. Z., Stone, D. L., Britton, K. E., and Elliott, A. T.,** Emission computerised tomography with ^{99m}Tc-pyrophosphate in myocardial infarction, *Nucl. Med. Commun.,* 2, 140, 1981.
91. **Goris, M. L., Daspit, S. G., McLaughlin, P., and Kriss, J. P.,** Interpolative background subtraction, *J. Nucl. Med.,* 17, 744, 1976.
92. **Goris, M. L., Gordon, E., and Kim, D.,** A stochastic interpretation of thallium myocardial perfusion scintigraphy, *Invest. Radiol.,* in press.

93. **Kirch, D. L., Vogel, R. A., LeFree, M. T., Sklar, J., Hasegawa, B. H., and Steele, P. P.,** An Anger camera/computer system for myocardial perfusion tomography using a seven pinhole collimator, *IEEE Trans. Nucl. Sci.*, NS-27, 412, 1980.
94. **Chang, W., Lin, S. L., and Henkin, R. E.,** A rotatable quadrant slant hole collimator for tomography (QSH): a stationary scintillation camera based SPECT system, in *Single Photon Emission Computed Tomography and Other Selected Computer Topics*, Sorenson, J. A., Book Coordinator, The Society of Nuclear Medicine, New York, 1980, 81.
95. **Bailey, I. K., Griffith, L. S. C., Rouleau, J., Strauss, H. W., and Pitt, B.,** Thallium-201 myocardial perfusion imaging at rest and during exercise, *Circulation*, 55, 79, 1977.
96. **Lenaers, A.,** Thallium-201 myocardial perfusion scintigraphy during rest and exercise, *Cardiovas. Radiol.*, 2, 195, 1979.
97. **Massie, B. M., Botvinick, E. H., and Brundage, B. H.,** Correlation of thallium-201 scintigrams with coronary anatomy: factors affecting region by region sensitivity, *Am. J. Cardiol.*, 44, 616, 1979.
98. **Ritchie, J. L., Trobaugh, G. B., Hamilton, G. W., Gould, K. L., Narahara, K. A., Murray, J. A., and Williams, D. L.,** Myocardial imaging with thallium-201 at rest and during exercise, *Circulation*, 56, 66, 1977.
99. **Ritchie, J. L., Zaret, B. L., Strauss, H. W., Pitt, B., Berman, D. S., Schelbert, H. R., Ashburn, W. L., Berger, H. J., and Hamilton, G. W.,** Myocardial imaging with thallium-201: a multicenter study in patients with angina pectoris or acute myocardial infarction, *Am. J. Cardiol.*, 42, 345, 1978.
100. **Verani, M. S., Marcus, M. L., Razzak, M. A., and Erhardt, J. C.,** Sensitivity and specificity of thallium-201 perfusion scintigrams under exercise in the diagnosis of coronary artery disease, *J. Nucl. Med.*, 19, 733, 1978.
101. **Albro, P. C., Gould, K. L., Westcott, R. H., Hamilton, G., Ritchie, J., and Williams, D.,** Noninvasive assessment of coronary stenoses by myocardial imaging during pharmacologic coronary vasodilatation, *Am. J. Cardiol.*, 42, 751, 1978.
102. **Francisco, D., Go, R., Van Kirk, O., Erhardt, J., and Marcus, J.,** Tomographic thallium-201 perfusion scintigrams following maximal coronary vasodilatation with dipyridamole, *Circulation*, 50 (Abstr.), 174, 1979.
103. **Harris, D. N. F., Taylor, D. N., Ackery, D. M., and Conway, N.,** Imaging for myocardial ischemia with dipyridamole, ^{201}Tl, and gated wall motion, *Nucl. Med. Commun.*, 1, 74, 1980.
104. **Gould, K. L., Westcott, R. J., Albro, P. C., and Hamilton, G. W.,** Noninvasive assessment of coronary stenoses by myocardial imaging during pharmacological coronary vasodilation. Clinical methodology and feasibility, *Am. J. Cardiol.*, 41, 279, 1978.
105. **Raff, U., Kirch, D. L., and Hendee, W. R.,** Seven pinhole tomography, clinical protocols. Tomographic methods in nuclear medicine, in *CRC Handbook*, Ahluwalia, B., Ed., 1985.
106. **Lebowitz, E., Greene, M. W., Bradley-Moore, P., Atkins, H., Ansari, A., Richards, P., and Belgrave, E.,** ^{201}Tl for medical use, *J. Nucl. Med.*, 14, 421, 1973.
107. **Lebowitz, E., Greene, M. W., Fairchild, R., Bradley-Moore, P. R., Atkins, H. L., Ansari, A. N., Richards, P., and Belgrave, E.,** Thallium-201 for medical use, *J. Nucl. Med.*, 16, 151, 1975.
108. **Mueller, T. M., Marcus, M. I., Erhardt, J. C., Chaudhuri, T., and Abboud, F. M.,** Limitations of thallium-201 myocardial perfusion scintigrams, *Circulation*, 54, 640, 1976.
109. **Kawana, M., Krizek, H., Porter, J., Lathrop, K. A., Charleston, D., and Harper, P. V.,** Use of ^{199}Tl as a potassium analog in scanning, *J. Nucl. Med.*, 11 (Abstr.), 133, 1970.
110. **Strauss, H. W., Harrison, K., Langan, J. K., Lebowitz, E., and Pitt, B.,** Thallium for myocardial imaging: relation of thallium-201 to regional myocardial perfusion, *Circulation*, 51, 641, 1975.
111. **Cook, D. J., Bailey, I., Strauss, H. W., Rouleau, J., Wagner, H. N., Jr., and Pitt, B.,** Thallium-201 for myocardial imaging appearance of the normal heart, *J. Nucl. Med.*, 17, 583, 1976.
112. **Weich, H. F., Strauss, H. W., and Pitt, B.,** The extraction of thallium-201 by the myocardium, *Circulation*, 56, 188, 1977.
113. **Strauss, H. W. and Pitt, B.,** ^{201}Thallium as a myocardial imaging agent, *Sem. Nucl. Med.*, 7, 49, 1977.
114. **Lederer, C. M., Hollander, J. M., and Perlman, I.,** *Tables of Isotopes*, 6th ed., John Wiley & Sons, Inc., New York, 1967.
115. **Hoffman, E. J.,** 180° compared with 360° sampling in SPECT, *J. Nucl. Med.*, 23, 745, 1982.
116. **Ritchie, J. L., Larsson, S., Israelson, A., Schnell, P. O., Holmgren, A., Williams, D. L., and Thorell, J. I.,** Single photon tomographic imaging of a standard heart phantom with ^{201}Tl: a gamma camera based system, *Eur. J. Nucl. Med.*, 7, 254, 1982.
117. **MacIntyre, W. J., Go, R. T., Houser, T. S., Sufka, B., Napoli, C., and Cook, S. A.,** Evaluation of 180-deg reconstruction of the heart by transaxial tomography with thallium-201, in *Emission Computed Tomography: Current Trends*, Esser, P. D., Ed., Society of Nuclear Medicine, New York, 1983, 197.
118. **Lewis, M. H., Bonte, F. J., Lewis, S. E., and Stokely, E. M.,** Work in progress: A comparison of data collection protocols for single-photon emission tomography: 180° versus 360°, *Radiology*, 145, 501, 1982.

119. **Tamaki, N., Mukai, T., Ishii, Y., Fujita, T., Yamamoto, K., Minato, K., Yonekura, Y., Tamaki, S., Kambara, H., Kawai, C., and Torizuka, K.,** Comparative study of thallium emission myocardial tomography with 180° and 360° data collection, *J. Nucl. Med.*, 23, 661, 1982.
120. **Coleman, R. E., Jaszczak, R. J., and Cobb, F. R.,** Comparison of 180° and 360° data collection in thallium-201 imaging using single-photon emission computerized tomography (SPECT): concise communication, *J. Nucl. Med.*, 23, 655, 1982.
121. **Chang, W. and Henkin, R. E.,** Photon attenuation in Tl-201 myocardial SPECT and quantitation through an empirical correction, in *Emission Computed Tomography: Current Trends*, Esser, P. D., Ed., Society of Nuclear Medicine, New York, 1982, 123.
122. **Axelsson, B., Msaki, P., and Israelson, A.,** Subtraction of Compton-scattered photons in single-photon emission computerized tomography, *J. Nucl. Med.*, 25, 490, 1984.
123. **Jaszczak, R. J., Greer, K. L., Floyd, C. E., Jr., Harris, C. C., and Coleman, R. E.,** Improved SPECT quantification using compensation for scattered photons, *J. Nucl. Med.*, 25, 893, 1984.
124. **Hamilton, G. W., Narahara, K. A., Yee, H., Ritchie, J. L., Williams, D. L., and Gould, K. L.,** Myocardial imaging with thallium-201: effect of cardiac drugs on myocardial images and absolute tissue distribution, *J. Nucl. Med.*, 19, 10, 1978.
125. **Gottschalk, S. C., Salem, D., Lim, C. B., Binhim, D., and Wake, R. H.,** SPECT resolution and uniformity improvements by noncircular orbit, *J. Nucl. Med.*, 24, 822, 1983.
126. **Stern, D. M.,** Personal communication, Research Systems, Inc., Denver.
127. **Borrello, J. A., Clinthorne, N. H., Rogers, W. L., Thrall, J. H., and Keyes, J. W., Jr.,** Oblique-angle tomography: a restructuring algorithm for transaxial tomographic data, *J. Nucl. Med.*, 22, 471, 1981.
128. **Maublant, J., Cassagnes, J., Veyre, A., and Meyniel, G.,** Myocardial emission tomography with thallium-201, *Eur. J. Nucl. Med.*, 6, 289, 1981.
129. **Maublant, J., Cassagnes, J., Le Jeune, J. J., Mestas, E., Veyre, A., Jallut, H., and Meyniel, G.,** A comparison between conventional scintigraphy and emission tomography with thallium-201 in the detection of myocardial infarction: concise communication, *J. Nucl. Med.*, 23, 204, 1982.
130. **Ritchie, J. L., Williams, D. L., Harp, G., Stratton, J. L., and Caldwell, J. H.,** Transaxial tomography with thallium-201 for detecting remote myocardial infarction, *Am. J. Cardiol.*, 50, 1236, 1982.
131. **Kirsch, C-M., Doliwa, R., Buell, U., and Roedler, D.,** Detection of severe coronary heart disease with Tl-201: comparison of resting single photon emission tomography with invasive arteriography, *J. Nucl. Med.*, 24, 761, 1983.
132. **McIntyre, W. J., Go, R. T., and Cook, S. A.,** Comparison of stress and redistribution 201-thallium imaging with a single photon transaxial tomographic technique, in *Nuclear Medicine and Biology*, Raynaud, D., Ed., Pergamon, Paris, 1982, 1281.
133. **Raff, U., Spitzer, V. M., Klingensmith, W. C., and Hendee, W. R.,** Optimal myocardial SPECT imaging parameters, *J. Nucl. Med.*, 24, 67, 1982.
134. **Caldwell, J. H., Williams, D. L., Hamilton, G. W., Ritchie, J. L., Harp, G. D., Eisner, R. L., Gullberg, G. T., and Nowak, D. J.,** Regional distribution of myocardial blood flow measured by single-photon emission tomography: comparison with in vitro counting, *J. Nucl. Med.*, 23, 490, 1982.
135. **Keyes, J. W., Jr., Brady, T. J., Leonard, P. F., Svetkoff, D. B., Winter, S. M., Rogers, W. L., and Rose, E. A.,** Calculation of viable and infarcted myocardial mass from thallium-201 tomograms, *J. Nucl. Med.*, 22, 339, 1981.
136. **Garcia, E. V., Van Train, K., Maddahi, J., Prigent, F., Friedman, J., Areeda, J., Waxman, A., and Berman, D. S.,** Quantification of rotational thallium-201 myocardial tomography, *J. Nucl. Med.*, 26, 17, 1985.
137. **Holman, B. L., Jones, A. G., Lister-James, J., Davison, A., Abrams, M. H., Kirshenbaum, J. M., Tumeh, S. S., and English, R. J.,** A new Tc-99m labeled myocardial imaging agent, hexakis(t-butyl-isonitrile)-technetium(I)[Tc-99m TBI]: initial experience in the human, *J. Nucl. Med.*, 25, 1350, 1984.
138. **Mullani, N. A., Gould, K. L., and Gaeta, J. M.,** Tomographic imaging of the heart with thallium-201: seven-pinhole or rotating gamma camera?, *J. Nucl. Med.*, 22, 925, 1981.
139. **Moore, M. L., Murphy, P. H., and Burdine, J. A.,** ECG-gated emission computed tomography of the cardiac blood pool, *Radiology*, 134, 233, 1980.
140. **Philippe, L., Itti, R., Lorgeron, J. M., Demeyer, J. F., and Raynaud, P.,** Thick slice emission tomography for quantitative assessment of cardiac function, *J. Nucl. Med.*, 23 (Abstr.), 61, 1982.
141. **Maublant, J., Bailly, P., Mestas, D., Cassagnes, J., Lasson, J. R., Zurowski, S., Huffer, E., Veyre, A., Jallut, H., and Meyniel, G.,** Feasibility of gated single-photon emission transaxial tomography of the cardiac blood pool, *Radiology*, 146, 837, 1983.
142. **Tamaki, N., Mukai, T., Ishii, Y., Yonekura, Y., Yamamoto, K., Kadota, K., Kambara, H., Kawai, C., and Torizuka, K.,** Multiaxial tomography of heart chambers by gated blood-pool emission computed tomography using a rotating gamma camera, *Radiology*, 147, 547, 1983.
143. **Barat, J. L., Brendel, A. J., Colle, J. P., Magimel-Pelonnier, V., Ohayon, J., Wynchank, S., Leccia, F., Besse, P., and Ducassou, D.,** Quantitative analysis of left-ventricular function using gated single photon emission tomography, *J. Nucl. Med.*, 25, 1167, 1984.

144. **Ingels, N. B., Daughters, G. T., Stinson, E. B., and Alderman, E. L.**, Evaluation of methods for quantitating left ventricular segmental wall motion in man using myocardial markers as a standard, *Circulation*, 61, 966, 1980.
145. **Holman, B. L., Kirsch, C.-M., and Zielonka, J. S.**, The heart, in *Computed Emission Tomography*, Ell, P. J., Ed., Oxford University Press, New York, 1982, chap. 17.
146. **Tamaki, N., Mukai, T., Ishii, Y., Yonekura, Y., Kambara, H., Kawai, C., and Torizuka, K.**, Clinical evaluation of thallium-201 myocardial emission tomography using a rotating gamma camera: comparison with seven-pinhole tomography, *J. Nucl. Med.*, 22, 849, 1981.
147. **Khan, O. and Ell, P.**, Liver and spleen, in *Computed Emission Tomography*, Ell, P. J. and Holman, B. L., Eds., Oxford University Press, New York, 1982, chap. 16.
148. **Jaszczak, R. J., Whitehead, F. R., Lim, C. B., and Coleman, R. E.**, Lesion detection with single-photon emission computed tomography (SPECT) compared with conventional imaging, *J. Nucl. Med.*, 23, 97, 1982.
149. **Strauss, L. G., Clorius, J. H., Frank, T., and van Kaick, G.**, Single photon emission computerized tomography (SPECT) for estimates of liver and spleen volume, *J. Nucl. Med.*, 25, 81, 1984.
150. **Dendy, P. P., Keyes, W. I., Reid, A., Undrill, P. E., Smith, F. W., Mallard, J. R., and MacDonald, A. F.**, A clinical trial of the value of a tomographic section view to identify liver abnormalities by radionuclide imaging, with special reference to metastatic disease, *Eur. J. Nucl. Med.*, 6, 51, 1981.
151. **Berche, C., Aubry, F., Langlais, C., Vitaux, J., Parmentier, C., and Di Paola, R.**, Diagnostic value of transverse axial tomoscintigraphy for the detection of hepatic metastases: results on 53 examinations and comparisons with other diagnostic techniques, *Eur. J. Nucl. Med.*, 6, 435, 1981.
152. **Strauss, L., Bostel, F., Clorius, J., Raptou, E., Wellman, H., and Georgi, P.**, Single-photon emission computed tomography (SPECT) for assessment of hepatic lesions, *J. Nucl. Med.*, 23, 1059, 1982.
153. **Croft, B. Y. and Teates, C. D.**, Experience with single photon emission computed tomography of the liver, in *Emission Computed Tomography: Current Trends*, Esser, P. D., Ed., Society of Nuclear Medicine, New York, 1983.
154. **Gyves, J. W., Ziessman, H. A., Ensminger, W. D., Thrall, J. H., Niederhuber, J. E., Keyes, J. W., Jr., and Walker, S.**, Definition of hepatic tumor microcirculation by single photon emission computerized tomography (SPECT), *J. Nucl. Med.*, 25, 972, 1984.
155. **Tauxe, W. N., Soussaline, F., Todd-Pokropek, A., Cao, A., Collard, P., Richard, S., Raynaud, C., and Itti, R.**, Determination of organ volume by single-photon emission tomography, *J. Nucl. Med.*, 23, 984, 1982.
156. **Taplin, G. V., Dore, E. K., Johnson, D. E., and Kaplan, H. S.**, Scientific Exhibit on Colloidal Radioalbumin Aggregates for Organ Scanning, 10th Annual Meeting, Society of Nuclear Medicine, Montreal, June 26—29, 1963.
157. **Wagner, H. N., Jr., Sabiston, D. C., Jr., McAfee, J. G., Tow, D. E., and Stern, H. S.**, Diagnosis of massive pulmonary embolism in man by radioisotope scanning, *New Engl. J. Med.*, 271, 377, 1964.
158. **Taplin, G. V. and Poe, N. D.**, A dual lung scanning technique for evaluation of pulmonary function, *Radiology*, 85, 365, 1965.
159. **Wagner, H. N., Jr.**, The use of radioisotope techniques for the evaluation of patients with pulmonary disease, *Am. Rev. Respir. Dis.*, 113, 203, 1976.
160. **Alderson, P. O., Rujanavech, N., Seckler-Walker, R. H., and McKnight, R. C.**, The role of ^{133}Xe ventiliation studies in the scintigraphic detection of pulmonary embolism, *Radiology*, 120, 633, 1976.
161. **Taplin, G. V., Tashkin, D. P., Chopra, S. K., Anselmi, O. E., Elam, D., Calvarese, B., Coulson, A., Detels, R., and Rokaw, S. N.**, Early detection of chronic obstructive pulmonary disease using radionuclide lung imaging procedures, *Chest.*, 71, 567, 1977.
162. **Macey, D. J. and Marshall, R.**, The lungs, in *Computed Emission Tomography*, Ell, P. J. and Holman, B. L., Eds., Oxford University Press, New York, 1982.
163. **Maeda, H., Itoh, H., Ishii, Y., Mukai, T., Todo, G., Fujita, T., and Torizuka, K.**, Determination of the pleural edge by gamma-ray transmission computed tomography, *J. Nucl. Med.*, 22, 815, 1981.
164. **Osborne, D. R., Jaszczak, R. J., Greer, K., Roggli, V., Lischko, M., and Coleman, R. E.**, Detection of pulmonary emboli in dogs: comparison of single photon emission computed tomography, gamma camera imaging, and angiography, *Radiology*, 146, 493, 1983.
165. **Pulouse, K. P., Reba, R. C., and Wagner, H. N., Jr.**, Characterization of the shape and location of perfusion defects in certain pulmonary diseases, *New Engl. J. Med.*, 279, 1020, 1968.
166. **Taplin, G. V. and Hayes, M.**, Lung imaging with radioaerosols for the assessment of airway disease, *Sem. Nucl. Med.*, 23, 1980.
167. **Philipson, K.**, Radioisotope labeling of aerosols for the study of lung function, *Chest (Suppl.)*, 80, 818, 1981.
168. **Garrard, C. S., Gerrity, T. R., Schreiner, J. F., and Yeates, D. B.**, The characterization of radioaerosol deposition in the healthy lung by histogram distribution analysis, *Chest (Suppl.)*, 80, 840, 1981.
169. **Brain, J. D. and Valberg, P. A.**, Deposition of aerosol in the respiratory tract, *Am. Rev. Resp. Dis.*, 120, 1325, 1979.

170. **Donaldson, R. M., Kahn, O., Raphael, M. J., Jarritt, P. H., and Ell, P. J.,** Emission tomography in embolic lung disease: angiographic correlations, *Clin. Radiol.*, 33, 389, 1982.
171. **Le Jeune, J. J., Maublant, J., Lahellec, M., and Veyre, A.,** Emission computed tomography vs. perfusion scanning in lung disease, *Eur. J. Nucl. Med.*, 7, 171, 1982.
172. **Line, B. R., Hunninghake, G. W., Keogh, B. A., Jones, A. E., Johnston, G. S., and Crystal, R. G.,** Gallium-67 scanning to stage the alveolitis of sarcoidosis: correlation with clinical studies, pulmonary function studies and brochoalveolar lavage, *Am. Rev. Respir. Dis.*, 123, 440, 1981.
173. **Line, B. R., Fulmer, J. D., Reynolds, H. Y., Roberts, W. C., Jones, A. E., Harris, E. K., and Crystal, R. G.,** Gallium-67 citrate scanning in the staging of idiopathic pulmonary fibrosis: correlation with physiologic and morphologic features and bronchoalveolar lavage, *Am. Rev. Respir. Dis.*, 118, 355, 1976.
174. **Dubovsky, E. V., Diethelm, A. G., Balch, C. M., and Tauxe, W. N.,** Differentiation of cell-mediated and humoral rejection by orthoiodo-hippurate kinetics, *Arch. Intern. Med.*, 137, 738, 1977.
175. **Tauxe, W. N., Todd-Pokropek, A., Soussaline, F., Raynaud, C., and Kellershohn, C.,** Estimates of kidney volume by single photon emission tomography: a preliminary report, *Eur. J. Nucl. Med.*, 8, 72, 1983.
176. **Britton, K. E.,** Adrenal imaging, in *Clinical Nuclear Medicine,* Maisey, M. N., Britton, K. E., and Gilday, D. L., Eds., Chapman and Hall, London, chap. 6, 1983.
177. **Britton, K. E., Shapiro, B., and Hawkins, L. A.,** Emission tomography for adrenal imaging, *Nucl. Med. Comm.*, 1, 37, 1980.
178. **Hawkins, L. A., Britton, K. E., and Shapiro, B.,** ^{75}Se selenomethylcholesterol. A new agent for quantitative functional scintigraphy of the adrenals: physical aspects, *Br. J. Radiol.*, 53, 920, 1980.
179. **Shapiro, B., Rigby, L., and Britton, K. E.,** The assessment of thyroid volume with single photon emission tomography, *Nucl. Med. Comm.*, 1, 3, 1980.
180. **O'Connor, M. K., Cullen, M. J., and Malone, J. F.,** The value of tracer doses in predicting the kinetics of therapeutic doses of ^{131}I in thyrotoxicosis, *Br. J. Med.*, 52, 719, 1979.
181. **Smith, R. N. and Wilson, G. M.,** Clinical trials of different doses of ^{131}I in treatment of thyrotoxicosis, *Brit. Med. J.*, 1, 129, 1967.
182. **Rassmussen, S. N. and Hjorth, L.,** Determination of thyroid volume by ultrasonic scanning, *J. Clin. Ultrason.*, 2, 143, 1974.
183. **Pavel, D. G., Syrota, A., Soussaline, F., Todd-Pokropek, A., and Kellershohn, C.,** Single photon emission tomography in diagnosis of liver metastases, *J. Nucl. Med.*, 22, 31, 1981.
184. **Mortelmans, L. A. and DeRoo, M. J. K.,** Diagnostic value of SPECT in a case of lower neck uptake on bone scan, *Clin. Nucl. Med.*, 8, 616, 1983.
185. **Shapiro, B., Britton, K. E., Hawkins, L. A., and Edwards, C. R. W.,** Emission tomography of the pituitary, *Nucl. Med. Comm.*, 1, 150, 1980.

Chapter 6

POSITRON EMISSION TOMOGRAPHY IMAGING SYSTEMS AND APPLICATIONS

B. Ahluwalia

TABLE OF CONTENTS

I. INTRODUCTION

A. Imaging Strategies

Most of the existing imaging modalities such as radiography, X-ray transmission computed tomography, and ultrasound provide anatomical information. Some of the nuclear medicine procedures, which use conventional radiopharmaceuticals, also provide functional information. The use of positron-emitting radiopharmaceuticals is promising for the study of physiologic function as well as anatomy in organ imaging. The potential of positron imaging has been known since the 1950s. Clinical applications have been limited, however, because of slow developments in various essentials, such as production of radionuclides, appropriate radiopharmaceuticals, and high resolution imaging devices. Small cyclotrons are now available for use in clinical facilities. A variety of radiopharmaceuticals have been developed and have proven useful for physiological studies. Imaging instruments, known as positron cameras, are now commercially available.

B. Principle of Positron Emission Tomography

As the positrons emitted by radionuclides slow down, they are captured by an electron. This process leads to their mutual annihilation and the emission of two 511-keV photons which come out at 180° relative to each other. The distribution of these photons is isotropic from the point of annihilation of the positron. This property of back-to-back emission of gamma rays is utilized in conjunction with coincidence counting for the positron imaging instrument. The first practical device used a pair of sodium iodine detectors and was developed by Brownell and Sweet,[1] and ^{74}As was the radionuclide used for study of brain tumors and abscesses. Based on this concept, more sophisticated positron imaging systems have been developed at the Massachusetts General Hospital (MGH), Boston.[2,3] Subsequently, positron imaging systems have been developed at Washington University in St. Louis, Donner Laboratory at Berkeley, and at the University of Chicago in collaboration with Searle Radiographics (later acquired by Siemens).

II. DETECTION OF ANNIHILATION RADIATION IN POSITRON IMAGING

Consider two detectors linked in coincidence with a medium of thickness, d, in between. The coincidence system will give a signal only when both the detectors record the arrival of a photon within some finite resolving time. One can show that the sensitivity with which an annihilation event is detected, is constant along the coincidence line. This is unlike conventional radionuclide imaging with gamma cameras where the probability of detection depends upon the distance from the face of the crystal. Assuming two photons escape from a point, the medium thicknesses from this point to the detectors are x and d − x, respectively. The probability of detection of both events is the product of the individual probabilities of detection by each detector;

$$P = e^{-\mu x} \, e^{-\mu(d - x)}$$

$$P = e^{-\mu d}$$

This evidently depends only upon d, the thickness of the medium along the line of coincidence. The medium thickness could be different for different coincidence lines, as in actual organ imaging. Unlike conventional imaging, however, this nonuniformity can be readily measured and a sensitivity correction matrix can be obtained from transmission measurements.

The coincidence signal coming out from the two will depend upon the resolving time (t) and the system dead time (T). The resolving time (t) is proportional to the signal decay time divided by the total light output per pulse. Dead time is the time required in which most of the light collected by the scintillation detector is processed. For sodium iodide NaI(Tl), T is on the order of a 1 μs and t is on the order of 10 to 20 ns.

The coincidence rate (CR) depends upon the annihilation rate (N), the geometric solid angle factor (G), and the efficiency (E).

$$CR = 2N\ (G1E1)(G2E2)$$

The subscripts 1 and 2 refer to crystal 1 or 2. The accidental rate (AR) is given by the following:

$$AR = 2t\ (2GNE)^2$$

where t is the coincidence resolving time. Considering G, N, and E to be equal for both crystals, the accidental to coincidence ratio is given by the following:

$$AR/CR = 4tN$$

The ratio of the accidental to coincidence rate depends upon the source strength and is independent of the detector efficiency. The accidental fraction can be reduced by a smaller coincidence resolving time or by lowering the singles rate.

III. PHYSICAL ASPECTS OF POSITRON IMAGING

A. Gantry and Couch

The mechanical gantry of most of the research and commercially developed instruments consists of an assembly which holds the detector system, head shielding, and septa. The instrument opening is on the order of 55 to 60 cm for whole body and smaller for ring instruments dedicated to brain imaging. Most of the instruments have provisions so that the gantry can be tilted. In some instruments, the detectors ''wobble'' or oscillate over a present distance, which adds to the sampling. The patient couch is similar to those used in diagnostic transmission computerized tomography. Some systems have capabilities for monitoring the position of both couch and gantry with a computer.

B. Lead Shielding and Septa

Lead septa are used between detectors for interplane shielding in multiring detector systems. Lead sides surround the detector systems in between crystals on the ring sides. This reduces the radiation from outside the section under examination.

C. Radiation Detection and Scintillators

The detectors are the heart of the positron camera system. Various types of scintillator materials are used. A detector assembly consists of scintillator, photomultiplier tube, and amplifier. The scintillator converts the annihilation gamma radiation into light while the photomultiplier tube changes the light energy into electrons. Signal gain is provided in the photomultiplier tube and the amplifier.

The scintillators used in positron imaging equipment include: sodium iodide NaI(Tl), barium fluoride (BaF_2), bismuth germanate (BGO), and gadolinium orthosilicate (GSO). BGO is better for slower imaging where sensitivity and resolution linearity are of major interest. BaF_2 is a faster detector and is appropriate for time-of-flight instruments.

D. Resolution

Three types of resolution are of concern in positron imaging: radial, tangential, and axial. The radial resolution is also called in-slice resolution and is best at the center and poorer at the periphery of the field of view. Tangential resolution is measured in-plane tangential to a radial line at different radial distances. This quantity is also the best in the center and poorer at larger distances away from the center. Axial resolution is measured along the axis and depends upon the detector size, interdetector spacing in the axial direction, and the diameter of the detectors. Axial resolution also depends upon the type of collimation in the frame of the detector.

The spatial resolution in any of the three dimensions is defined by full width at half maximum (FWHM). Cho et al.,[4] Phelps et al.,[5] and Derenzo and Budinger[6] have measured FWHM for various positron-emitting radionuclides. The measured values of FWHM for ^{18}F, ^{15}O, and ^{82}Rb were found to be 2.04, 2.98, and 3.38 mm, respectively.[7] These values were obtained from the line spread function (LSF) and represent radial resolution.

An image consists of true counts and some signals resulting from false coincidences. The false coincidence component tends to degrade the image. Major components of the noise in positron imaging are the statistical fluctuation of the recorded events and the scattered photons which may lead to false coincidences. In conventional nuclear medicine imaging, the scattered contribution is controlled by energy discrimination. However, the energy discrimination in positron imaging reduces coincidence sensitivity by a factor of 4 to 25. For this particular reason, some sort of slit or iris collimator is essential to reduce random and scattered coincidence events.

E. Sensitivity

The camera sensitivity depends upon the type of scintillator, scintillator size and resolution with the number of rings or the number of crystals. BGO has 30% higher photon sensitivity than a BaF_2 crystal. The comparison of this factor for different instruments depends upon the design, whether sensitivity is expressed for the straight on slice alone or whether interplane cross coincidence is considered. Some multiring cameras also use the second, third, and possibly the fourth cross-plane coincidence information. The use of such cross-plane coincidences enhances the sensitivity of the cameras employing this technique.

F. Scatter

A low-level window is set so as to achieve reasonable coincidence sensitivity. Compton scattering in the patient increases the scatter component. This component can be reduced with a geometrical design and shields. Scatter is a component which deteriorates image resolution and quantitative positron imaging. Due to the high density and higher relative photo fraction, BGO has less scatter contribution than BaF_2. The scatter reduction is on the order of 20 to 30% in BGO over BaF_2.

G. Attenuation Correction

Positron emission tomography requires a correction for attenuation so that the results can be quantitated. This is accomplished by applying an attenuation correction factor to each scan projection. One method for attenuation correction factors employs measurements of transmission attenuation with an external source. Transmission scan data are collected in a manner similar to that of emission scan data. Workers at UCLA[8] have shown that random noise in transmission measurements can seriously increase the noise level in positron tomography. The noise level can be reduced by filtering; the amount of reduction is limited, however, because excessive filtering will introduce image distortions.[9] In order to obtain low-noise transmission data, one has to increase the scan time, which can lead to distortions due to patient motion. A second method is based on calculations from simple shapes that approximate the attenuation media. Correction factors based on the geometric shape have limitations as no organ can be treated exactly by geometric shapes. A third method, called the boundary method for attenuation correction, has been developed by Huang and coworkers.[9] This technique can provide accurate attenuation correction from transmission images.

In the boundary method, the transmission images are used to provide the key features of attenuation in the region of interest. Transmission data with built-in high noise levels are utilized to reconstruct the transmission image. After this image is smoothed, edge-finding techniques are used to find boundaries between tissues. After boundaries are established, each region is enclosed by a boundary and assigned a uniform attenuation coefficient equal to the average value within that region. Attenuation correction factors for all angular views can be calculated from the quantized image. The boundary method is effective in reducing random noise in transmission measurements; for example, transmission imaging time can be reduced by a factor of 3 to 10 when this method is employed for attenuation correction.

H. Positron-Emitting Radionuclides

The application of positron radionuclides in imaging has been quite limited for a while. Since the mid-1970s a variety of compounds have been labeled with positron emitters. Extensive work has been done with positron imaging in evaluation of a variety of neurological functions. The positron emitting radionuclides which have been in extensive clinical usage are short-lived. Most of these are produced in a cyclotron. Elements such as carbon, nitrogen, oxygen, and fluorine, which make up the biological molecule, are of great interest. The positron-emitting radionuclides of these elements are ^{11}C, ^{13}N, ^{15}O, and ^{18}F; their half-lives are 20, 10, 2, and 110 min, respectively. Short-lived radionuclides are used in precursor-labeled compounds. Numerous workers[10-12] have reviewed the labeling aspects of short-lived radionuclides. These radiotracers do not disturb the structure and metabolism of the compound.

1. Generator-Produced Radionuclides

Some radionuclides with larger half-life are available from a generator system. The most commonly used radionuclide which belongs to this class is ^{68}Ga, obtained from a ^{68}Ge-^{68}Ga generator. Production of ^{68}Ga and generator description are provided by Loc'h and coworkers.[13] ^{68}Ga-radiopharmaceuticals have been used extensively as a bone-seeking agent,[14] in cerebral imaging,[15] and in liver and kidney imaging.[16] Another generator produced positron emitter of interest is ^{82}Rb (half-life 1.25 min), obtained from a ^{82}Sr-^{82}Rb generator. The details of the ^{82}Rb generator are described by Yano and Roth.[17] ^{82}Rb is analogous to ^{38}K for myocardial uptake.

2. Cyclotron-Produced Radionuclides

^{15}O, ^{13}N, ^{11}C, and ^{18}F radionuclides are short half-lived radionuclides produced in a cyclotron by bombardment of accelerated particles on stable compounds. Numerous hospitals have a cyclotron on the premises for clinical use. In 1955, the first cyclotron was installed at Hammersmith Hospital in London for the research and medical use of short-lived radionuclides. Within 10 years after the installation of the first medical cyclotron, Washington University, Mallinckrodt Institute of Radiology, MGH and Sloan-Kettering Cancer Institute acquired a cyclotron for production of positron emitters. In the early 1970s there were less than a dozen cyclotrons in medical institutions, whereas now there are over 50 dedicated cyclotrons all over the world. There are over 24 medical cyclotrons in North America, 20 in Europe, the rest are in Japan, South America, and Saudi Arabia. Different energy cyclotrons are available, the cyclotron energy limits being the production mechanism. In general, protons, deutrons, ^{3}He, or ^{4}He particles are accelerated in the cyclotron. A cyclotron can be a fixed energy or a variable energy machine. Figure 1 shows a Cyclotron Corporation

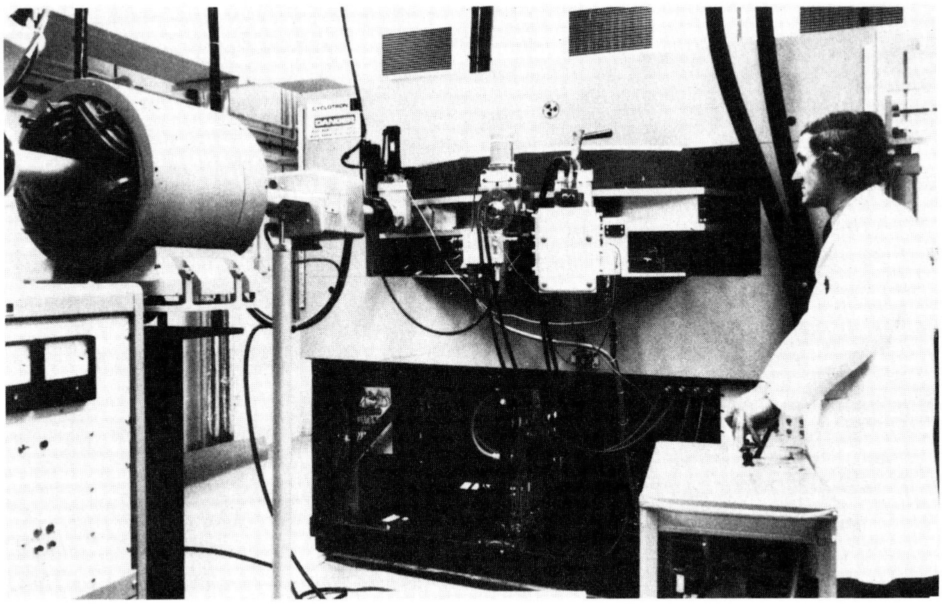

FIGURE 1. Cyclotron Corporation Model CS30 cyclotron installed in a medical facility. (Courtesy of Cyclotron Corporation.)

Model CS30 fixed energy cyclotron, installed in a hospital. A variety of small and large cyclotrons are now available for production of positron emitters. Some small cyclotrons are quite compact and have built in shielding. Large cyclotrons require special shielding considerations.

The production of these short-lived radionuclides has been described by Welch and Ter-Pogossian[18] and Wolf and Jones.[19] Institutions have developed automated production of some of the gaseous radionuclides. In the case of gaseous radionuclides, the target comes in contact with continuous flow of the parent gas. The system can easily be switched from the production of one type to a different type of radionuclide by changing the inlet gas. Similarly, the product will be switched automatically to a different route depending upon the radionuclide and the specific processing. Machine down-time in switching is insignificant. In the 1970s, some of the cyclotrons occasionally required replacement of the target. In some cyclotrons, the target replacement can be performed remotely. Remote handling, automatic switching and automated chemistry procedures help to reduce the radiation exposures to personnel. Radioactive gases can be piped directly into an imaging room or to a radiopharmaceutical processing room. These radionuclides have been used to label a variety of molecules. A few of the organic molecules which have shown clinical importance are described here. ^{11}C,^{18}F-labeled deoxyglucose has been utilized to measure glucose metabolism.[20] Amino acids labeled with ^{11}C, ^{13}N, and ^{18}F have demonstrated use for detection of metabolic abnormalities.[21] ^{11}C-palmitic acid has been extensively used by Sobel et al.[22] for evaluation of remote myocardial infarction. Table 1 provides a summary of nuclear reactions and different products of various biological positron emitters. Daughter products of all the emitters listed in Table 1 are stable and do not disturb the metabolism. Table 2 provides a summary of some of the positron-emitting radiopharmaceuticals used for imaging and physiological study in humans. A review of the clinical application of the positron-emitting radiopharmaceutical is given in a subsequent section of this chapter.

Table 1
POSITRON-EMITTER RADIONUCLIDES AND CHARACTERISTICS

Isotope	^{11}C	^{13}N	^{15}O	^{18}F
Half-life (min)	20.4	9.96	2.07	109.7
Reaction	$^{14}N(p,\alpha)$	$^{12}C(d,n)$ $^{16}O(p,\alpha)$	$^{14}N(d,n)$	$^{20}Ne(d,\alpha)$
Produced form	$^{11}CO_2$ ^{11}CO	$^{13}N_2$	$^{15}O_2$ $C^{15}O_2$ $C^{15}O$	$^{18}F_2$
Daughter	^{11}B	^{13}C	^{15}N	^{18}O

Table 2
SOME POSITRON-EMITTING RADIOPHARMACEUTICALS USED FOR IMAGING AND METABOLIC FUNCTION

Labeled compound	Application
^{11}C Carboxyhemoglobin	Blood volume
^{11}C 2D-deoxyglucose	Glucose metabolism
^{18}F 2D-deoxyglucose	Glucose metabolism
^{13}N ammonia	Perfusion
^{13}N gaseous	Ventillation
^{11}C thymidine	DNA synthesis
^{11}C amino acids	Transport, tumor localization
^{11}C, ^{13}N amino acids	Metabolism, tumor localization
^{11}C glucose	Glucose metabolism
^{11}C palmitic acid	Fatty acid, metabolism
^{15}O Co, CO_2, O_2	Oxygen utilization
^{15}O H_2O, CO	Extra vascular lung water
^{68}Ga adenosinetriphosphate	Brain
^{68}Ga citrate	Bone
^{68}Ga ferric hydroxide	Lung
^{68}Ga albumin microaggregates	Lung
^{68}Ga red cells	Blood pool
^{68}Ga platelets	Thrombus
^{68}Ga colloid	Kidney and spleen

IV. POSITRON CAMERAS

Basically, there are two types of positron-imaging devices. These have either planar arrays or ring arrangement of crystals. Sometimes it is important to view the entire organ in a short temporal study. This aspect is particularly important for the evaluation of rapidly metabolized agents. Besides planar views, these systems can provide multiple transverse sections if the system is capable of rotating around the organ. The MGH positron camera, University of Chicago (Searle) camera, and University of California, San Francisco, multiwire proportional systems are examples of this class of device. Some of the instruments of the planar array and the ring arrangement are reviewed in the following.

A. Planar Positron Imaging System

1. MGH Planar Positron Cameras

It is of historical importance to mention that the first positron scanner was developed at MGH in 1970. This scanner, designed for brain imaging used two rows of nine detectors in each. The image could be electronically focused on parallel planes lying between the two rows of detectors. Subsequently, MGH whole body cameras PCI and PCII were developed using this concept. The PCI camera used 2 banks of 127 NaI(Tl) detectors coded to 72 photomultiplier tubes. The solid angle for each detector is such that the crystal viewed 25 crystals of the opposite bank in coincidence. Each crystal was in coincidence with 25 crystals in the opposite bank. PCI employed a total of 2549 coincidence circuits. Images could be focused electronically on planes lying between and parallel to the detector banks. PCI design, however, required the rotation of the patient.

A modified imaging instrument, PCII,[23] was developed with rotation around the patient. PCII had 2 detector banks with 12 × 12 arrays of 1 × 3.8 cm NaI (Tl) detectors coded to 82 photomultiplier tubes in each bank. Each detector is viewed by two photomultiplier tubes. A coincidence event occurs when two adjacent photomultiplier tubes in each bank record signals. For this system, the radial resolution is 1 cm and the sensitivity per plane is 4500 per μCi/cm^3 in a 20 cm diameter phantom.[22] Emission images are taken with detector banks rotating and translating about the patient. Data are acquired at 30 angles with 6° steps. Imaging time for each angle is 3 s. A transmission image is obtained with an external plane source. From the set of emission or transmission-corrected emission images, 23 images spaced at 1.4 cm or 12 images spaced at 2.8 cm can be obtained. The instrument is linear to within +5% for quantitation of activity. Based on the PCII concept, Cyclotron Corporation has produced a commercial instrument.[24] This system has been studied with shielding to depths of 4, 9, and 14 cm. The scatter to true ratio for these distances was 0.71, 0.39, and 0.22, respectively. Clearly, the scattering contribution becomes smaller as the shielding depth increases. Such rejection is important as far as quantitation is concerned. This instrument has been used extensively for human organ imaging since 1975.

2. Multiwire Proportional Chamber Positron Camera

Similar to the concept of the planar MGH positron system, the University of California, San Francisco, has developed a multiwire proportional chamber positron camera[25] consisting of large area parallel detectors. The sensitive area is 48 × 48 cm. Each planar detector bank consists of two wire chambers coupled to honeycomb lead converters. High energy electrons are liberated from the lead surface location where the incident gamma interacts. The detector chamber is filled with a 70% argon and 30% methane gas mixture and has three grids of wire mesh. The center wire mesh is the anode. When an electron reaches the anode plane, signal multiplication occurs and an induced signal is developed at the two outer grid meshes. The signal location is determined by the time it takes to reach the end of the X, Y delay lines coupled to each mesh. The system has resolution of about 6 mm FWHM for positron annihilation near the center plane. The system sensitivity is 1000 Hz/min/μCi and radial resolution is 7 mm for objects placed in a 15 cm diameter.

B. Positron Crystal Ring Imaging System

A multiple ring system is more suited for simultaneous whole organ imaging and multislice capability. Figure 2 shows a multiring ECAT II scanner developed by Ortec, presently installed at UCLA. This figure shows a patient in the scanner, operator control booth, and display system.

1. University of Stockholm and Scanditronix Positron Camera

A system dedicated for brain imaging has been developed by Scanditronix in collaboration with scientists at the University of Stockholm and the Karolinska Hospital.[26] This device consists of four rings, each containing 12 sector-shaped cassettes. A single cassette has eight radially positioned BGO crystals. Thus, there are a total of 384 crystals which are separated radially by lead. The ring diameter is 48 cm with an aperture of 27 cm. The four-ring system

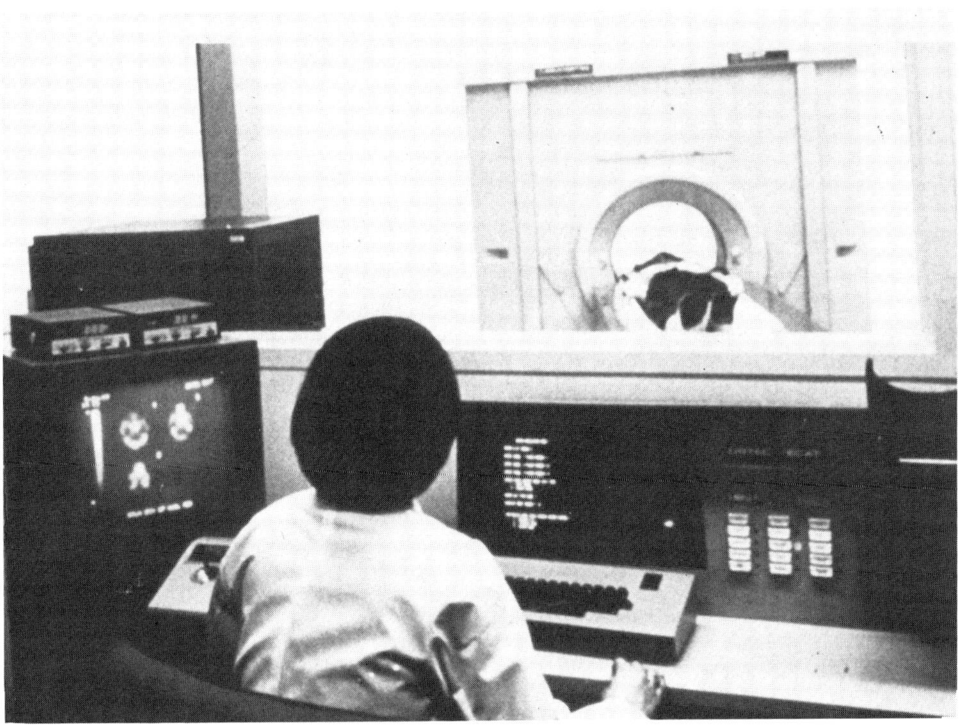

FIGURE 2. ECAT II Positron camera installed at the University of California, Los Angeles. (Courtesy of Computer Technology and Imaging, Inc.)

covers an axial range of 10 cm. Each BGO crystal is mapped by a photomultiplier tube. The signals from the photomultiplier tubes are fed to a discriminator to remove the background noise. Then corresponding coincidence is established. A specific crystal in a ring is coupled in coincidence with a number of crystals on the opposite side of its own ring. Similarly, it is coupled to opposing crystals on other rings. A total of seven transverse sections, four from the rings and three from the in-between rings, is obtained. The coincidence and the single count rate data are simultaneously stored. Random coincidences are calculated from the single count rates of the individual detectors. Considering N_i and N_j are the dead-time corrected single count rates, then for a 2t coincidence time window, the random rate is given by

$$CRij = 2t\ Ni\ Nj$$

A scatter contribution is estimated by fitting the outer channels of the projection data to estimated scatter distributions obtained with a semiempirical method. The calculated scatter contribution and the random contribution are subtracted from the dead-time corrected coincidence counts. The net true coincidence counts are then normalized and attenuation corrected, considering the head to be an ellipse, by the edge-detection algorithm or by use of transmission data. The projections are normalized, filtered and back-projected onto a 128 $\times$ 128 (or 64 $\times$ 64 or 32 $\times$ 33) image matrix. Figure 3 provides brain images taken with this device using ^{68}Ga EDTA. The seven images show the uptake of ^{68}Ga EDTA at the region of an infarction.

2. Washington University, St. Louis, PETT Systems

A series of positron emission transaxial tomography instruments, commonly referred to as PETT systems, has been developed by Ter-Pogossian and co-workers at Washington

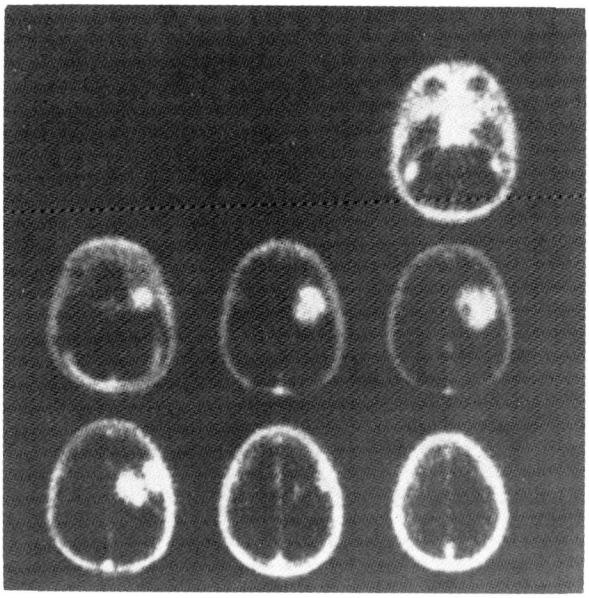

FIGURE 3. Seven transverse section scintigrams of the brain showing ^{68}Ga EDTA uptake in right parietal area of infarction. Images utilized Scanditronix multiring camera at the University of Stockholm. (Courtesy of Scanditronix, Inc.)

University.[27,28] A commercial version of PETT III known as ECAT has been marketed by Ortec.

The ECAT consists of a hexagonal array of 66 NaI(Tl) detectors (3.8 cm diameter × 7.6 cm). Each crystal in each bank is in coincidence channels. Two scanning motions are performed: a short linear axial motion over a 3-cm distance, and gantry rotation through a 5° angle. After each rotation, the linear scanning is repeated in the opposite direction. The crystal ring is also capable of rectilinear scanning so that ECAT can provide simultaneous AP and oblique views. The system rotates through a full angle of 60° and provides a section diameter of 50 cm. The system employs different shields which affect the resolution and sensitivity. Optimal resolution (FWHM) is 0.95 cm and without shields the resolution is 1.85 cm. Minimum scan time is on the order of 10 s per set of slice. For an object having a 20 cm diameter, sensitivity of the system is 29,000 Hz for 1 μCi/cm^3. The Ortec ECAT system has been described more completely by Phelps et al.[28]

Computer Technology and Imaging, Inc. has modified the basic Ortec scanner design. The rectangular detectors are now arranged in a circular geometry of 512 BGO crystals per ring. Commercial systems can have any number of rings ranging from 1 to 4. Each crystal has front and rear side shielding. This shielding limits the solid angle of acceptance by shielding the detectors from radiation originating outside the plane of interest. There are shielding plates in between the rings. Their position can be adjusted to improve the imaging resolution in the axial direction. The reconstructed spatial resolution is 5 mm FWHM, axial resolution varies between 5 to 18 mm. Efficiency for direct counts is 50,000 Hz/s/μCi/ml. The ECAT scanner has been used extensively for human organ imaging at the University of California, Los Angeles. UCLA ECAT II multiring system is shown in Figure 2. Phelps and co-workers[30,31] have extensively studied glucose metabolism with the use of 2-fluoro-2 deoxy-D-glucose (FDG).

3. PETT IV and PETT V

PETT IV, the Washington University camera, is a multislice version of its predecessor

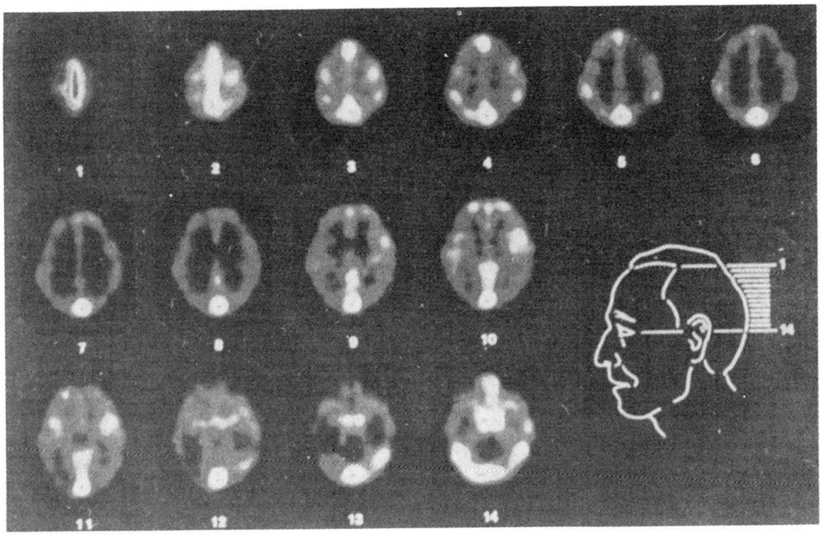

FIGURE 4. Transverse section images showing uptake of ^{15}O carboxyhemoglobin in the brain taken with PETT IV system at Washington University, St. Louis. (Courtesy of Nucleotronix, Inc.)

PETT III. It has six banks of eight crystals each. Each crystal is in coincidence with all crystals of the opposite bank. The crystal is viewed at each end by a phototube. Depending upon the light output in the two phototubes, the computer places the event on one of the four planes. This plane localization is similar to the logic in a conventional Anger camera. The slice thickness is 16 mm FWHM. The resolution of PETT IV depends upon the collimator; the best resolution is 12 mm FWHM. The sensitivity of the system is 47,300 Hz for 1 $\mu Ci/cm^3$ of tissue in a head size object. PETT V, an improvement of PETT IV, has 64 crystals on a ring. The localizing in PETT V in different planes is the same as in PETT IV. Figure 4 shows the image of the brain. These scans were performed with the use of ^{15}O-carboxyhemoglobin and the PETT IV system at the Washington University.

4. PETT, SUPER PETT, and TOF Systems

Nucleotronix is marketing positron imaging systems based on the designs of the systems developed at the Washington University, St. Louis. A variety of systems such as PETT 600 and SUPERPETT 2000 with different rings are available. PETT 600 is a system dedicated for the head. Patient aperture is 29.3 cm diameter and has 4 rings of 72 cesium fluoride crystals. Seven slices can be obtained simultaneously. SUPER PETT 2000 is a whole body and head scanner with a 47 cm diameter aperture. It has 4 rings of 96 cesium fluoride crystals on each ring and the gantry can rotate through + 90°. The SUPER PETT system also utilizes time-of-flight (TOF) for resolution improvement. The first application of TOF was developed by Ter-Pogossian and co-workers.[32,33] Figure 5 shows the SUPER PETT developed by Ter-Pogossian and co-workers at the Washington University. Figure 6 shows the transverse section images of the brain with ^{11}C-carboxyhemoglobin and SUPER PETT TOF system.

There are advantages and disadvantages of TOF positron emission tomography (TOFPET) as compared with the conventional non-TOFPET.[34] In non-TOFPET, the bismuth germanate (BGO) detector has high efficiency and high spatial and temporal resolution; it has low signal-to-noise ratio, however, relative to the TOFPET. The TOFPET can handle high count rate detection and the accidental rates are reduced relative to the non-TOFPET. The efficiency of the detectors in TOFPET is small due to the available sizes. The spatial resolution of the TOFPET systems is limited and can be improved with smaller and efficient crystal-phototube detectors.

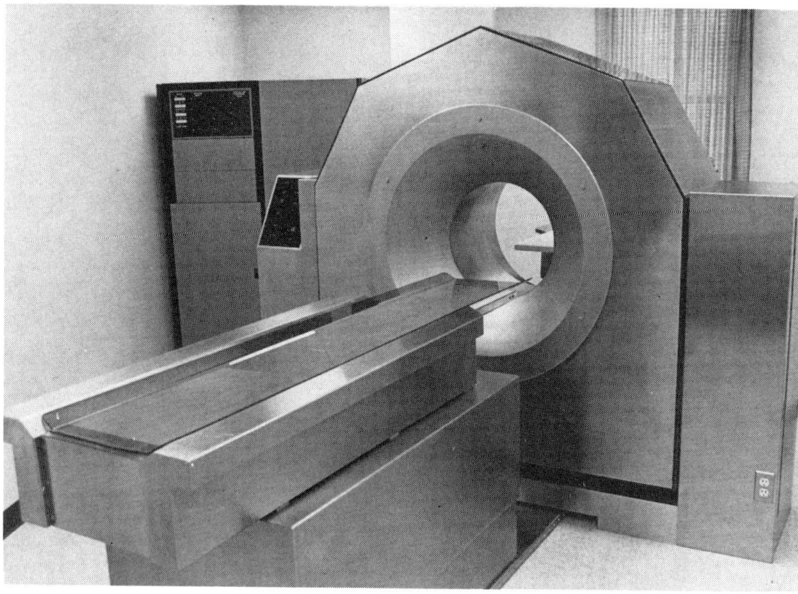

FIGURE 5. SUPER PETT 1 of Washington University, St. Louis. (Courtesy of Michel Ter-Pogossian, St. Louis.)

5. Donner Laboratory Crystal Ring System

Derenzo and co-workers[35] at Donner Laboratory of the University of California at Berkeley have also developed a crystal ring imaging system with 280 NaI crystals. The resolution of the system varies from 8 mm at the center to 11 mm at the radius of 10 cm. The system sensitivity is 10,000 Hz for 400 μCi in a phantom of 20 cm diameter with 1 cm thickness.

6. Posicam Camera

Positron Corporation markets a Posicam Camera, which is a modular system and can incorporate up to a six rings configuration with either barium fluoride (BaF_2) or bismuth germanate (BGO). The barium fluoride detectors can be operated with or without TOF operation for fast dynamic imaging with short-lived tracers such as ^{15}O and ^{82}Ru. The radial resolution of the system varies from 12 to 16 mm depending upon the slice spacing and number of cross-planes coincidence used in reconstruction. Resolution can be further improved to 6 mm when special lead collimators are used. The sensitivity for barium fluoride and BGO is 12,000 Hz and 16,000 Hz/s/μCi/s, respectively. Details of the TOF camera are described by Mullani et al.[36]

C. Imaging System Quality Control

Similar to the single photon emission tomography camera, uniformity and sensitivity correction can be carried out in positron transverse section tomography. The cylindrical phantom described in Chapter 2, consisting of lucite rods and spherical structures, is also used in positron system quality control. The phantom is filled with 2 to 3 mCi of ^{68}Ga. Images similar to Figure 4 (A, B, C) of Chapter 4 are taken to evaluate the uniformity and resolution. Regions of equal area are placed at different locations and the counts in each area are evaluated to express the regional variations in uniformity and sensitivity in the slice. Absolute sensitivity of the system should be evaluated on a routine basis with a known ^{68}Ga point source at the center. Similarly, the pixel size along the transverse section can be calibrated from the distance between two line sources placed in a plane. Spatial resolution is also evaluated from the line spread function of a line source. Full width at half maximum of the line source profile is the resolution limit. Resolution can also be evaluated from the

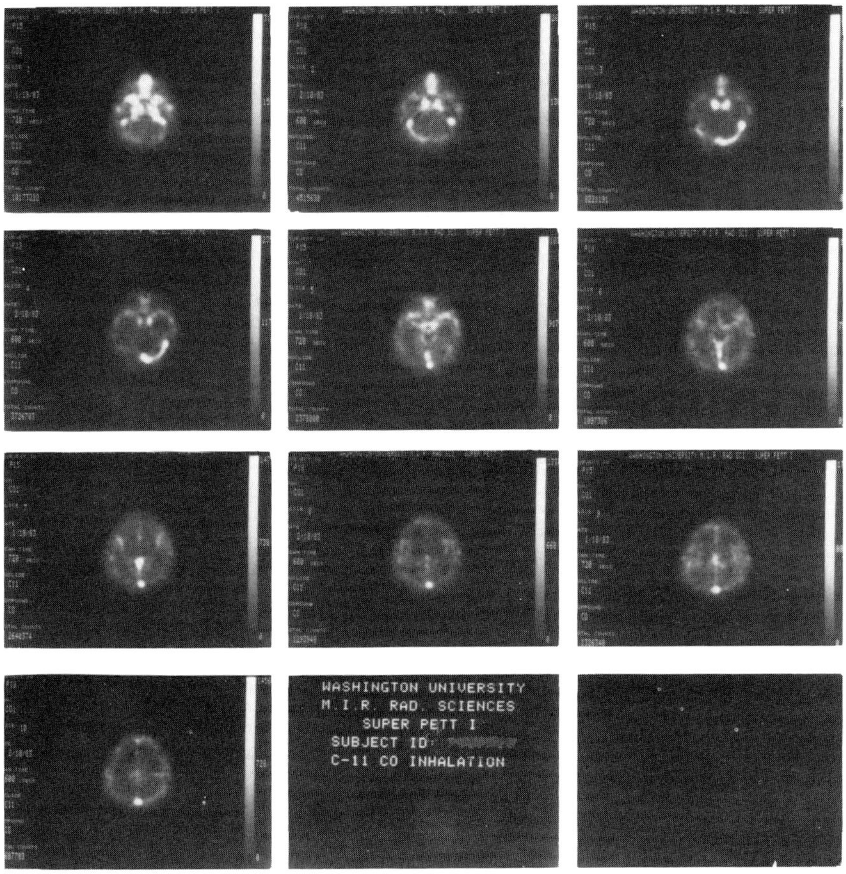

FIGURE 6. Transverse section images showing uptake of ^{11}C carboxyhemoglobin in brain taken with SUPER PETT 1 TOF System. (Courtesy of Michel Ter-Pogossian, Washington University, St. Louis.)

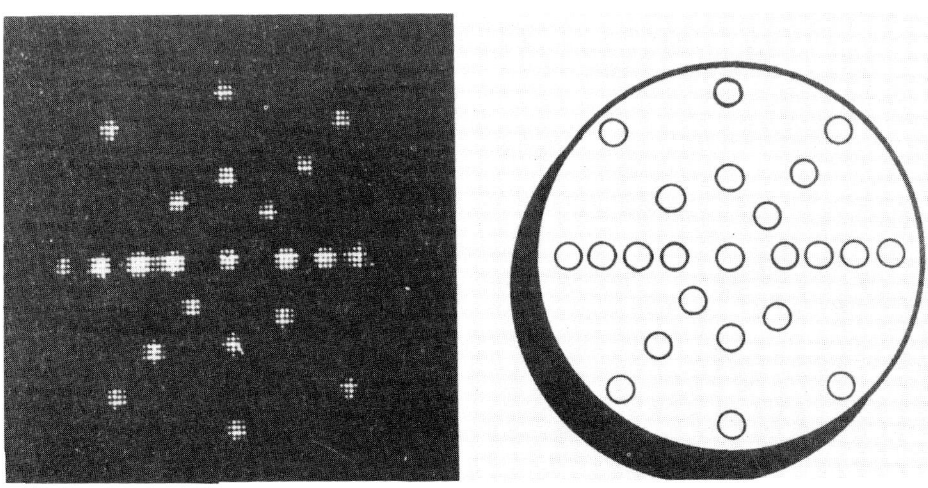

FIGURE 7. Resolution phantom. ^{68}Ga point sources spaced at 2, 3, 4, and 5 cm.

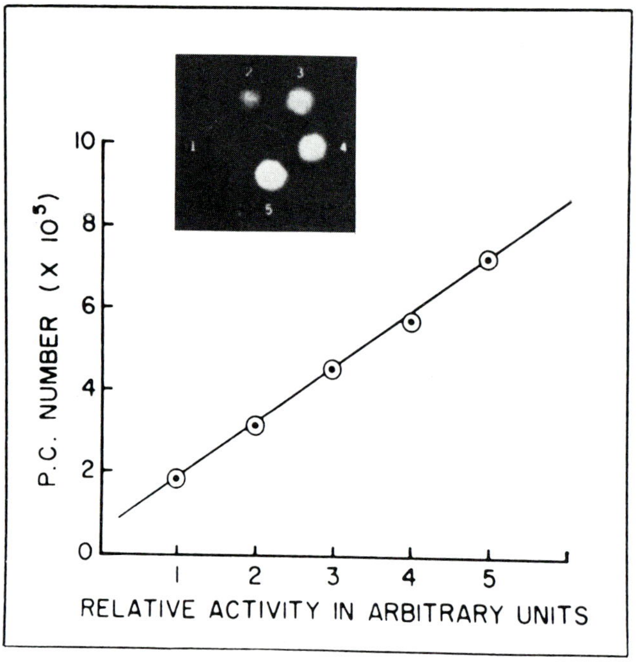

FIGURE 8. Intensity phantom. ^{68}Ga, five concentrations, in disc sources in 20 cm diameter water absorber.

image of the phantom similar to Figure 4 (C) of Chapter 4. Figure 7 shows the transverse section of a resolution phantom with ^{68}Ga point sources spaced at 2, 3, 4, and 5 cm.

System linearity response is very important for quantitation. A test to evaluate the linearity should be performed routinely. Figure 8 shows the transverse section image of a cylindrical phantom filled with water and containing five disc sources of ^{68}Ga. The discs have different concentrations. Figure 8 also gives the relative activity of each disc and corresponding positron image density (P.C.) count number. The straight line signifies the linearity of the system.

V. ORGAN IMAGING APPLICATIONS: BRAIN AND HEART

Positron emitters have been used extensively in pathophysiological studies of the various organs for about the last 15 years. The progress has not been quite constant due to slow developments in the instrumentation for imaging and developments of radiopharmaceuticals. Positron imaging has been credited, however, for noninvasive imaging of the brain and heart for metabolic function studies. A review of the important applications for brain and heart imaging is summarized in the following.

Positron emission tomography imaging has been extensively utilized in study of metabolic brain functions by Reivich,[37,38] Brownell,[39] Phelps,[40-42] Ackerman,[43-45] and Lenzi[46] and other workers at Hammersmith Hospital.[46,47] The most utilized positron emitters for brain function imaging are ^{11}C, ^{15}O, and ^{18}Fl.

For measurement of local cerebral metabolic rate for glucose, ^{18}F-fluorodeoxyglucose (^{18}F-FDG) or ^{11}C-deoxyglucose (^{11}C-DG) is intravenously administered. Glucose and ^{18}F-FDG or ^{11}C-DG compete for, or share a common carrier for transport between plasma and brain tissue. Once transported to the brain, they also compete for a common carrier for transport back from brain to plasma or for hexokinase phosphorylation to the respective hexose-6-phosphatase. The ^{18}F-FDG_6-PO_4 or ^{11}C-DG_6-PO_4, once formed, is fixed or trapped in the tissue and is not metabolized. The regional activity of the tracer is measured with PET imaging. Specific activity of ^{18}F-FDG or ^{11}C-DG in plasma is also measured with time. With the knowledge of rate constants for the transport from plasma to the tissue precursor pool, for the transport back from tissue to plasma, for the phosphorylation of deoxyglucose in the tissue, and the tracer activity, the local regional metabolic rate of the consumption of glucose has been obtained by Phelps and co-workers.[40-42] The ^{18}F-fluorodeoxyglucose imaging has been used for the study of Alzheimer's disease[48] and also by Di Chiro[49] for study of metabolic changes in brain stem and spinal cord.

Regional cerebral blood flow and oxygen utilization has been investigated by Lenzi et al.[46] and Ito et al.[47] Positron emitters as gaseous ^{15}O labeled carbon dioxide and oxygen-labeled ^{15}O were continuously inhaled by subjects and brain images were taken at equilibration. Continuous inhalation of carbon dioxide gas labeled with ^{15}O tracer has been noninvasively used by Ackerman et al.[43-45] to study stroke patients. Tracer activity patterns were observed in areas of ischemic injury.

Positron imaging has been of great value for noninvasive measurements of regional myocardial blood flow, regional myocardial metabolism, and mechanical function. Positron imaging offers the potential for an improved understanding of regional and global pathophysiology. Carbon monoxide labeled with ^{11}C or ^{15}O, or red cells labeled with ^{68}Ga are used as a blood pool imaging agents. Blood flow indicators are ^{68}Ga-labeled microspheres, ^{38}K, ^{81}Ru, ^{82}Ru, or ^{13}N-ammonia. Similarly, the metabolism indicators are ^{11}C-labeled fatty acids (palmitate), $^{18}F_2$-deoxyglucose, or ^{13}N-labeled amino acids (glutamic acid).

Tracer concentration in the tissue can be quantitated. PET underestimates indicator tissue concentrations in structures smaller than the system resolution. ^{13}N ammonia administered intravenously is distributed in proportion to the blood flow and completely clears from the blood into the myocardium where it is trapped. According to Schelbert et al.,[50] the tracer concentration in the myocardium are linearly related to the myocardial blood flow. Except for extreme changes in arterial plasma pH levels, trapping of ^{13}N ammonia in the myocardium is unaffected by changes in metabolic and functional states of the heart. Positron imaging with ^{13}N ammonia may be a possible agent for quantification of regional myocardial blood flow. Beller et al.[51] has validated the use of ^{81}Ru for evaluation of regional myocardial perfusion.

In vivo methods for study of regional myocardial metabolism have been quite unsatisfactory. It is in this area where the positron emission computed tomography has unique potential. ^{11}C palmitate has been used as a myocardial imaging agent[22,52] and for sizing myocardial infarcts in human beings. There is homogeneous uptake of ^{11}C-palmitate in all sections of the heart in normal subjects. In patients who have ischemia, there is an impaired fatty acid uptake and defects in the accumulation of palmitate. One could also distinguish between reversible and irreversible injury. In the case where the injury is reversible, the defect in the palmitate image will disappear, so a sequential palmitate imaging is performed to determine whether the lesion is reversible.

In the use of ^{11}C-palmitate for metabolic rate measurement in animal studies, a bolus of ^{11}C-palmitate was injected into the coronary arteries and time activity curves were obtained. The curve consisted of three monoexponential components. The slope of the first component reflects the washout of the tracer through the coronary venous effluent. The second clearance represents the redistribution and washout of the combined interstitial fluid and the vascular spaces. The last phase is the clearance of the ^{11}C-palmitate and represents the turnover rate of the fatty acid that has been incorporated into the cell. The slope of this clearance is related to the rate of metabolic oxidative activity of the cell or rate of oxidation of the fatty acids released from triglycerides. Thus, one could distinguish areas of the myocardium and their relative metabolic activity. Figure 9 shows the myocardial tomographic images with uptake of ^{11}C-palmitate in a normal patient. These scintigrams have been taken with the SUPER PET 1 system at Washington University.

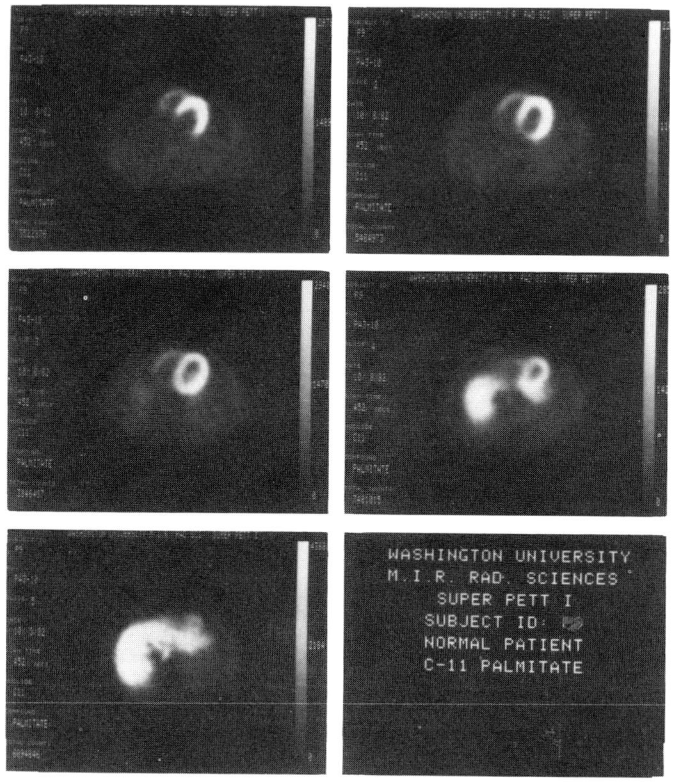

FIGURE 9. Scintigrams showing uptake of ^{11}C-palmitate in a normal subject. (Courtesy of Michel M. Ter-Pogossian, Washington University, St. Louis.)

Measurement of regional glucose utilization rates with ^{18}F-deoxyglucose is similar to the measurements of the brain. FDG is administered intravenously and serial samples of venous blood are drawn. At the steady state, cross sectional images are taken. Plasma levels of glucose and FDG are also measured. Thus, by knowing the rate constants for forward and reverse transport across the capillary and cell membrane, and the rate constants for phosphorylation and dephosphorylation between FDG and FDG_6-PO_4, as in the brain studies, one could calculate the glucose utilization rates of regions of the myocardium.

VI. CONCLUSIONS

Positron emission computed tomography uses unique biological tracers. It has the potential for measurement of blood flow and metabolism. For brain studies it is specific for detection of lesions, evaluation of stroke, epilepsy, Huntington's disease, and dementia. Similarly, it provides specific information of tissue viability, degree of injury, and specific biochemical defects as far as myocardial imaging is concerned.

Studies performed at UCLA, Washington University, MGH, Brookhaven National Laboratory, University of Pennsylvania Hospital, and Memorial Sloan-Kettering Cancer Center provide great evidence, significance of the new contributions, and promise for positron tomography. Small cyclotrons have been introduced in various hospitals and major institutions. There is no doubt that this diagnostic modality is being applied more and is receiving wider recognition.

REFERENCES

1. **Brownell, G. L. and Sweet, W. H.,** Localization of brain tumors with positron emitters, *Nucleonics,* 11, 40, 1953.
2. **Burnham, C. A. and Brownell, G. L.,** A multicrystal positron camera, *IEEE Trans. Nucl. Sci.,* NS-19, 3, 1972.
3. **Brownell, G. L., Burnham, C. A., Ahluwalia, B., Alpert, N. M., Chesler, D. A., Cochavi, S., Correia, J. A., and Deveau, L. A.,** Positron imaging instrumentation, *IEEE Trans. Nucl. Sci.,* NS-24, 914, 1977.
4. **Cho, Z. H., Chan, J. K., Eriksson, L., et al.,** Positron imaging obtained from biomedically important positron emitting radionuclides, *J. Nucl. Med.,* 16, 1174, 1975.
5. **Phelps, M. E., Hoffman, E. J., Huang, S. C., et al.,** Effect of positron range on spatial resolution, *J. Nucl. Med.,* 16, 649, 1975.
6. **Derenzo, S. E. and Budinger, T. F.,** Resolution limit for positron imaging devices, *J. Nucl. Med.,* 16, 491, 1977.
7. **Colombino, P., Fiscella, B., and Trossil, A.,** Study of positronium in water and ice from 20- to 144 degree centigrade by annihilation quantum measurements, *Nuovo Cimento,* 38, 707, 1965.
8. **Huang, S. C., Carson, R. E., Phelps, M. E., et al.,** A boundary method for attenuation correction in positron computed tomography, *J. Nucl. Med.,* 22, 627, 1981.
9. **Huang, S. C., Hoffman, E. J., Phelps, M. E., and Kuhl, D. E.,** Quantitation in positron emission computed tomography, effect of inaccurate attenuation correction, *J. Comput. Assist. Tomogr.,* 3, 804, 1979.
10. **Ferrieri, R. A. and Wolf, A. P.,** The chemistry of positron emitting nucleogenic (hot) atoms with regard to preparation of labeled compounds of practical utility, *Radiochim. Acta,* 34, 69, 1983.
11. **Fowler, J. S. and Wolf, A. P.,** The Synthesis of Carbon-11, Fluorine-18, and Nitrogen-13 Labeled Radiotracers for Biomedical Applications, Nucl. Sci. Ser., NAS-NS-3201, National Academy of Sciences, Washington, D.C., 1982.
12. **Welch, M. J., Kilbourn, M. R., Mathais, C. J., Mintun, M. A., and Raichel, M. E.,** Comparison in animal models of F-18-spiroperdol and F-18-haloperidol: potential agents for imaging the dopamine receptor, *Life Sci.,* 33, 1687, 1983.
13. **Loc'h, C., Maziere, B., and Comar, D.,** A new generator for ionic gallium-68, *J. Nucl. Med.,* 21, 171, 1980.
14. **Dewanjee, M. K., Hnatowich, D. J., and Beh, R.,** New ^{68}Ga labeled skeletal imaging agent for positron scintigraphy, *J. Nucl. Med.,* 19, 1003, 1976.
15. **Hoop, B., Hnatowich, D. J., Brownell, G. L., et al.,** Technics for positron scintigraphy of brain, *J. Nucl. Med.,* 17, 473, 1976.
16. **Schuhmacher, J., Maier-Borst, W., and Wellman, H. N.,** Liver and kidney imaging with Ga-68 labeled dihydro-anthraquinone, *J. Nucl. Med.,* 21, 983, 1980.
17. **Yano, Y. and Roth, E. P.,** An alumina column ^{82}Rb generator, *Int. J. Appl. Rad. Isotopes,* 30, 382, 1979.
18. **Welch, M. J. and Ter-Pogossian, M.,** Preparation of short-lived radioactive gases for medical studies, *Rad. Res.,* 36, 580, 1968.
19. **Wolf, A. P. and Jones, W. B.,** Cyclotrons for biomedical radioisotope production, *Radiat. Chim. Acta,* 34, 1, 1983.
20. **Kuhl, D. E., Phelps, M. E., Kowell, A. P., et al.,** Effects of stroke on local cerebral metabolism and perfusion; mapping by emission computed tomography of ^{18}FDC and ^{13}NH, *Ann. Neurol.,* 8, 47, 1980.
21. **Kirchner, P. T., Ryan, J., Zalutsky, M. R., et al.,** Positron emission tomography for the evaluation of pancreatic disease, *Semin. Nucl. Med.,* 10, 374, 1980.
22. **Sobel, B. E., Weiss, E. S., Welch, M. J., et al.,** Detection of remote myocardial infarction in patients with position-emission transaxial tomography and intravenous C-11-palmitate, *Circulation,* 35, 853, 1977.
23. **Brownell, G. L., Correia, J. A., and Zamenhof, R. G.,** Positron instrumentation in *Recent Advances in Nuclear Medicine,* Vol. 5, Lawrence, J. H. and Budinger, T. F., Eds., Grune & Stratton, New York, 1978, 1.
24. **Carroll, L. R.,** Design and performance characteristics of a production model positron imaging system, *IEEE Trans. Nucl. Sci.,* NS-25, 606, 1978.
25. **Lim, C. B., Chu, D., Kaufman, L., Perez-Mendez, V., et al.,** Initial characterization of a multi-wire proportional chamber position camera, *IEEE Trans.,* NS-22(1), 388, 1975.
26. **Bohm, C., Eriksson, L., Bergstrom, M., et al.,** A computer assisted ring detector positron camera system for reconstruction tomography of brain, *IEEE Trans,* NS-25(1), 624, 1978.
27. **Ter-Pogossian, M. M., Phelps, M. E., Hoffman, E. J., et al.,** A positron emission transaxial tomography for nuclear imaging (PETT), *Radiology,* 114, 89, 1975.

28. **Hoffman, E. J., Phelps, M. E., Mullani, N. A., Higgins, C. S., and Ter-Pogossian, M. M.,** Design and performance characteristics of a whole body transaxial tomography, *J. Nucl. Med.*, 17, 493, 1976.
29. **Phelps, M. E., Hoffman, E. J., Huang, S. C., and Kuhl, D. E.,** ECAT: a new computerized tomographic imaging system for positron-emitting radiopharmaceuticals, *J. Nucl. Med.*, 19, 635, 1978.
30. **Phelps, M. E., Huang, S. C., Hoffman, E. J., Selinc, A., et al.,** Tomographic measurements of local cerebral glucose metabolic rate in humans with (F-18) 2 fluoro-2 deoxy-D-glucose: validation of method, *Ann. Neurol.*, 6, 37, 1979.
31. **Huang, S. C., Phelps, M. E., Hoffman, E. J., et al.,** Noninvasive determination of local cerebral metabolic rate of glucose in man, *Am. J. Physiol.*, 238, E69, 1980.
32. **Mullani, N., Markham, J., and Ter-Pogossian, M.,** Feasibility of time-of-flight reconstruction in positron emission tomography, *J. Nucl. Med.*, 21, 1095, 1980.
33. **Ter-Potossian, M. M., Mullani, N. A., Ficke, D. C., et al.,** Photon time-of-flight-assisted positron emission tomography, *J. Comput. Assist. Tomogr.*, 5, 227, 1981.
34. **Budinger, T. F.,** Time-of-flight positron emission tomography: status relative to conventional PET, *J. Nucl. Med.*, 24, 73, 1982.
35. **Derenzo, S. E.,** Positron ring cameras for emission-computed tomography, *IEEE Trans. Nucl. Sci.*, NS-24(2), 881, 1977.
36. **Mullani, N., Gaeta, J., Yeriam, K., et al.,** Dynamic imaging with high resolution time of flight PET camera TOFPET-I, *IEEE Trans. Nucl. Sci.*, NS-31(1), 609, 1984.
37. **Reivich, M., Alavi, A., Wolf, A., et al.,** Use of 2-deoxy-D-(1-11C) glucose for the determination of local cerebral glucose metabolism in human: variation with and between subjects, *J. Cereb. Blood Flow Metab.*, 2, 307, 1982.
38. **Reivich, M. and Alavi, A.,** Positron emission tomographic studies of local cerebral glucose metabolism in humans in physiological and pathophysiological conditions, *Adv. Metab. Disorders,* 10, 135, 1983.
39. **Brownell, G. L., Ackerman, R. H., Strauss, H. W., et al.,** Preliminary imaging results with 18-F-2-fluoro-2-deoxy-D-glucose, *J. Comput. Assis. Tomogr.*, 4, 473, 1980.
40. **Phelps, M. E., Huang, S. C., Hoffman, E. J., et al.,** Tomographic measurement of cerebral glucose metabolic rate in human with (F-18) 2-fluoro-2-deoxy-D-glucose. Validation of method, *Ann. Neurol.*, 6, 371, 1979.
41. **Phelps, M. E., Huang, S. C., Hoffman, E. J., et al.,** Tomographic measurement of cerebral blood volume with C-11 labelled carboxy-hemoglobin, *J. Nucl. Med.*, 20, 328, 1979.
42. **Phelps, M. E., Mazziotta, J. C., and Huang, S. C.,** Study of cerebral function with positron computed tomography, *J. Cereb. Blood Flow Metab.*, 2, 113, 1982.
43. **Ackerman, R. H., Subramanyam, R., Correia, J. A., et al.,** Positron imaging of cerebral blood flow during continuous inhalation of O-15 carbondioxide, *Stroke,* 11, 45, 1980.
44. **Ackerman, R. H., Correia, J. A., Alpert, N. M., et al.,** Positron imaging in ischaemic stroke disease using compounds labeled with oxygen-15, *Arch. Neurol.*, 38, 537, 1981.
45. **Ackerman, R. H., Alpert, N. M., Correia, J. A., et al.,** Clinical aspects of positron emission tomography (PET), *Radiol. Clin. North Am.*, 20, 9, 1982.
46. **Lenzi, G. L., Frackowiak, R. S. J., and Jones, T.,** Cerebral oxygen metabolism and blood flow in human cerebral ischaemic infarction, *J. Cereb. Blood Flow Metab.*, 2, 321, 1982.
47. **Ito, M., Lammertsma, A. A., Wise, R. J. S., et al.,** Measurement of regional cerebral blood flow and oxygen utilization in patients with cerebral tumors using O-15 and positron emission tomography: analytical technique and preliminary results, *Neuroradiology,* 23, 63, 1982.
48. **Benson, F. D., Kuhl, D. E., Hawkins, R. A., et al.,** The fluorodeoxyglucose 18-F scan in Alzheimer's disease and multi-infarct dementia, *Arch. Neurol.*, 40, 711, 1983.
49. **Di Chiro, G., Oldfield, E., Bairamian, D., et al.,** Metabolic imaging of the brainstem and spinal cord: studies with positron emission tomography using 18-F-2-deoxyglucose in normal and pathological cases, *J. Comput. Assist. Tomogr.*, 7, 937, 1983.
50. **Schelbert, H. R., Phelps, M. E., Hoffman, E., et al.,** Regional myocardial blood flow, metabolism and function assessed noninvasively with positron emission tomography, *Am. J. Cardiol.*, 46, 1269, 1980.
51. **Beller, G. A., Cochavi, S., Smith, T. W., and Brownell, G. L.,** Positron emission tomographic imaging of myocardium with Rb-81, *J. Comput. Assist. Tomogr.*, 6, 341, 1982.
52. **Ter-Pogossian, M. M., Klein, M. S., Markham, J., et al.,** Regional assessment of myocardial metabolic integrity in vivo by positron-emission tomography with C-11 labeled palmitate, *Circulation,* 61, 242, 1980.

Chapter 7

FOCAL PLANE DUAL HEAD LONGITUDINAL TOMOGRAPHY

M. W. Groch, A. Ali, W. D. Erwin, and E. W. Fordham

TABLE OF CONTENTS

I. PHYSICAL ASPECTS OF LONGITUDINAL TOMOGRAPHY

A. Introduction

The purpose of tomography in nuclear medicine is to produce images of the distribution of radioactivity in a target organ at a given depth. Improvement in image contrast in the tomographic plane is achieved by blurring or removing information from outside the plane of interest. Early forms of tomography achieved this improvement in contrast solely by blurring planes above and below a plane of interest, which was visualized in focus. Early scanning devices produced sharp images in only a very thin plane due to a short depth of focus.[1] The amount of blurring achieved for planes outside the plane of interest was severe and although this could be of some advantage when imaging thin organs, these scanners did not provide for large organ imaging. Further, survey scanning, whole-body or otherwise, when the lesion locations in depth are unknown, could not be performed by such scanners. A device to overcome these limitations and suitable for whole-body scanning was developed at Donner Laboratory.

A rectilinear scanning device capable of simultaneously producing images from multiple longitudinal tomographic planes was described by H. O. Anger in 1966.[2] The images produced by this scanner represent a series of planes oriented longitudinally parallel to the long axis of the patient's body. Using Anger's tomographic scanner (ATS), multiple tomographic planes could be read out simultaneously, greatly enhancing the scanning efficiency of the system while providing a suitable method for survey scanning. A commercial version of ATS was produced by a company then known as Searle Radiographics, Inc. (now Siemens Gammasonics, Inc., Des Planes, IL), which was marketed under the trade name Pho/Con™.

Later Siemens Gammasonics, Inc. introduced an improved version of the original Pho/Con model 1792 scanner known as the Pho/Con model 192 (Figure 1).[3-5] The Pho/Con-192 utilizes the basic principle of ATS but has been improved in terms of image performance.

B. Historical Perspectives

After theoretical description by Anger in 1966, the ATS was prototyped at Donner Laboratories and underwent clinical trials.[6-8] The single-detector tomographic scanner built at Donner Laboratories showed clinical promise and a dual-headed version of the ATS was designed and released by Searle Radiographics Incorporated in 1974 (Pho/Con model 1792). Popularity of the system grew through the middle 1970s and an improved version of the ATS was released in December 1979 (Pho/Con model 192). A comparison of the Pho/Con model 1792 and Pho/Con model 192 is provided in Table 1.[9] In essence, the improved tomographic scanner provided increased system spatial resolution and increased system sensitivity by enlarging the crystal size. Also incorporated were improvements in tomoplane separation and plane offset flexibility.

Since 1980, with the increasing popularity of single-photon emission computed tomography (SPECT), the clinical applications for longitudinal tomography imaging have declined, but the ATS still provides a viable method for whole-body survey scanning and is particularly useful for ^{67}Ga imaging. Since most SPECT systems (General Electric-400A, Siemens Orbitor, etc.), utilize light, low-energy gamma camera heads, they are not ideal for conventional ^{67}Ga imaging, nor for gallium-emission computed tomographic imaging. The ATS, by virtue of its three analyzer windows, is able to perform triple-peak ^{67}Ga scanning efficiently, and the ATS is well shielded for high-energy protopeaks.

C. Principles of Longitudinal Tomography

The ATS simultaneously produces 12 images on X-ray film from two detectors with focusing collimators, which scan the area of interest in synchronism. Each image represents a selected plane that is orthogonal to the detector's central axis. Generally, the tomoplanes

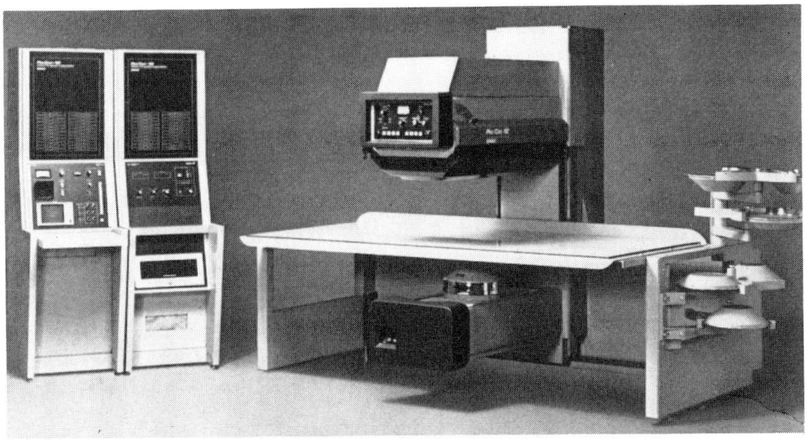

FIGURE 1. The Anger tomographic scanner. (Pho/Con™ model 192, courtesy of Siemens Gammasonics Inc., Des Planes, IL.)

Table 1

Feature	Pho/Con 1792	Pho/Con 192	Advantage
Crystal	1 in. thick	$^1/_2$ in. thick	Increased resolution
Crystal size	8.5 in.	9.25 in.	Increased sensitivity
Photo-Multiplier tubes	7—3 in. tubes	19—2 in. tubes	Increased resolution
Isotope control	4 separate analyzers—2 for each detector	3 analyzers for each detector	Able to perform triple peak studies-^{67}Ga
Isotope control	Each analyzer had to be peaked separately for each detector	11 preset isotope buttons for automatic peaking of both probes at the same time; 1 manual isotope button for any manual setting	Automatic peaking less time involved; peaking more accurate
Window width	5—40% (increments of 5)	1—99%	More variable lower energy isotopes
Speed control	9-preselected settings	Any setting from 65—1065 cm/min	Variable to achieve the highest quality of images
Plane separation	Chart setting dependent on patient size, format, and collimator; settings are 0.2—10.0 cm; cannot be set independently	1.0—4.0 (increments of 0.5)	Can now independently set any separation for any patient and any probe
Plane offset	Dependent on plane separation settings	2, 4, 5, 6, 10, 12, 14 cm	Now variable to compensate for patient size and organ position

are spaced evenly around the collimator's geometrical focal plane, with separation between tomoplanes being adjustable by the user. Emission of γ-rays from each individual tomoplane are sharply focused, and the best resolution is obtained near the focal point of the collimator. Out of plane information is contained in each tomoplane, but is out of focus.

A schematic representation of the longitudinal tomographic scanner is shown in Figure 2. To understand the principle of longitudinal tomographic scanning, consider what happens when a focused collimator (Figure 3) scans through its focal plane. At the focal point, all the collimator holes will receive γ-ray events, flooding the detector. If the number of the events is displayed as an intensity value on X-ray film, the CRT will deposit an intense

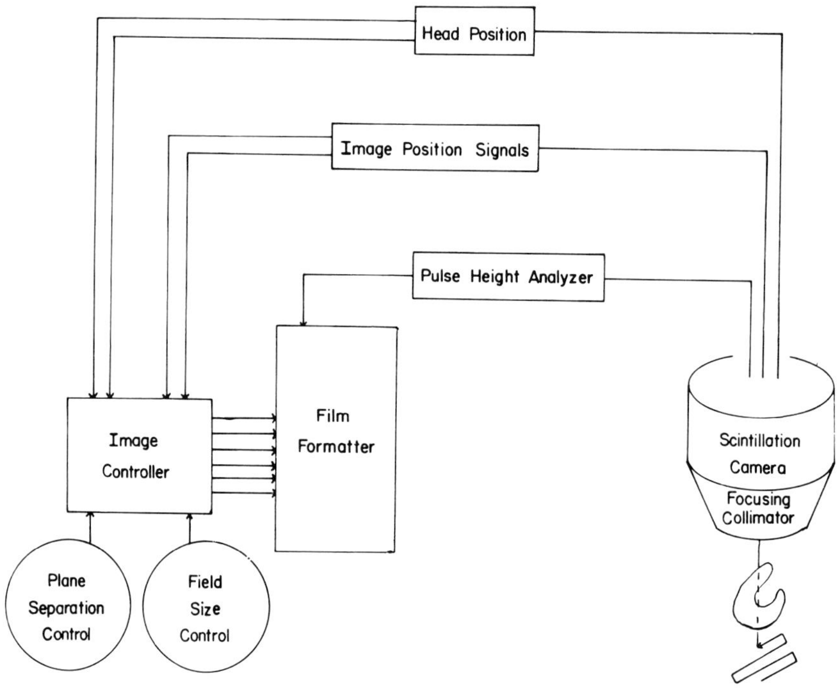

FIGURE 2. Schematic representation of the Anger tomographic scanner showing 3 major signals from the scintillation camera detector: detector head position, camera image position signals, and pulse height analyzers.

pinpoint event at the appropriate x and y scan coordinates of the detector head. Let us consider, for simplicity, a single-detector longitudinal tomographic scanner as depicted in Figure 4. If we again consider scanning through the focal point, events will be detected through all the collimator holes while events emanating from plane A near the face of the detector will be seen by only a fraction of the collimator holes. In plane A, events will be seen first by the leading holes and then by succeeding holes as the detector is scanned. The intensity of the events on the X-ray film will be less than events emanating from the focal plane and will be proportional to the length of time the point in plane A is seen by the detector. Further, events from plane A will appear on the films as a blur, being out of focus for a plane selected through the focal plane of the system.

In order for plane A to be perceived in sharp focus, a method must be devised to keep events in plane A relatively motionless across the detector face. One way to accomplish this is depicted in Figure 4. In this case, the CRT beam is used to register events from multiple planes onto films. Concurrently with the scanning motion, the films representing the focal plane and plane A are moved with appropriate speed to maintain the focal plane events in focus with plane A blurred, and the focal plane events blurred with plane A in focus.

Moving films at different speeds will provide multiple longitudinal tomographic scans with one plane of interest in focus and other planes out of focus, but this is not practical. The identical effect can be achieved by adjusting the dots on the CRT electronically instead of moving the film. In the ATS, a constant mathematical correction is assigned to the y axis for each plane (Figure 5). Using this correction, an event occurring in plane A moving across the collimator is registered at only one point on the film for as long as it appears anywhere in the detector. This provides, in effect, a longer length of exposure and ensures that an image intensity will be recorded in plane A equal to that recorded by focal plane events.

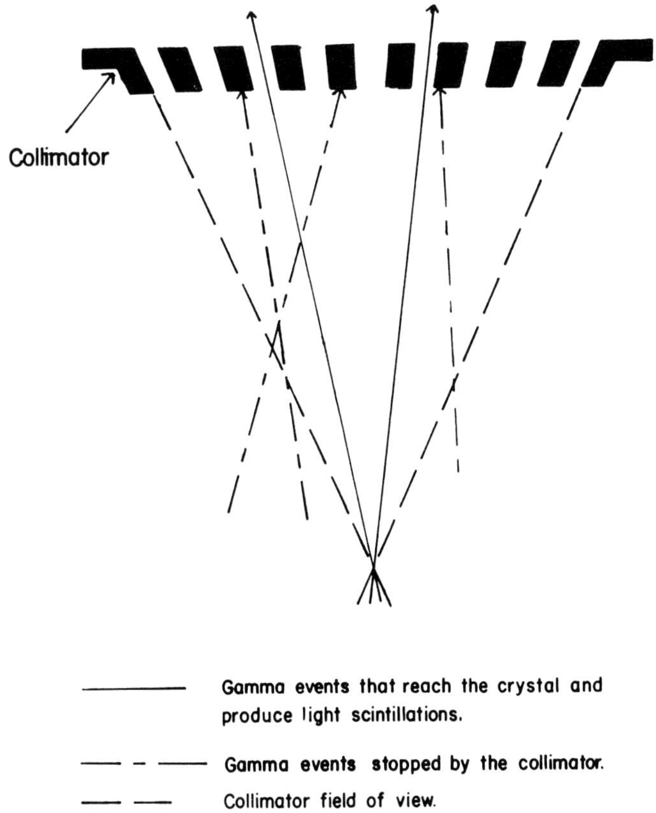

FIGURE 3. Focusing collimator used on the Anger tomographic scanner.

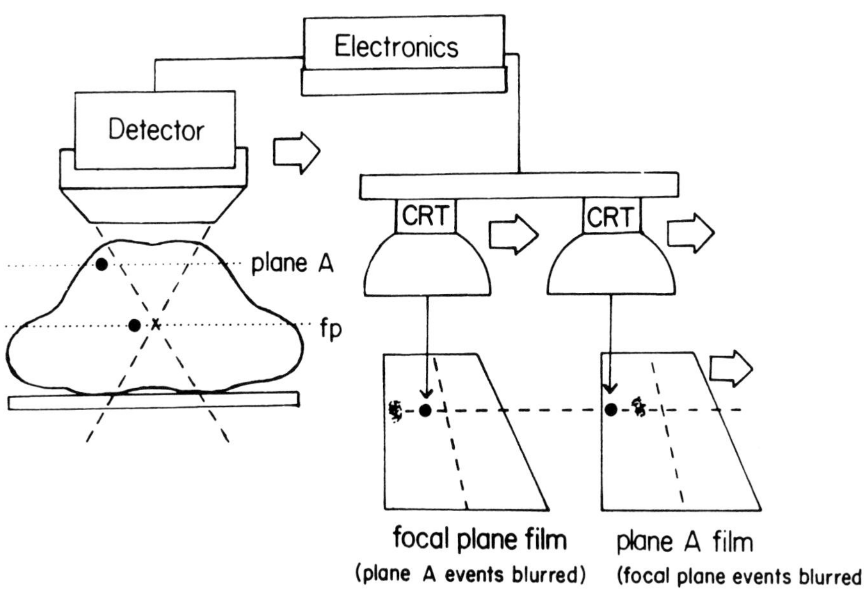

FIGURE 4. Tomographic scanning of the events in the focal plane and events in plane A, above the focal plane (single detector shown for simplicity).

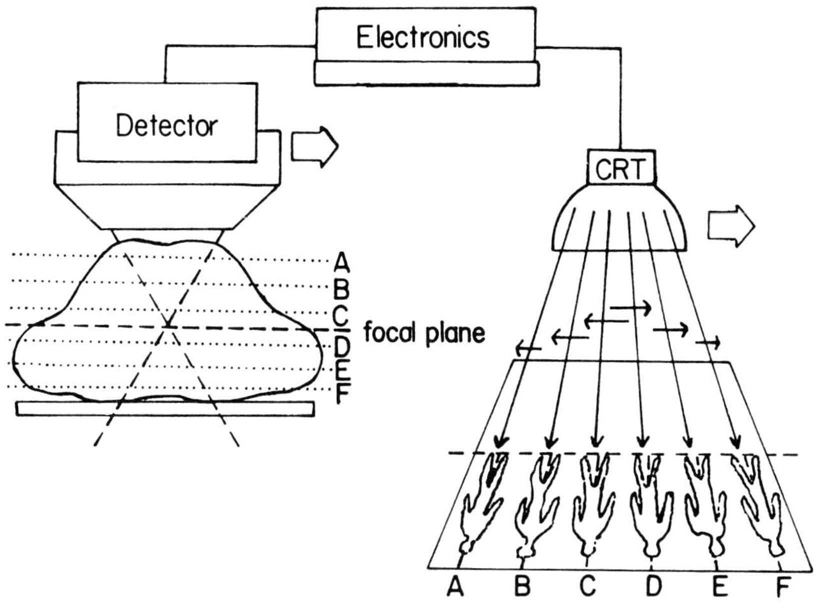

FIGURE 5. Multiple plane readout by electronic corrections of CRT dot position for each tomoplane.

As depicted in Figure 5, several planes can be imaged utilizing this method. Geometrically, events in plane B will move across the collimator face at a faster speed than in plane A, and likewise events in plane C will move faster than in plane B. Unique mathematical corrections are required for each plane, with planes below the focal plane imaged by the same method; the direction of movement, however, and hence the mathematical correction is reversed. In the case shown in Figure 5, six planes (excluding the focal plane) are depicted through the subject being imaged. The commercial ATS, Pho/Con™, utilizes 2 detector heads and 6 planes are selected for each, with 1 detector head imaging the anterior 6 of 12 planes through the patient and the second detector imaging the posterior 6 of the 12 through the patient. In the time it would take to scan 1 tomographic plane, 12 longitudinal tomographic planes are obtained under identical clincial imaging conditions.

D. Electronic Image Reconstruction for Tomoplanes

To maintain good sensitivity and resolution in tomoplanes outside the focal plane of the scanner, each event incident in the detectors is electronically corrected for the particular tomoplane of interest by appropriate electronic X,Y offsets which will reconstruct each tomoplane in a manner analogous to the moving film technique. The γ-ray events detected by the upper and lower detectors of the ATS produce signals which contain data on each event's energy and the position of its image in the scintillation detector. For each point detected in the scintillation cameras, an event is placed in each of the tomoplanes using a correction factor, or offset, appropriate for the tomoplane level relative to the focal point.

The geometry for tomoplane reconstruction is illustrated in Figure 6.[10] Consider a point source in a plane a distance h from an X,Y,Z coordinate system. The focal length of the ATS is given by F, and the detector sits a height H away from the X,Y axis. Xdc and Ydc signals are generated dependent on the coordinate of the X-ray scanning probe as it scans in rectilinear fashion over the patient. The method whereby these Xdc, Ydc coordinates are generated are discussed in detail in the instrumentation section. Next, the position of the γ-ray event within the detector $X\gamma$, $Y\gamma$ is determined. The origin of the second set of coordinates ($X\gamma$, $Y\gamma$) is located at the center of the scintillation camera.

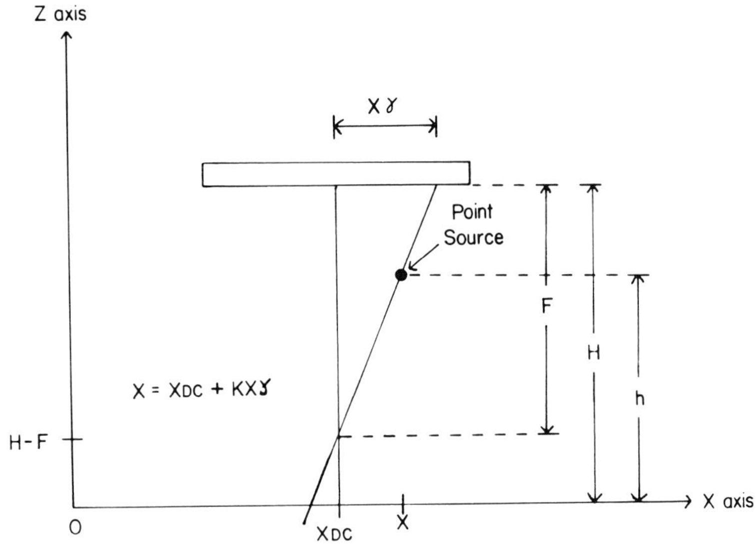

FIGURE 6. Point source image reconstruction geometry. X = the X location of original gamma ray event; Xdc = the X location of the detector's center (from shaft encoder); Xγ = the x location of the detector ray event in the crystal; F = the distance from the crystal to the geometric focal points; H = height above the X, Y plane; (H − F) = height of the geometric focal plane above the X, Y plane; h = height of the plane of interest (tomoplane) from the X, Y plane k = (h − H + F) 1/F derived from geometry of the figure.

As detectors scan the patient, each scintillation event will be stored in each of the tomoplanes produced by the system. The location of each scintillation event (X,Y) is different for each tomoplane, except in the special case where the scintillation occurs exactly in the center of the detector probe, where Xγ and Yγ are equal to zero. The point at which the events are stored in each tomoplane (kth) is given by the following equations:

$$
\begin{aligned}
X &= Xdc + kX\gamma \\
Y &= Ydc + kY\gamma
\end{aligned}
\qquad (1)
$$

where X and Y are coordinates stored in each tomoplane, Xdc, Ydc the detector centers' locations, and Xγ, Yγ are the locations of the scintillation event in the crystal (relative to the crystal center). K is a constant whose value is determined by the tomoplane location, i.e., the distance of the plane from the geometric focal plane of the collimator. The correction factor applied, k, is derived from the geometry of Figure 6. Consider a single point source in a plane sitting a distance h from a fixed coordinate system. By inspection of the geometry in Figure 6 the correction factor can be derived as:

$$k = (h - H + F)/F \qquad (2)$$

The location at which an event is positioned in a particular tomoplane varies as h changes from near the detector to the focal point, and the correction factor becomes negative as the distance of the tomoplane, h, becomes less than H − F (that is, the plane is lower than the focal plane of the collimator). At the focal plane of the collimator, h is equal H − F and the correction factor, k, is equal to 0. Thus, at the focal plane, the location of the event X,Y is simply the location of the detector probe, Xdc, Ydc. For center points in each of the planes at any h, where $X\gamma = Y\gamma = 0$, the coordinate of the event is also the location of the detector probe.

II. INSTRUMENTATION

A. Dual-Headed, Dual Analyzer System

The ATS consists of two sodium iodide detector probes which are, in essence, small-field-of-view Anger cameras. In the latest configuration, $^1/_2$ in. thick sodium iodide crystals are used for the detector probe which has a diameter of $9^1/_4$ in. In the Pho/Con™ model 192, 19 2-in. photomultiplier tubes are utilized; thus the detector is similar to a small-field-of-view gamma camera but has slightly poorer intrinsic spatial resolution than current state of the art cardiac or small-field-of-view gamma cameras, which generally contain 37 photomultiplier tubes and $^1/_4$ in. crystals. Due to the unique principle of the ATS and its collimator characteristics, intrinsic spatial resolution is not as important a factor in image formation as in conventional gamma camera imaging. In fact, although the NEMA specification for intrinsic spatial resolution of the detector heads is 6.0 mm, the effective intrinsic resolution with a low-energy collimator using ^{99m}Tc is 0.0 mm at the geometric focal plane and 2.1 mm at 17.8 cm from the collimator face.[11] The effective intrinsic resolution is excellent due to a large magnification provided by the highly converging collimator. At the geometric focal point, the intrinsic resolution contribution to the system resolution is 0 and only the collimator resolution affects the system resolution.

B. Detector Probe Location Spatial Encoding

The Pho/Con™ uses shaft encoders to determine the location of the detector over the patient (the Xdc, Ydc components). A shaft encoder is a device which produces an output signal each time the shaft rotates through one revolution. The shaft is a worm gear which moves the detector over to the scanning area. Two shaft encoders are required, one for the transverse motion (Xdc-direction) and one for the longitudinal direction (Ydc-direction). For patient scanning, the Ydc-direction is defined as the step location from the patient's head to his feet, and the Xdc-direction is across the patient. The shaft encoders provide information about the position of the probe detectors which is supplied to the CRT display to determine the ultimate X and Y location of the event as previously described.

The outputs of each of the photomultiplier tubes in the detector probes are summed together to produce an output pulse which is proportional to the energy deposited in the detector. The sum pulse is then sent to the pulse height analyzer (PHA), which produces an output pulse only when the energy criteria of the PHA are met. In the latest Pho/Con model, three PHAs are provided for simultaneous triple photopeak detection from both detectors; however, each analyzer can be independently set to incorporate a particular photopeak energy in the window for each individual detector.

The characteristics of the Pho/Con™ are provided in Table 1. Spatial linearity of the system is 3.5% and full-width half-maximum-energy resolution for ^{99m}Technetium is 14%. The system is capable of handling a count rate of 100,000 counts/s (the sum from both detectors) and detector uniformity is $\pm 6\%$.

C. Multiplane Readout

The tomoplane separation in plane offsets can be selected by the user. The plane separation can be selected independently for either probe from 1 to 4 cm, in increments of 0.5 cm. Plane offset from 2 to 14 cm can be selected to encompass the patient or organ size on the study. Figure 7 illustrates the spacing of the tomoplanes between the upper and lower detector probes for 2 cm plane separation for both the lower and upper probes, with an upper probe offset of 2 cm and a lower probe offset of 4 cm. The tomoplane separation depicted in

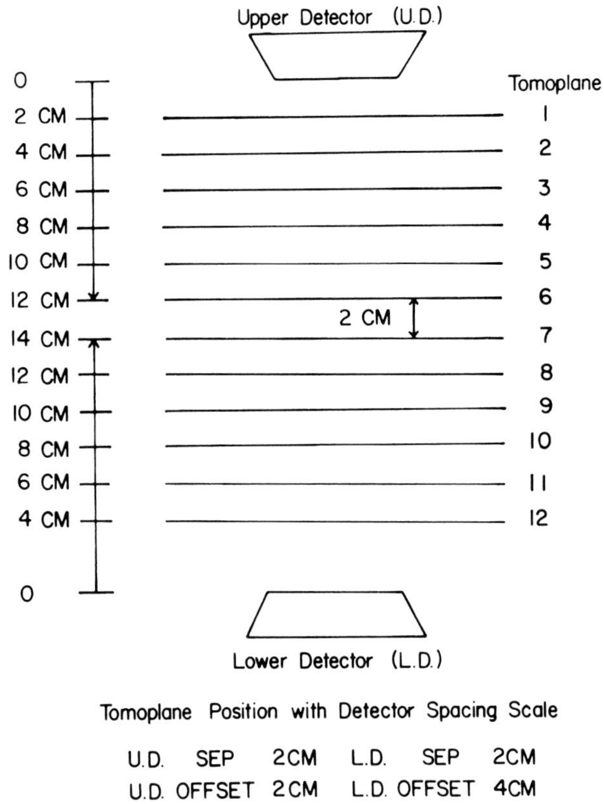

FIGURE 7. Tomoplane separation for uniform, 2 cm plane spacing, 2 cm from the upper detector, and 4 cm from the lower detector.

Figure 7 typically is used when uniform plane separation is required throughout the patient as the lower detector probe is farther from the patient than the upper detector probe. Alternatively, plane separation from the upper detector can be adjusted to provide more closely spaced tomoplanes, while the lower detector plane separation can be set to provide more widely spaced tomoplanes, if the organ under study happens to lie closer to the upper detector probe (more anteriorly).

D. Collimators and Characteristics

The ATS is provided with both low-energy ^{99m}Tc collimators and high-energy ^{67}Ga collimators. Typically, the Pho/Con is supplied with two collimators designed for low photopeak energy, a low-energy all-purpose (LEAP) and a high-resolution collimator. In addition, a medium energy, 300 keV collimator is supplied for ^{67}Ga imaging. A plot of the system resolution vs. distance from collimator face for the low-energy collimators is shown in Figure 8. Figure 8 compares the system resolution from the original Pho/Con model 1792 (Pho/Con I) to the system resolution of the improved Pho/Con model 192 (Pho/Con II). The best overall system resolution is provided by the ultrahigh resolution collimator (not commercially supplied by the manufacturer). Note the difference in shape of the curves between the Pho/Con I and Pho/Con II. The LEAP collimator for the Pho/Con II (-line) is significantly better than the LEAP collimator system resolution (long- and short-lines) for the original Pho/Con model 1792. Also note the more linear change in resolution at depth for the Pho/Con II collimator. The Pho/Con LEAP collimator exhibits a more parabolic shape as this collimator was more highly convergent than the current LEAP and high-resolution Pho/Con collimators.

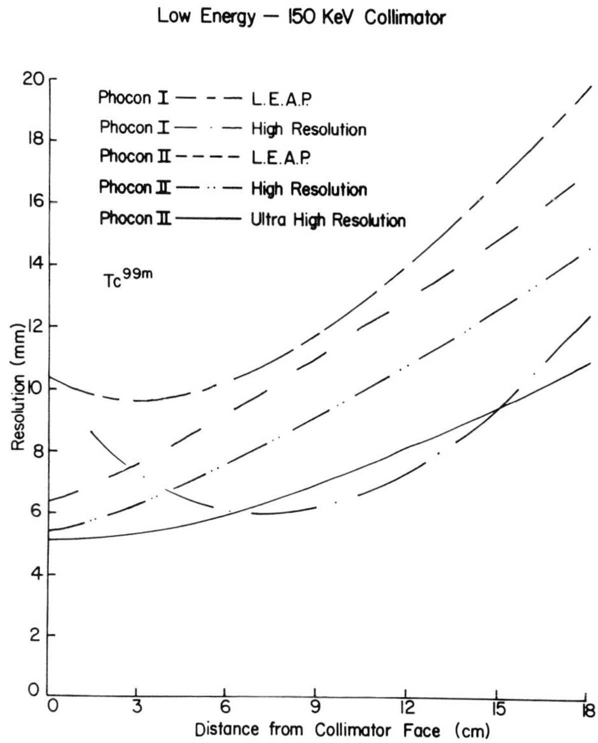

FIGURE 8. System spatial resolution (mm) vs. distance from collimator face (cm) for ^{99m}Tc for various collimators from Pho/Con 1792 (Pho/Con I) and Pho/Con 192 (Pho/Con II).

This effect is particularly noticeable for the high-resolution collimator for the original Pho/Con which had extremely nonlinear resolution response at depth compared with the current high-resolution collimator.

The system resolution for the ATS is approximately 9.0 mm at 10 cm from the collimator face for the high-resolution collimator. The system resolution for the current ATS is comparable to current state of the art gamma cameras operating in a conventional imaging mode, and the images from the ATS are tomographic. At 15 cm from the collimator face, however, the system resolution is approximately 12.5 cm, which is improved over current state of the art Anger gamma cameras. Thus, the ATS offers better resolution at larger patient distances, providing an advantage for whole-body survey imaging or the entire width of the patient is imaged.

A plot of resolution vs. distance from collimator face for the medium energy Ga collimator is shown in Figure 9. These results were obtained using ^{67}Ga imaging only the 184 and 296 keV photopeaks (−) and for data acquired using the 296, 184, and 93 keV photopeaks (− − −). The results for dual- and triple-photopeak acquisition are similar, with slightly better system resolution obtained when three peaks of ^{67}Ga were utilized. Of note is the system resolution at 10 cm using Ga. When the system resolution is compared with Tc, the results are fairly comparable to ^{99m}Tc imaging. That is, a system resolution of approximately 10.0 mm is obtained at 10 cm from the collimator face for ^{67}Ga, comparing well with system resolution obtained at ^{99m}Tc energies (9.0 mm with the high resolution collimator and 11.0 mm obtained with the LEAP collimator for Tc). Thus, the ATS provides excellent ^{67}Ga images and significantly improved system resolution over Ga studies performed using conventional Anger cameras with medium energy collimators. Typically, with medium energy

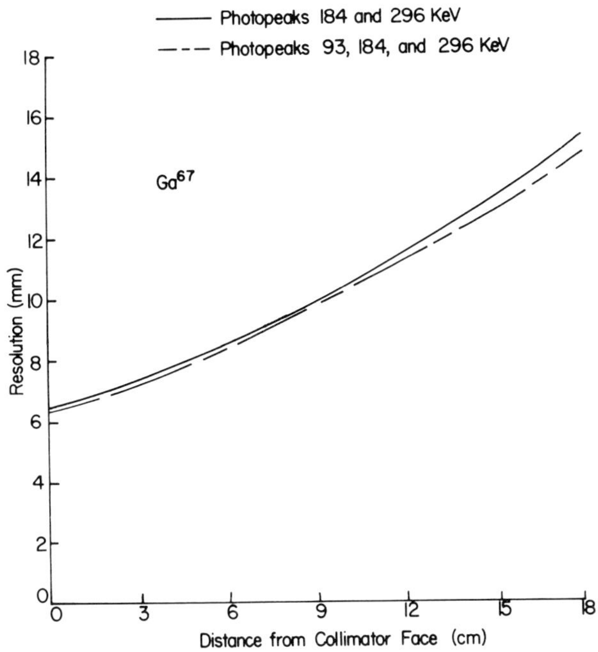

FIGURE 9. System resolution (mm) vs. distance from collimator face (cm) for medium energy (300 keV) collimator from Pho/Con 192 shown for acquisition incorporating 2 photopeaks (184 and 296 keV) and 3 photopeaks (93, 184, and 296 keV).

collimators on an Anger camera, system resolution (Siemens ZLC™) is in the range of 15.0 mm at 10 cm from the collimator. The ATS is well suited for Ga imaging and provides improved image quality over conventional imaging with stationary gamma cameras.

As quoted by Anger,[12] the overall resolving distance R_o can be calculated from the equation:

$$R_o = (R_C^2 + R_P^2 + R_b^2)^{1/2} \tag{3}$$

where R_C is the resolving distance of the central channel of the collimator, R_P is the resolving distance due to the parallax of the collimator channels at a particular readout plane, and R_b is the intrinsic resolving distance of the detector probe referred to the particular readout plane. This relationship indicates that intrinsic resolution of the detector probe is of less importance than the intrinsic resolution of a conventional gamma camera as the collimator itself is the primary factor for the ATS that determines the overall system spatial resolution.

III. QUALITY ASSURANCE

A. System Performance Evaluation

Since the ATS is a relatively complex device incorporating detector scintillation cameras, scanning mechanisms, reconstruction electronics, and image display electronics, the best quality control measure is one that evaluates the overall operation of the system. The best phantom, therefore, to evaluate overall system performance is the so-called "clock phantom." The clock phantom is a paired double-helix of 0.38-mm tubing wound at a slope of approximately 45° over a cylindrical canister of a diameter 128 mm and a height of 180 mm. The clock phantom is centered in the ATS with the center diameter of the phantom aligned accurately to the y axis of the scanner. The offset for the upper and lower detectors is set to 2 cm with a slice separation of 2 cm. The phantom is scanned with a speed adjusted to obtain an adequate image intensity on the film. After acquisition for each plane, the angle of best focus is plotted to obtain the vertical positions of the planes. The resolution observed on the film is noted and compared to previous checks.

To measure the angle for each plane, mark the upper and lower limits of the resolve lines in each image and connect vertically the phantom center points on the film to form the 0° index. Each angle is measured as the angle formed by the 0° index and the upper and lower limits seen on each image. The number of degrees measured for each angle is equal to the number of millimeters of depth from the top of the phantom. The slice width and its position in space can then be calculated.

B. Detector Scintillation Camera Quality Control

Quality control of the detector scintillation head is performed in a manner similar to conventional gamma cameras (as per NEMA standards). Most important is field-flood uniformity, which can be obtained by removal of the ATS collimator and flooding of the detector heads. To perform a proper flood without a collimator, move the upper detector to the upper limit and the lower detector to the lower limit. Place a source of ^{99m}Tc on the table (usually 0.5 mCi) and set the tomograph separation to 10, press the scan control and record a flood.

To evaluate detector uniformity with the collimators, a flood-source activity must be used or an assembly constructed to hold a point source at the focal distance of the collimator. Tomoseparation should be set at 10, slide the protective shroud back, press "SYNC", and activate the scan mode for sufficient time to get a good image set. Note that the scan heads will not move.

Obtaining flood uniformity without the collimator is performed more readily but is less consistent. Flood uniformity obtained with the collimator provides a more consistent image set in flood-field size, and shape can be evaluated. Perhaps the most important quality control check for flood acquisitions is evaluation of tomoplane size and shape. For this, the manufacturer provides a template illustrating the appropriate size of the flood for each tomoplane. Image size should be checked periodically to insure distortion-free scanning. In our experience, we have found that image size changes occur much more frequently than other performance indices. Depending on the age of the scanner, weekly or monthly checks for image size, shape, and uniformity should be performed.

C. Multiple Window Spatial Registration

The procedures outlined for flood uniformity should be evaluated for each analyzer on the ATS. Frequently, correct image size will be obtained for one analyzer, but not for another.

D. Scanning Mechanism

The scan speeds may be checked by timing the scans with a stopwatch and comparing them with a dial setting. The measurement of scan speed in this manner will, of course, give only average speed and would not diagnose scan speed fluctuations.

E. Reconstruction Electronics and Image Display

Reconstruction electronics and image display must be checked as part of the overall system performance, preferably with the clock phantom.

F. System Resolution and Linearity

System resolution and linearity can be obtained by scanning an appropriate phantom as illustrated in Figure 10. Figure 10 illustrates the use of the dual-line phantom, which consists

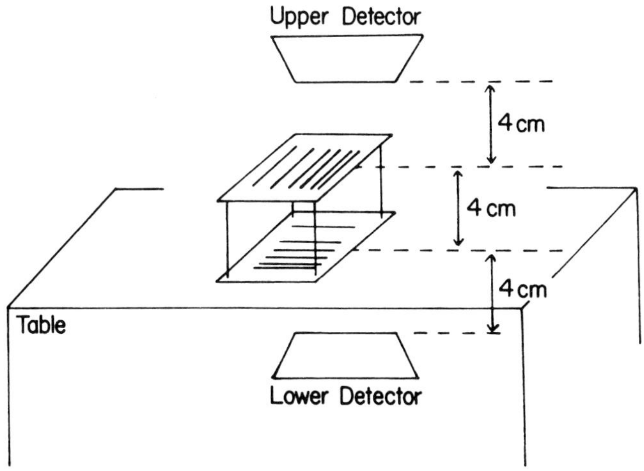

FIGURE 10. Pho/Con phantom for assessment for system spatial resolution and linearity. Lines indicate tubing filled with isotope with intervals of decreasing distance (20 to 3 mm separation).

of two pieces of plexiglass with tubing at intervals of decreasing distance. The upper tube set is perpendicular to the lower set, and line spacing is in a range from 20 to 3 mm. This phantom also demonstrates focal plane definition and directional tomographic capabilities. An example of an image set obtained using this phantom is shown in Figure 11.

IV. NEW INSTRUMENTATION DEVELOPMENTS

A. Focal Plane Scanning for Retrospective Reconstruction

Several investigators have interfaced the ATS to minicomputers. The advantage of computer interfacing is that plane separation and plane thickness can be selected retrospectively rather than prospectively. Retrospective selection allows the operator to: (1) better define tomoplanes over the organ of interest, (2) control image display intensity, and (3) allow for image processing such as, image smoothing, background thresholding, etc. Chang et al.[13] have mathematically defined an algorithm by which out of focus background can be removed from a collection of tomographic planes.

Garcia and Diaz[14] have reported on a method to obtain five improved longitudinal and transverse SPECTs using the ATS. After computer interface, digital images were acquired and recorded on magnetic disks on an event by event basis (list mode). Serial mode acquisition was utilized to create a list of the positional coordinates and the probe which recorded the events. A reconstruction algorithm converted the conventional tomogram, which contained out of focus information from other planes, into a computed tomogram providing a single-slice presentation without the blurring associated with out of focus activity. The method, a form of limited-angle reconstructive techniques, utilized a backprojection method with "cone beam geometry". By choice of an appropriate filter (one calculated to appropriately fit the reconstruction geometry), each scintillation event was filtered as it was received and the result backprojected. This created a deblurred image by cancelling contributions from lines of intersection, in contrast to simple backprojection which is strictly an additive process. The filter decreases out of focus contributions with an increase in contrast as more events are filtered and projected.

This reconstruction method was applied to liver images and ^{99m}Tc-PYP bone scanning. Images could be reconstructed in longitudinal or transverse projections. Garcia reported an increase in contrast in the deblurred images compared to the uncorrected tomographs.

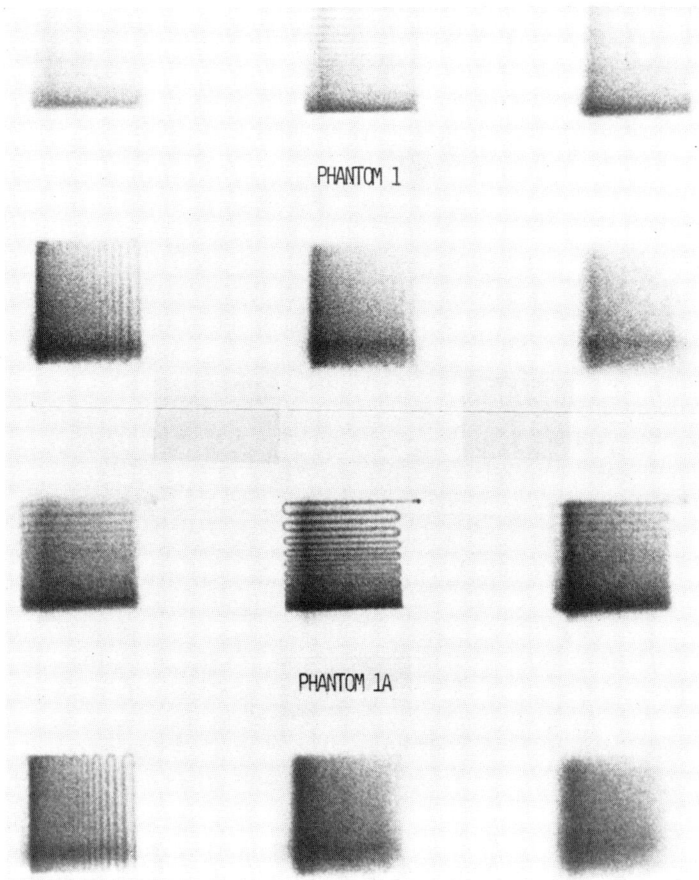

FIGURE 11. Image obtained from phantom shown in Figure 10 using tomoplane spacing similar to Figure 7, but with identical 2 cm offsets from both the upper and lower probes. Phantom 1 images are obtained from the upper detector and phantom 1A images are from the lower detector.

Pickens et al.[15] at Vanderbilt University utilized the method of Chang and compared images reconstructed in longitudinal and transverse sections to conventional multiplane images from the Pho/Con™ model 192. Their results on phantoms, bone scans, and ^{201}Tl myocardial images showed an improvement in image sharpness for the reconstructed sections. The group reported sharpened images in the planes where the distribution of activity actually existed, while removing almost all traces from other planes.

With all the reported techniques, computer reconstruction can improve image quality and does remove a part of the out of plane information. The ATS provides only limited-angle reconstruction and some out of plane information propagates into the plane of interest.

B. Adaptation of the Tomographic System for Positron Imaging

The ATS has been adapted for positron imaging in our institution by Silverstein et al.[16] The ATS was modified for imaging with positron emitters by providing coincidence detection of the positron annihilation radiation. Coincidence electronics was added externally to the system and additions and modifications were made to the internal electronics of the ATS to allow positron data collection by the existing acquisition system. Positron mode or normal, single-photon mode operation is selectable. Positron mode coincidence operations were performed with an advanced coincidence resolving time of 20 ns with coincidence losses of

13%. The system sensitivity was determined to be 3.6 × 10^3 counts/min/μCi with the detectors 60 cm apart for a point source midway between the detectors. A full-width-half-maximum spatial resolution of 1.5 cm is obtained from the point spread function.

A valid positron event consisted of 2 simultaneous events lying within the ATSs 20% PHA centered at 511 keV. The positional signal X_u Y_u and X_l Y_l from the upper and lower detectors, respectively, appears at the inputs to the multiplex control board (Figure 12). This board has been modified to defeat the normal ATS logic and allow an upper-lower event pair to co-exist. Valid events as determined by the PHA for the upper and lower detectors are brought to a timing single-channel analyzer set at 511 keV (with a 20% window). The pulse from the fast coincidence is suitably shaped, delayed, and logically combined from the ATS energy analyzers generating a modified unblank signal. Since the positron event consists of two x,y pairs instead of a single pair from a single-photon event, a second slave-derandomizing buffer was added so that the data enter and leave in synchronization with the master derandomizing buffer used in the system. A schematic of the system is shown in Figure 12.

The output from the modified ATS is presented to a DEC PDP 11/20 computer in list mode format. The positron operation required is a three-word time-independent format. The first word contains digital shaft encoder information giving the position of the detectors, while the second and third words hold the coordinates of the event on the detector. Data analysis was performed by backprojection of the image events onto the desired image planes. Data reconstructed from phantoms indicated a significant improvement in each tomoplane with most out-of-plane information removed.[16]

Positron imaging holds future promise for metabolic and physiologic studies. Adaptation of existing imaging devices for positron scanning can provide a cost effective measure to take advantage of new positron radiopharmaceutical developments without necessitating an outlay of significant amount of funds. The cost of a dedicated positron detection system has been projected to exceed $1,300,000.[17]

V. CLINICAL APPLICATIONS

Since its introduction into the imaging field in 1972, the ATS has proven to be a useful clinical imaging instrument. It is, however, not the instrument of choice for most routine ^{99m}Tc clinical procedures performed in the field of nuclear medicine. The low-energy isotopes such as ^{99m}Tc are handled better by highly efficient and flexible scintillation gamma camera systems with high resolution. In skeletal imaging, for example, some lesions are seen to better advantage by tomographic scanner. The multiple images generated by ATS scanning, however, require more time and a greater degree of attention on the part of the observer in interpretation than those generated by scintillation cameras (Figures 13 to 22). Tomography, however, is very helpful in localizing the exact site and depth of the lesion. The improved resolution of system offers clear advantage over conventional rectilinear scans when high-energy radionuclides are used. We feel that gamma camera (with or without total-body capability) should routinely be the instrument of choice for any scintigraphy using low-energy radioisotopes such as ^{99m}Tc. The scintillation gamma camera system, however, is not as efficient when dealing with high-energy isotopes, primarily due to the thin scintillation crystal and collimators which are not optimized for high-energy isotopes. The tomographic rectilinear scanner can handle the high-energy isotopes extremely well due to the fact that the scintillation crystal is thick, collimators are coarse with thick septas, and appropriate heavy shielding is available to block any scattered photons.

The ATS reconstructs 12 focal planes with excellent spatial resolution maintained from the surface of the collimator to a short distance beyond the focal plane of the collimator. The information about lesion depth that is available from multiple tomographic planes greatly

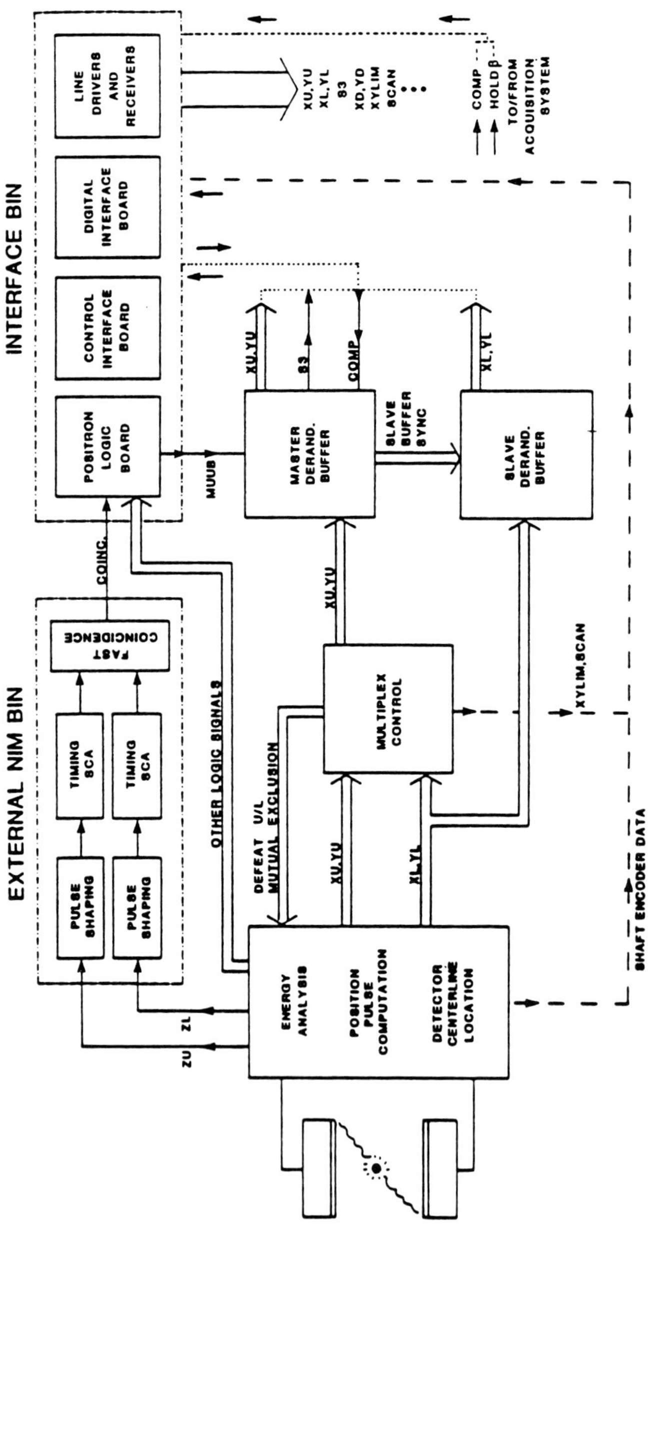

FIGURE 12. Schematic representation of the ATS system modified for positron imaging.

simplifies interpretation of images (Figure 18). The imaging can be performed in total-body or in one of several smaller formats viewing a specific area of the body. We routinely have been using ATS for total-body Ga, I, ^{52}Fe, and In leukocyte imaging. Parathyroid, pancreas, adrenal, and selected cases of radionuclide brain scans also are performed with ATS. The device is relatively inefficient in that it requires over 1 h to visualize head, trunk, upper arms, and thighs; complete imaging of the patient requires more than 2 h.

A. Brain Scanning

In 10 to 15% of cases it is difficult to distinguish foci of activity in bone and/or superficial soft tissues and blood vessels from lesions within the cranial cavity on standard gamma camera scintigrams. Turner et al.[18,19] have shown that ATS images improve observer performance in localizing the depth of lesions and in separating superficial from deep-seated lesions, when compared to the studies performed on a gamma camera. It should be noted, however, that it is rarely possible to see a focus of activity on tomographic images which was not seen also on the gamma camera image in the same projection.

The greater detectability of focal brain lesion with a tomographic scanner comes from the additional information the scanner provides regarding the location of the visualized foci of activity and tomographic display of images. Thus, it is particularly helpful in visualizing lesions obscured by activity in the overlying soft tissues, i.e., posterior fossa and supracellular region. The following illustrations will be helpful in understanding the importance of tomographic scanners in radionuclide brain imaging (Figures 13 to 15).

B. Scanning with ^{67}Ga, ^{52}Fe, ^{123}I, ^{131}I, and ^{111}In

Despite its nonspecificity, ^{67}Ga scintigraphy is a useful tool in the study of patients suspected of having occult site of infection or certain tumors. The detectability of sites of malignant lymphoma by ^{67}Ga is substantially better when the scans are performed with ATS than when performed with dual-probe rectilinear scan or most gamma cameras.[20] In Ga scintigraphy, the count density of the images can be improved by selecting more than one photopeaks and administering larger doses of ^{67}Ga (7 to 10 mCi) in patients with proven malignancy. Examples are shown (Figure 16) which highlight the importance of selecting more than one peak and the differences between low (3 mCi) and high dose (10 mCi) Ga scans done in the same patient. Beckerman et al.[21] reported the ATS to be the decisive choice for ^{67}Ga-citrate imaging of the lung. An ATS Ga scan is illustrated in Figure 17.

The ATS was compared with Ga-citrate imaging of the lung by conventional Anger camera and found to be superior to the gamma camera, with lateral views necessary when conventional gamma camera imaging was performed.

Hauser and Alderson[22] reported excellent results using the ATS for ^{67}Ga scans for intraabdominal inflammations, including subphrenic abscesses, post-op infections, pyelonephritis, or perinephric abscesses for peritonitis. The thickness of the abdomen and normal ^{67}Ga average structures, especially the colon, frequently make conventional Ga images difficult to interpret, whereas tomoscanning can provide information about the depth of the lesion (see Figure 18). These researchers reported that of 51 patients, 35 patients had equivalent results when comparing the ATS to the gamma camera, whereas 2 patients had lesions which were seen better by the gamma camera. In contrast, 12 patients had lesions that were seen better by the ATS and in 2 patients the lesion was seen only by the ATS. The overall sensitivity of Ga imaging was 87% with a 95% specificity vs. 73% sensitivity with 95% specificity for ultrasound.

Hauser and Gottschalk[23] compared the ATS and a large-field-of-view scintillation camera for Ga imaging. They studied 51 patients in which the ATS was preferred in 49% of the cases while the gamma camera was preferred in only 12% of the patients. Of the results, 39% were equivalent. They cited several theoretical advantages of the ATS over conventional

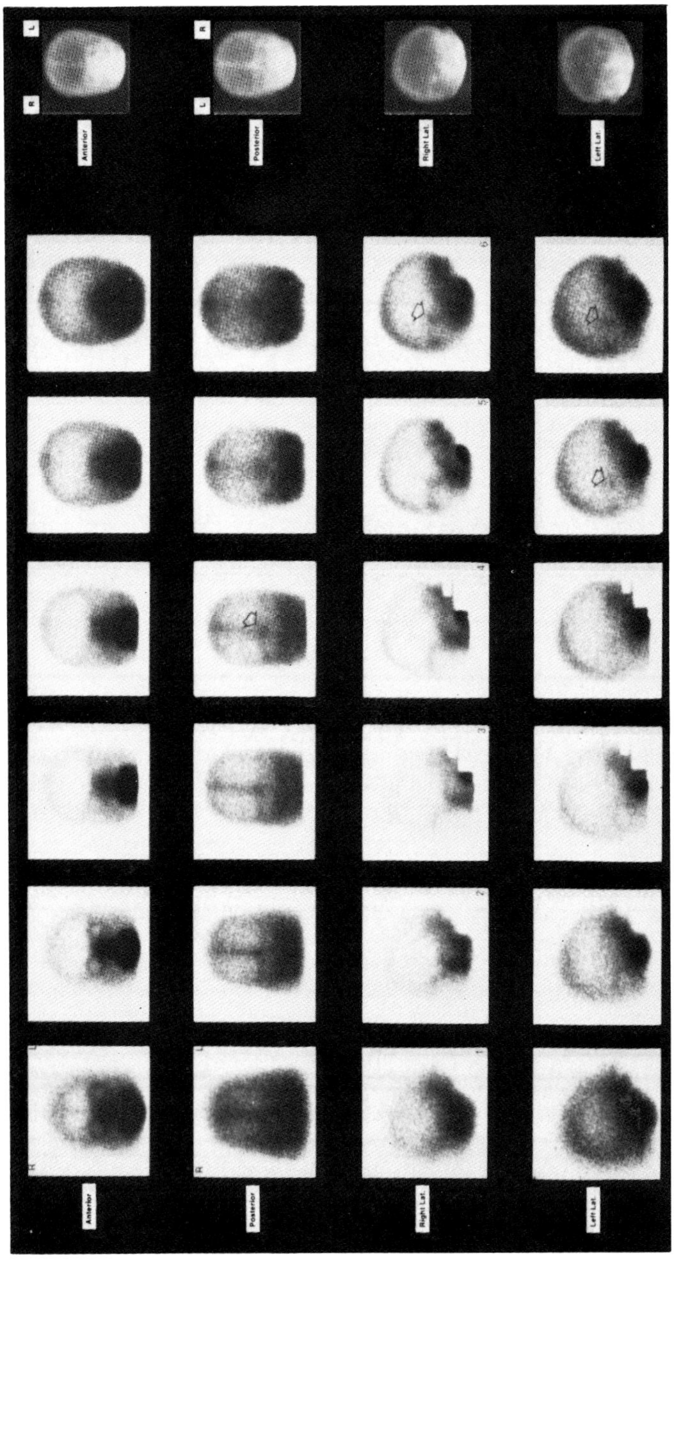

FIGURE 13. Note a lesion (arrows) in deep planes of right lateral and posterior tomographic images unobscured by dural sinuses. The gamma camera images demonstrate a prominent Torucula Herophili. Both camera and tomographic images were performed on the same day.

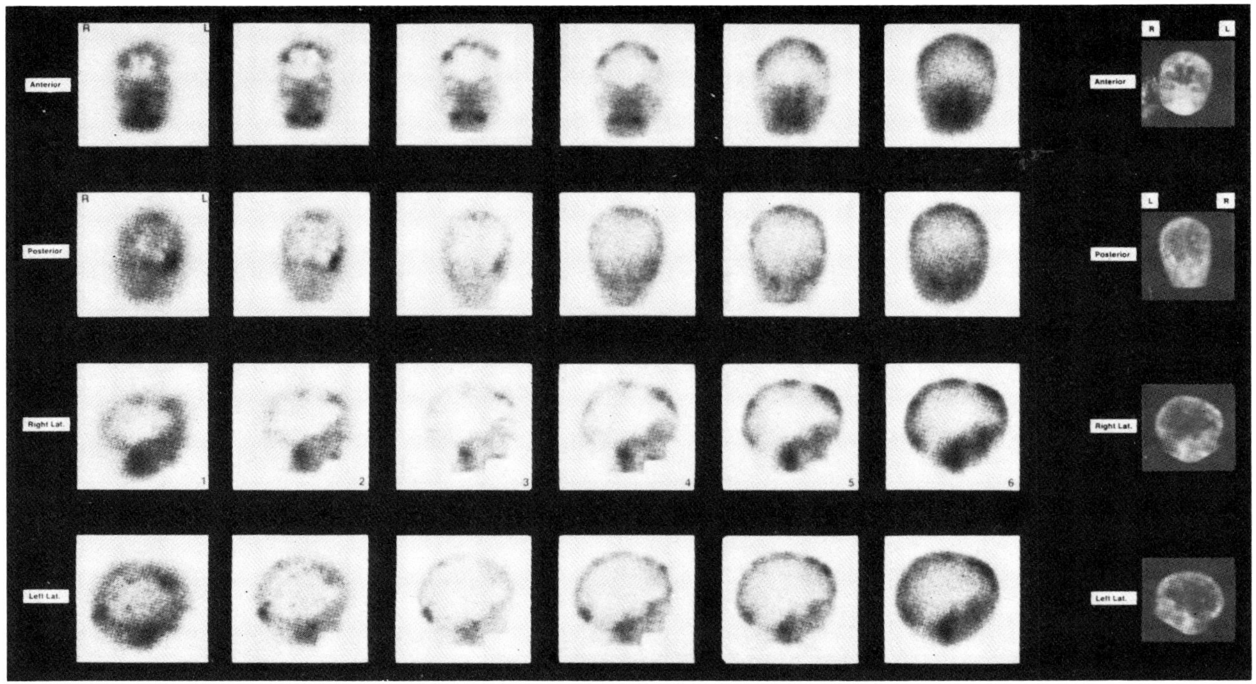

FIGURE 14. Anterior and right lateral tomographic images demonstrate multiple skull lesions. No intracerebral lesions are seen. It is impossible to exclude intracerebral abnormality on camera images.

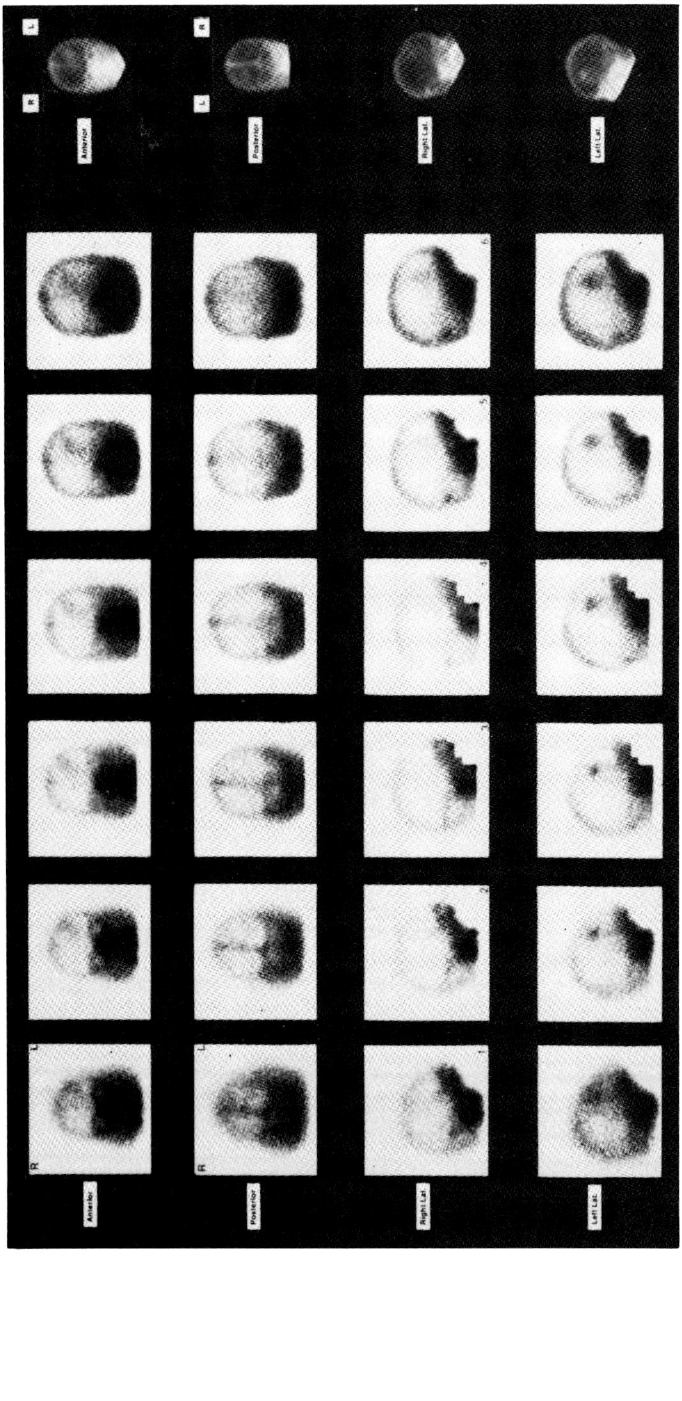

FIGURE 15. A lesion is clearly demonstrated on camera and tomographic images in left frontal lobe. Note depth of lesion is better appreciated on anterior and left lateral tomographic images.

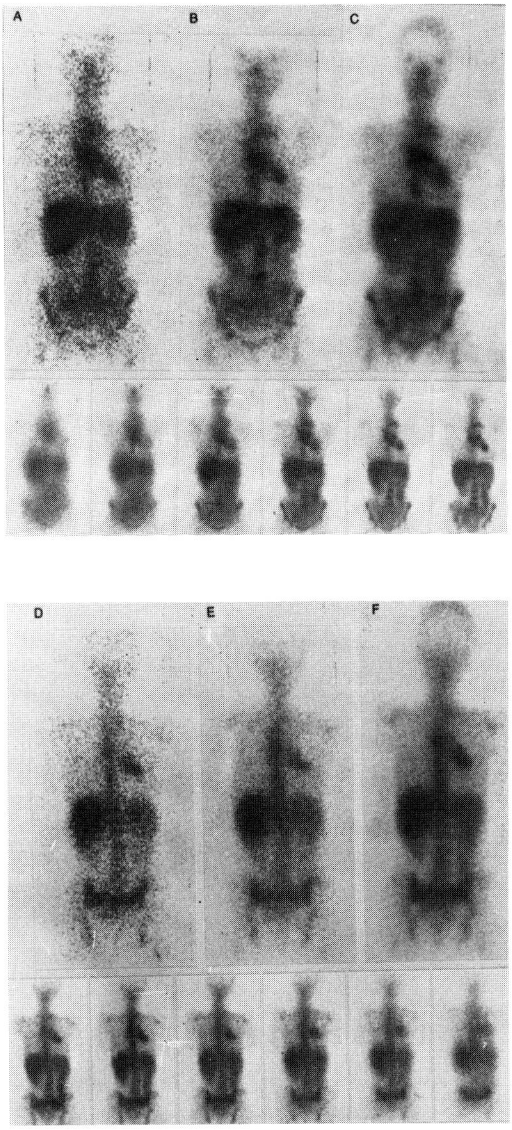

FIGURE 16. All the scans shown in this illustration are of the same patient, a young woman with Hodgkin's disease (nodular sclerosing type). Images A through F were performed on dual probe rectilinear scanner. Images A and D were obtained following intravenous injection of 3 mCi of Ga-citrate and using a single photopeak (184 keV). A single 250 keV integral "window" encompassing 184, 296, and 388 keV photopeaks was used for images B and E. Images C and F were done following injection of 10 mCi of Ga-citrate, using the same pulse height window as Figure B and E. Note improvement in count density when more than one photopeak is used (B and E). Further improvement in image quality is seen when 10 mCi of Ga were injected (C and F). The bottom row images were made on Anger multiplane tomographic scanner which reconstructs focal planes at 12 levels. Note that masses in left supraclavicular fossa and mediastinum are seen more discretely when compared to images obtained on rectilinear scanner (A through F). This shows improved spatial resolution of tomographic system.

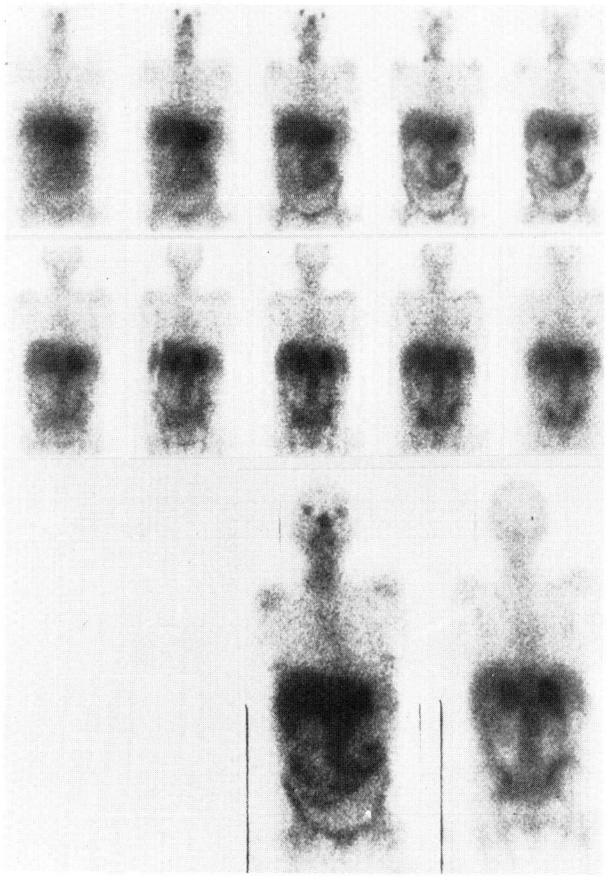

FIGURE 17. This 48-year-old female with a history of oat cell CA of the lung was treated with chemotherapy and radiation therapy over a few months. She was admitted for an evaluation of an ill-defined mass in the left upper quadrant of her abdomen. The rectilinear and tomographic images were performed on the same day. The tomographic images demonstrate lesions in right supraclavicular fossa, left upper quadrant of the abdomen anteriorly (seen in best focus on fourth anterior plane), and both adrenal glands. Note the clear separation of left adrenal gland lesion from the lesion in the left upper quadrant of the abdomen. It is almost impossible to separate these two lesions on rectilinear images. Moreover, the right neck lesion is not seen as clearly on rectilinear images. This case demonstrates the distinct advantage of tomographic scanners over conventional rectilinear scanners in defining the depth and location of the lesions.

gamma camera imaging: (1) the ATS enabled the delineation of deep structures despite the intervening superficial activity; (2) the ATS provided more precise localization of both normal and diseased structures; and (3) they reported an increased lesion detectability since the contrast is improved over a wide range of depths.

Imaging of erythropoietic marrow is accomplished most successfully with the use of ^{52}Fe. The physical characteristics of ^{52}Fe, however, are far from ideal. A special modification must be applied to make use of positron emission and to avoid a myriad of high-energy photons from associated contaminants, e.g., ^{55}Fe and other products. Although images of excellent resolution and information density can be obtained by using positron cameras, these devices are not readily available on a wide scale. Images of good quality have been obtained on the ATS. A lead shield placed around the interface between the collimator and

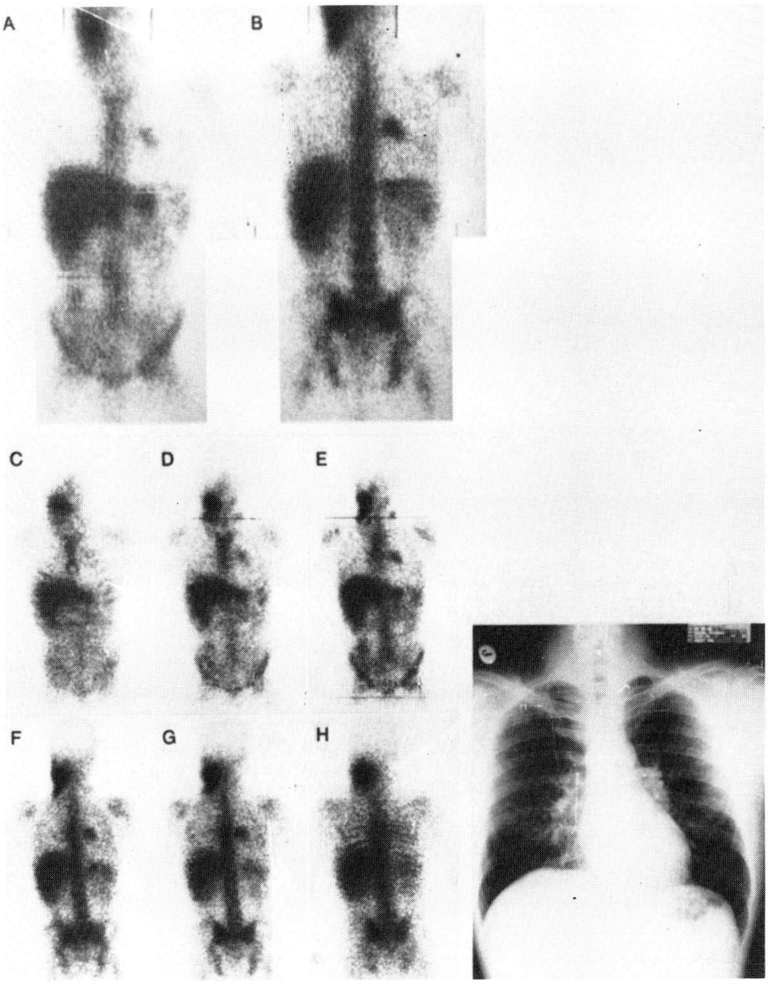

FIGURE 18. The depth information available from tomographic plane scans greatly simplify the interpretation of Ga images. There is the suggestion of a lesion in the lateral aspect of the left lobe of the liver on conventional rectilinear scans. This lesion is seen on a deep anterior plane (E) on tomographic images. This would place this lesion anterior to the spine in the retroperitoneal region and certainly not in the liver. The improved resolution of the system is again demonstrated by the clear visualization of a lesion in left supraclavicular fossa which is barely seen on the rectilinear images. Also note the excellent visualization of sternum and anterior ribs in plane C and posterior aspect of the ribs in plane H.

the detector housing would preclude any leakage or entry of scattered photons, which produces obvious improvement in the image contrast. A relatively inexpensive modification of the commercially available ATS with coincidence circuitry permits the more efficient use of positron emission, eliminating the need for efficiency-reducing collimation except for peripheral baffle. Initial testing of this device is extremely encouraging, and suggests that image quality can be increased sharply, while the administered dose can be lowered by one order of magnitude with a concomitant proportional reduction in radiation dose and subsequent related economic burden to the patient.

An ^{123}I whole body using the ATS is illustrated in Figure 19. Although ^{123}I can be used for imaging, it is currently expensive and can be difficult to obtain. ^{131}I is extremely useful in management of patients with papillary and/or follicular carcinoma of the thyroid gland.

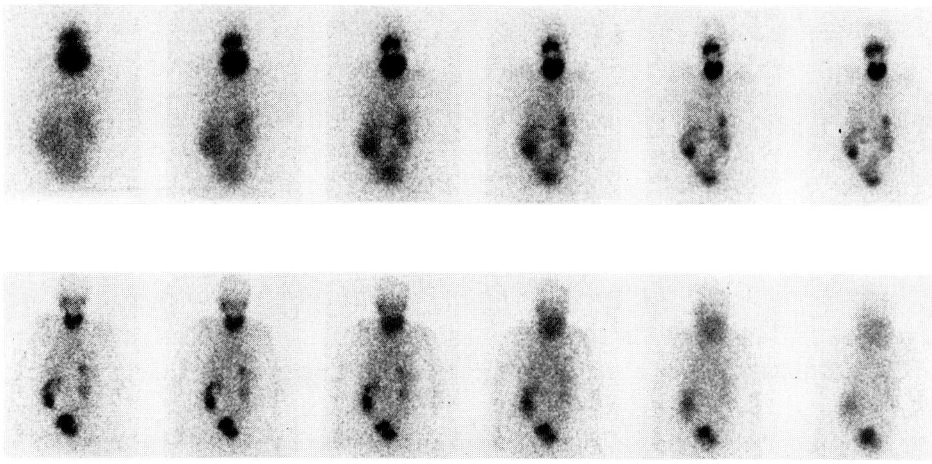

FIGURE 19. Total body ^{123}I scan in a patient who underwent partial thyroidectomy for follicular carcinoma of the thyroid gland several years ago. Patient was given 1 mCi of ^{123}I orally and the scan was obtained 24 h later.

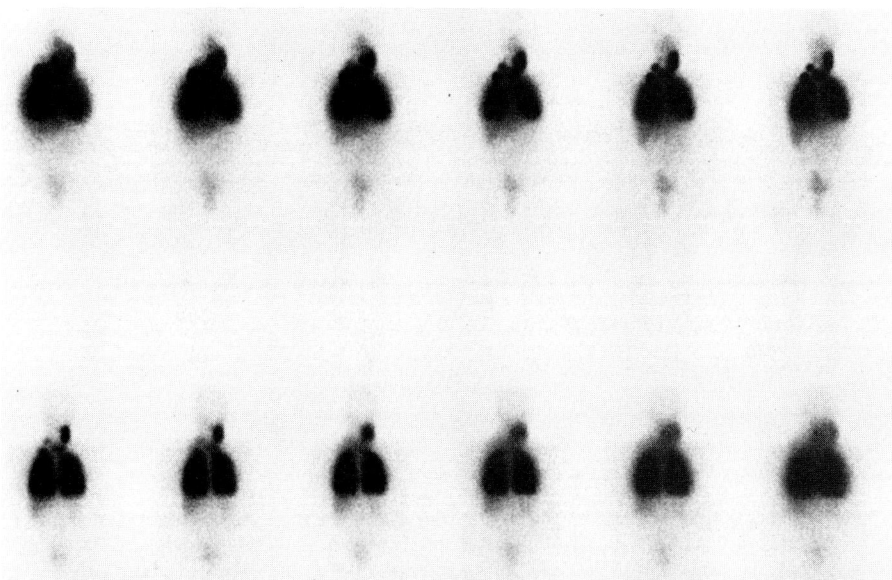

FIGURE 20. This 25-year-old male received 150 mCi of ^{131}I treatment of metastatic follicular and papillary carcinoma of the thyroid. The total body scan was obtained 10 d posttherapy. Note discrete lesions in anterior neck and diffuse increased uptake in both lungs.

It is used routinely in detecting sites of functioning metastatic thyroid tumor. We find ATS to be the instrument of choice for total-body imaging of patients who have received ^{131}I for diagnostic or therapeutic purposes. The main advantage of ATS is, again, its ability to handle efficiently the high-energy photons of this isotope. Examples are given in Figures 20 and 21.

^{111}In leukocyte imaging has now become very popular in detection of acutc infcctions (Figure 22). The energies of ^{111}In (173 and 247 KeV) can be handled by a gamma camera with a medium-energy collimator. We have found the total-body imaging using ATS to be more helpful since it allows the assessment of lesion depth and the location of the lesion with greater degree of confidence (Figure 23).

FIGURE 21. Note marked improvement in the lesions (Figure 20). This scan was obtained 1 year post-^{131}I therapy. Patient was given 10 mCi of ^{131}I orally and the scan was obtained 96 h later. Residual disease is noted in the left side of the neck anteriorly.

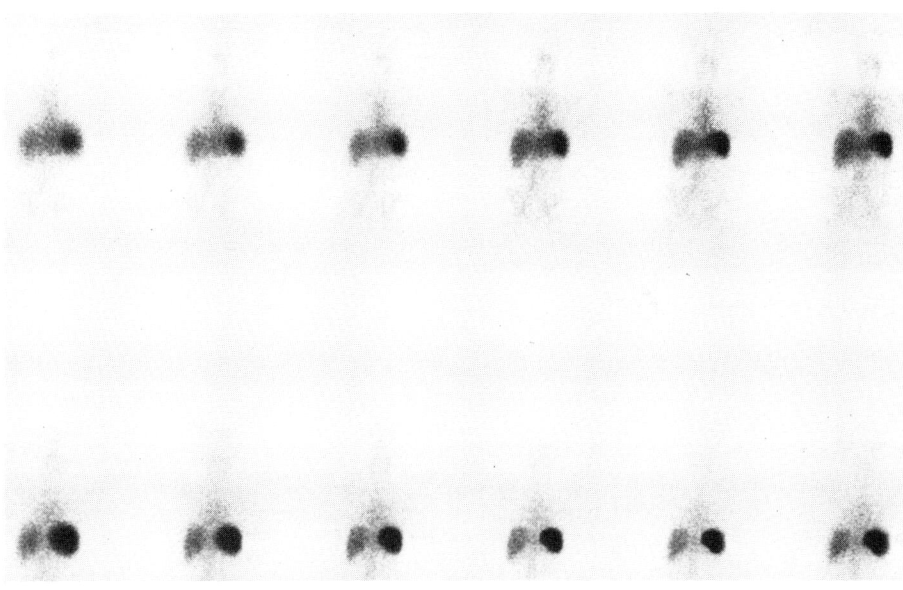

FIGURE 22. Normal total-body ^{111}In leukocyte scan.

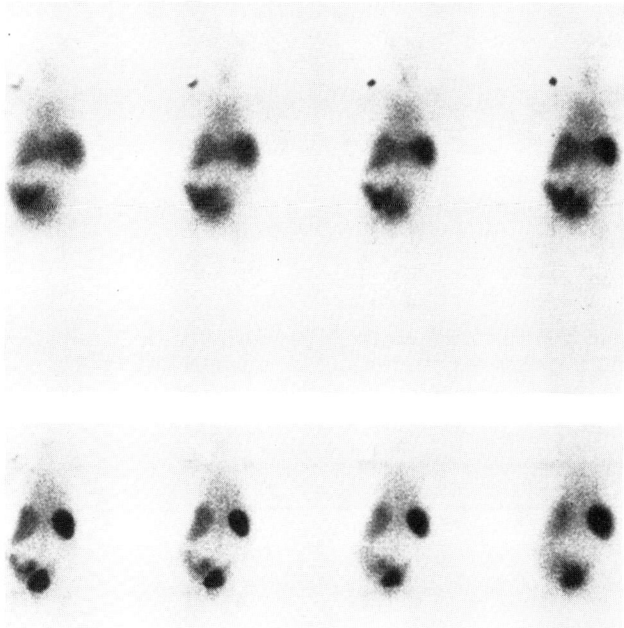

FIGURE 23. Abnormal ^{111}In leukocyte study. Note anterior and posterior location of abdominal abscesses. This indium leukocyte study was performed 18 h postinjection in a patient who presented with abdominal pain and fever of 5 d duration.

C. Adrenal Scanning

Brown et al.[24] using the ATS for adrenal scintigraphy reported that the ATS was preferred over the conventional camera. In general, no preference was associated with bilateral disease or normal adrenals, whereas in unilateral disease, the ATS demonstrated the asymmetry or resolved difficulties in separating the adrenal gland from overlapping liver or gallbladder.

Finally, Gaston et al.[25] using the ATS for imaging of the pancreas reported that the ATS was better able to resolve radionuclide concentrations at various steps in the pancreas, which is of particular advantage because the organ does not remain in the same plane throughout its longitudinal axis.

VI. CONCLUSIONS

In summary, the ATS can provide tomographic images for a number of clinical applications, particularly ^{67}Ga scanning. The ATS seems to be the instrument of choice for Ga scanning at this point and the tomographic capability is of use in a number of clinical procedures even though out-of-plane activity is contained in the tomoplane of interest. Theoretically, emission computed tomography using rotating gamma cameras has advantages over ATS imaging. It will be interesting to note over the coming years whether SPECT imaging will become the method of choice for ^{99m}Tc imaging procedures. It is doubtful that SPECT imaging will improve image interpretation and lesion detection significantly over the ATS for higher energy isotopes. The ATS is of direct clinical benefit in a number of imaging procedures as outlined. At this writing, the ATS is not commercially marketed. We feel the ATS provides a useful role in medical imaging, as outlined, and renewal of commercial availability would be welcomed.

ACKNOWLEDGMENTS

The authors would like to acknowledge Siemens Gammasonics, Inc., particularly Ms. Eileen Bergemann, for her cooperation providing Pho/Con information. We would also like to thank Helen Doktycz for graphic arts, Ruth Harris, and Toni Buckley for secretarial assistance, and our colleague, David A. Turner, M.D., for general assistance.

REFERENCES

1. **McAfee, J. G., Mosely, J. M., Natarajan, T. K., et al.,** Scintillation scanning with an eight-inch diameter Sodium Iodide (TL) Crystal, *J. Nucl. Med.*, 7, 521, 1966.
2. **Anger, H. O.,** Tomographic Gamma-ray Scanner With Simultaneous Readout of Several Planes, UCRL-16899 REV, Lawrence Radiation Laboratory, University of California Press, Berkeley, 1966.
3. **Turner, D. A., Fordham, E. W., Ramachandran, P., et al.,** The Anger Tomographic Rectilinear Scanner, Presbyterian-St. Luke's Hospital, Department of Nuclear Medicine, Chicago, 1974.
4. **Graham, L. S.,** Physical characteristics of longitudinal tomographic scanner, *Med. Phys.*, 2, 168, 1975.
5. **Graham, L. S. and Perez-Mendez, V.,** Special imaging devices, in *Nuclear Medicine Physics Instrumentation and Agents*, Rollo, F. D., Ed., C. V. Mosby, St. Louis, 271, 1977.
6. **Volpe, J. A., McRae, J., and Anger, H. O.,** Clinical experience with the multiplane tomographic scanner, *J. Nucl. Med.*, 12, 101, 1971.
7. **McRae, J. and Anger, H. O.,** Clinical results from the multiplane tomographic scanner, in *Tomographic Imaging in Nuclear Medicine*, Freedman, G. S., Ed., Society of Nuclear Medicine, New York, 1973, 240.
8. **McRae, J. and Anger, H. O.,** Tomographic imaging in nuclear medicine, in *Progress in Atomic Medicine, Vol. 4, Recent Advances in Nuclear Medicine*, Lawrence, J. H., Ed., Grune & Stratton, New York, 1974, 189.
9. **Bergemann, E.,** Private communication, Siemens Gammasonics Inc., Des Plaines IL.
10. Pho/Con Operations Manual, Siemens Gammasonics Inc., Des Plaines, IL.
11. Pho/Con-192 Specifications, Siemens Gammasonics Inc., Des Plaines, IL.
12. **Anger, H. O.,** Tomographic gamma-ray scanner with simultaneous readout of several planes, in *Fundamental Problems in Scanning*, Gottschalk, A. and Beck, R. N., Eds., Charles C Thomas, Springfield, IL, 1968, 195.
13. **Chang, L. T., MacDonald, D., and Perez-Mendez, V.,** Axial tomography and three dimensional image reconstructive, *IEEE Trans. Nucl. Sci.*, NS-23(No. 1), 568, 1976.
14. **Garcia, E. V. and Diaz, J. E.,** Improved longitudinal and transverse single-photon emission computed body tomography using an Anger tomographic scanner, in *Frontiers in Nuclear Medicine*, Hoist, W., Wagner, H. W., and Buchanan, J. W., Eds., Springer-Verlag, Berlin, 1980.
15. **Pickens, D. R., Price, R. N., Patton, J. A., et al.,** Simultaneous multiplane deconvolution in focal plane tomography, *J. Nucl. Med.*, 20, 666, 1979.
16. **Silverstein, E. A., Fordham, F. W., Chung-Bin, A., et al.,** Development of the computerized Anger tomographic scanner for positron imaging, *IAEA Proc.*, IAEA-Sm 247, Heidelberg, FRG, September 1980, 127.
17. **White, W.,** Private communication, Siemen's Gammasonics, Inc., Des Plaines, IL.
18. **Turner, D. A., Fordham, E. W., Pagano, J. V., et al.,** Brain scanning with the Anger multiplane tomographic scanner as a second examination, *Radiology*, 121, 115, 1976.
19. **Fordham, E. W. and Turner, D. A.,** Tomographic radionuclide brain imaging with the Anger tomoscanner, in *Noninvasive Brain Imaging: Computer Tomography and Radionuclides*, DeBlanc, H. J. and Sorenson, J. A., Eds., Society of Nuclear Medicine, New York, 1975, 81.
20. **Turner, D. A., Fordham, E. W., Ali, A., et al.,** Gallium-67 imaging in the management of Hodgkins disease and other malignant lymphomas, *Semin. Nucl. Med.*, 13, 205, 1978.
21. **Beckerman, C., Hoffer, P. B., Bitran, J. D., et al.,** Gallium-67 citrate imaging studies of the lung, *Semin. Nucl. Med.*, 10, 286, 1980.

22. **Hauser, M. and Alderson, P.,** Gallium-67 imaging in abdominal disease, *Semin. Nucl. Med.,* 13, 251, 1978.
23. **Hauser, M. and Gottschalk, A.,** Comparison of the Anger tomographic scanner and the 15 inch scintillation camera for gallium imaging, *J. Nucl. Med.,* 19, 1074, 1978.
24. **Brown, M. L., Wachnor, H. W., Hay, I. D., et al.,** Adrenal scintigraphy: comparison of the Anger tomographic scanner and the large-field gamma camera, *J. Nucl. Med.,* 21, 724, 1980.
25. **Gaston, E. L., Gaspard, C. L., Brooks, A. C., et al.,** Multiplane tomographic imaging of the pancreas, *J. Nucl. Med. Tech.,* 13, 28, 1980.

Chapter 8

LIMITED ANGLE SLANT-HOLE TOMOGRAPHY

John C. Lasher, Jack L. Lancaster, Wei Chang, and Ralph Blumhardt

TABLE OF CONTENTS

I. INTRODUCTION

Tomographic radiography was developed approximately 60 years ago[1] and is now a major clinical imaging modality. Many years lapsed, however, before Kuhl and Edwards applied similar tomographic principles to the problem of γ-ray image formation in medical radioisotope scanning in 1962.[2]

It was not until Anger invented the tomographic scanner in 1968 that widespread attention was directed to nuclear tomography.[3] The tomographic scanner is basically a large diameter rectilinear scanner which uses camera-like electronics to provide correction signals so that six images can be obtained simultaneously, each displaying a different plane in focus with all other planes out of focus. A tomographic scanner utilizing this concept was marketed later under the name of PHO/CON™.

Around 1970, gamma cameras equipped with slant-hole collimators began to be used for emission tomography.[4-6] Tomographic images of the brain[7] and liver[8] were obtained using analog reconstruction techniques. The application of digital techniques to tomography was described in 1973 by Freedman[9] using the slant-hole collimator and incremental rotation of the collimator during data acquisition. Even though the digital tomographic techniques had been worked out mathematically, software had not yet been written.

Since Freedman's original description of digital techniques, many changes have occurred in nuclear medicine instrumentation. Image processing computers have become commonplace and improvements have been made in the gamma camera's crystal size, resolution, linearity, and uniformity. These changes led to the development in 1976 and 1977 of several new systems utilizing various forms of emission computed tomography.[10-12]

None of these new systems seemed to capture much interest until 1978 when Vogel et al.[13] introduced the seven-pinhole tomographic imaging system. This system quickly found a home in the nuclear medicine community, partially because of the small investment necessary in additional hardware but mostly because of its initial clinical application to myocardial perfusion imaging with ^{201}Tl.[14] The seven-pinhole collimator, however, did not maintain its clinical acceptance because of major geometric problems and because of the high level of technical expertise required.[15]

Computerized slant-hole collimator tomography was developed in 1979 in an attempt to obviate some of the problems of the seven-pinhole tomographic system.[16-18] These slant-hole systems consisted of collimators capable of acquiring from one to four images simultaneously. When the system performance was studied,[19-21] it was found in most instances to be superior to seven-pinhole.[16,21,22]

II. HISTORY OF SLANT-HOLE TOMOGRAPHY

Radionuclide tomography using a gamma camera, a digital computer, and a special slant-hole collimator was described by Freedman.[9,23] In this system, the rotating slant-hole (RSH) collimator was mounted to a standard gamma camera. Images were acquired into a digital computer and stored on magnetic tape. The tomographic images were formed by replaying the tape into the computer where the data were rearranged to construct the plane of interest. This plane was displayed on an oscilloscope from which the images could be photographed.

The collimator was designed for ^{99m}Tc with parallel holes inclined 20° from perpendicular to the plane of the scintillation crystal. A motor was provided to rotate the collimator insert parallel to the plane of the crystal (Figure 1). The system was connected to the computer so that at the end of a predetermined time interval the motor would rotate the collimator 30° about an axis centered on and perpendicular to the crystal, repeating each time interval for a total of 12 stops. Digital images which were acquired into a 64 × 64 matrix during each time interval were transferred from the computer to magnetic tape storage for subsequent reconstruction of each tomographic plane of interest.

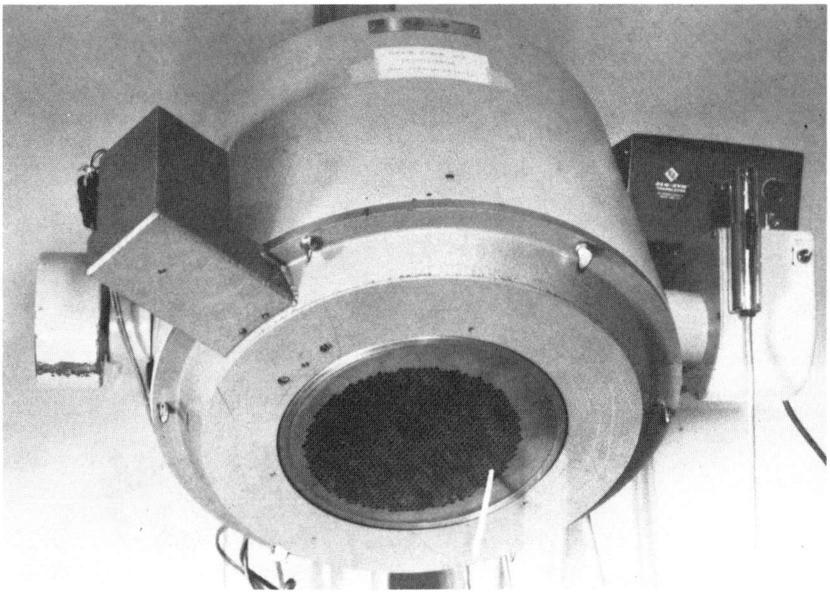

FIGURE 1. Top view of collimator showing drive mechanism. The extension from the collimator housing supports the motor drive which is connected to the computer. The white object protruding from the collimator is a drinking straw which is included to show the slant of the collimator channels. (Photo provided courtesy of Gerald S. Freedman.)

The collimator is shown in two positions 180° apart (Figure 2) illustrating that the intersection of projections of the collimator channels makes a series of planes A, B, and C. Digital images were obtained at each of the 12 positions and used to reconstruct each tomographic plane of interest.

The reconstruction process can be understood by a closer evaluation of Figure 3. All channels in the collimator are parallel to each other and slanted at an angle θ (in this case 20°) from the vertical. The initial 0° and 180° rotational angular positions of the collimator form a series of points such as 1, 3, 5, and 7 in plane A. Therefore, plane A can be reconstructed by selectively adding together counts from the channels that intersect to form all the points which determine this plane. Other planes can be reconstructed similarly with the end result being an intensification of the data in the plane of interest and a progressive blurring by systematic redistribution of data above and below the plane of interest.

One of the main disadvantages of this form of gamma camera tomography is that the useful cross-sectional area diminishes with depth (Figure 3). Points within the conical volume formed by the diminishing cross-sectional area are seen by all collimator projections and collectively called the common volume (CV). Although enlarging the crystal diameter would increase the CV, it was not feasible at that time since only 10-in. field-of-view cameras were available. A lower cost method of increasing the CV was to move the patient on a float-top table so that the patient remained within the CV, viewed by the angled collimator field.[4]

Muehllehner[24] increased the CV using a RSH collimator in conjunction with a table whose top moved in a circular motion (Figure 1). By using a modified CRT display, four tomographic scintiphotos were generated simultaneously, each showing a different plane in focus. A rotational speed of up to 4 rpm allowed scintiphotos to be obtained in as little as 15 s. The major difference between this device and the one described by Freedman was the use of the table to keep the patient within the field of view of the camera. These two methods were developed independently. The useful field of view for Freedman's system is approx-

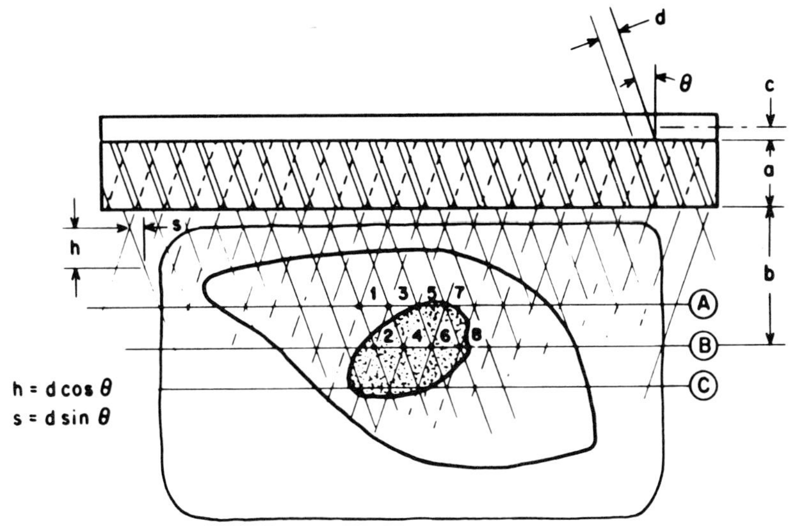

FIGURE 2. Collimators channels of diameter d are inclined 20° from vertical. When the collimator is rotated 180°, channels will be inclined in the opposite direction. Intersection of line of view of selected collimator channels form a series of points 1, 3, 5, and 7 in plane A, and 2, 4, 6, and 8 in plane B. To reconstruct the plane of interest, data from each view is shifted and added together, and the result is displayed as intensity on an oscilloscope. (From Freedman, G. S., *Tomographic Imaging in Nuclear Medicine,* Society of Nuclear Medicine, New York, 1973, 68.)

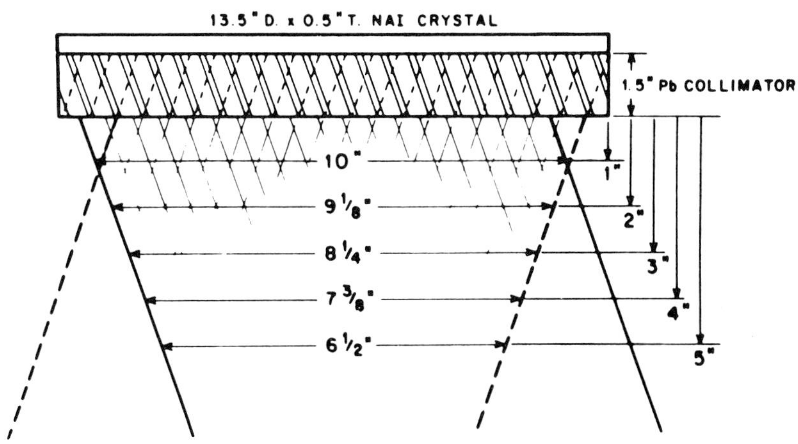

FIGURE 3. Loss of cross-sectional area as function of depth shows that at 5 in. using 20° collimator channel inclination, useful diameter is reduced by 50%. (From Freedman, G. S., *Tomographic Imaging in Nuclear Medicine,* Society of Nuclear Medicine, New York, 1973, 68.)

imately 6 in. at 4 in. from the face of the collimator. With Muehllehner's system the useful field of view can be increased to 10 in. by using the moving table. For a complete description of the system the reader is referred to an article written by Muehllehner.[5] These simple backprojection methods using the RSH collimator yielded a point spread function which had a "ring-like" appearance on planes away from the plane containing the point source. These rings were referred to as "halo" artifacts.[9]

The initial clinical experience using Freedman's method[9,23] showed it to be successful in demonstrating lesions not otherwise seen on conventional scans and especially helpful in determining the depth and the volume of those lesions.[25,26] That initial series consisted of patients who clearly showed lesions on conventional rectilinear scanning or on conventional gamma camera imaging. The difficulty in objectively determining whether the tomographic system was demonstrating lesions not seen by the conventional methods became apparent. In a few cases, however, the tomographic method did show the capability of demonstrating lesions not seen during conventional radionuclide imaging and did improve the characterization of the lesion in many cases. From these studies it was determined that when the tomographic capability exists, it should be used selectively to evaluate uncertain cases as a complementary alternative and not as a replacement for conventional methods.

Clinical experience using the tomographic system developed by Muehllehner[27] was obtained with the brain, pancreas, and liver.[7,28] The results suggested that tomographic imaging is of definite benefit to a certain group of patients which represents only a small percentage of the total patient workload in a nuclear medicine laboratory. This brought up the question of economical feasibility in proportion to its relatively limited usefulness. At the time the additional cost was $15,000 for this method and approximately $9000 for Freedman's method which did not require the special table.

At the end of these studies, the clinical interest in slant-hole tomographic methods diminished. It seemed that the performance of these RSH tomographic methods had such a slight edge over conventional means that thousands of clinical studies would have to be collected to make valid decisions regarding their clinical usefulness. Because overlying radioactivity is not removed but merely ''blurred'' by these methods of tomography, artifacts from radioactivity distribution could also be interpreted falsely as ''new'' lesions.[29] Methods were needed that improved lesion detectability and eliminated artifactual information.

During the period from 1973 to 1977, a revolution of technological advancements occurred in all fields of radiology. Digital image processing systems became commonplace as well as gamma cameras with improved sensitivity, resolution, linearity, and a larger field of view. Many tomographic image reconstruction algorithms were also developed for the numerous computerized tomographic X-ray units being sold to virtually all large radiology departments by the end of 1977. It was not surprising, therefore, to see an increased interest in scintillation camera single-photon emission tomography (SPECT).

The first of the new SPECT systems was the seven-pinhole tomographic system introduced by Vogel et al.[13] This system elicited great interest within the nuclear medicine community, partially because of the small investment necessary in additional hardware and the excellent initial clinical results when this system was applied to myocardial perfusion imaging utilizing ^{201}Tl.

Within 1 year after the introduction of seven-pinhole tomographic systems, RSH collimator systems began to surface. These new systems made use of the newer cameras which usually had larger crystal diameters than those used in the past. They also all used tomographic digital reconstruction algorithms which had some form of error correction that reduced off-plane activity and ''halo'' artifacts.

Gottschalk et al.[16] very nicely described tomographic reconstructions with RSH and seven-pinhole collimators on Anger cameras utilizing both phantoms and clinical studies. The seven-pinhole data were acquired on a Technicare SIGMA 410 wide-field-of-view camera and the RSH data were acquired on a Technicare SIGMA 420 small-field-of-view mobile camera. The RSH collimator had a 25°-slant angle. The authors' results showed that neither the seven-pinhole nor RSH collimators are strictly quantitative. The seven-pinhole system was found to have difficulties in locating large defects, accepted large amounts of scatter, had a narrow depth of usable reconstruction, was difficult to position, had poor resolution, and was unable to image large organs. In contrast, the RSH collimator could locate easily large defects, had much lower scatter acceptance, had a large depth of usable reconstructions,

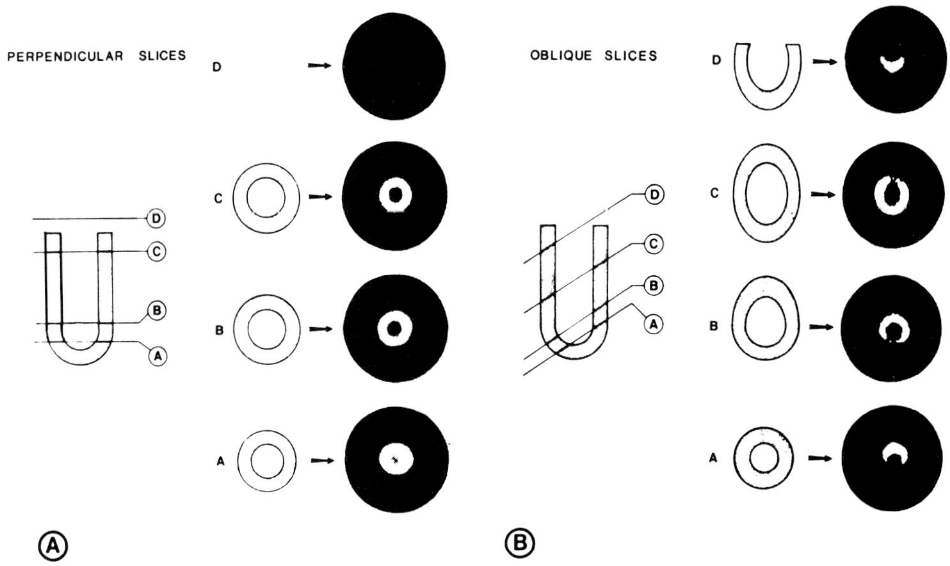

FIGURE 4. Schematic drawing of image planes through heart phantom, the expected cross-sectional images, and actual tomographic images for (A) perpendicular and (B) oblique slices. (From Ratib, O., Henze, E., Hoffman, E., et al., *J. Nucl. Med.*, 23, 34, 1982.)

was not as sensitive to lateral patient mispositioning as seven-pinhole, had better resolution, and could image large organs. This group also felt that the RSH system demonstrated an increased quality of reconstructed images. In addition, the larger field of view and resultant ease of positioning of the RSH collimator offered considerable advantages for clinical use.

The performance of the rotating single slant-hole collimator for the detection of myocardial perfusion abnormalities was reported by Ratib et al.[20] They evaluated the RHS collimator's performance with phantom studies. Perfusion defects of variable size, location, and tracer concentration were simulated and imaging was performed using both a conventional parallel-hole collimator and the RSH collimator. Their results showed RSH tomography to be more sensitive than planar imaging in detecting simulated myocardial defects; however, a possible weakness due to off-axis viewing of the ventricular phantom was observed (Figure 4).

Quantification of myocardial infarct size was estimated experimentally by Lewis et al.[30] using three methods in dogs injected with ^{99m}Tc-pyrophosphate (^{99m}Tc-PYP) 24 and 48 h following coronary ligation. All transmural infarcts were detected by all three imaging techniques. Rotating slant-hole tomography was superior to both four pinhole tomography and planar imaging for the detection of nontransmural infarction. Infarcts as small as 1.0 g were detected.

Herfkens et al.[31] developed a RSH system which they felt was clinically useful and offered certain advantages over seven-pinhole systems. It clearly defined ischemia and infarcted areas on ^{201}Tl images and was also useful with ^{99m}Tc-PYP as well as gated blood pool imaging. In another report from the same university, Shosa et al.[32] described motivating reasons for further development of the RSH approach to tomography. Their investigation extended to large cameras in the 38 to 53 cm range. They found that, in most cases, RSH systems can be designed which will yield comparable spatial resolution, comparable or superior sensitivity, and superior perspective angle relative to seven-pinhole designs. With large-field-of-view cameras the prospects of increased imaging efficiency using multiple-segment slant-hole collimators looked very promising.

A two segment RSH collimator tomographic system was described first by Nalcioglu et al.[17,19] This system consisted of a dual-segment slant-hole (Bilateral) collimator, a gamma

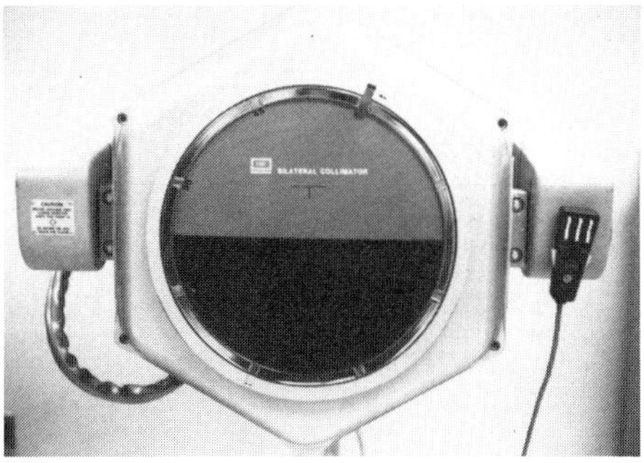

A

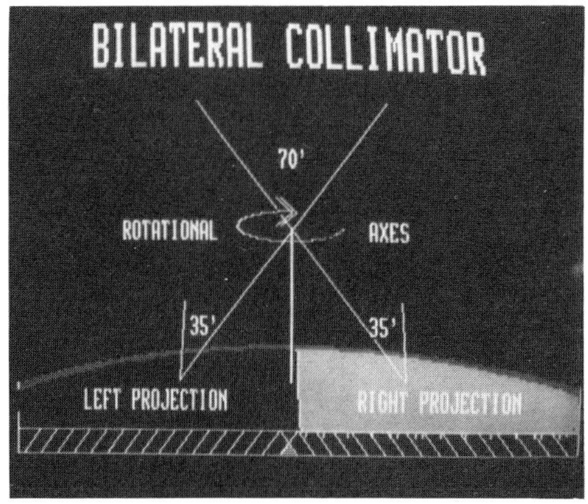

B

FIGURE 5. (A) Photograph of commercial 35° bilateral rotating slant-hole collimator for large field-of-view camera. (B) Geometry of the 35° bilateral rotating slant-hole collimator.

camera, and a minicomputer. The Bilateral collimator is capable of acquiring two spatially unique images (projections) of an object simultaneously (Figure 5). The collimator then can be rotated about an axis perpendicular to and centered on the crystal to form two additional projections at a new angle. After a sufficient number of projections are acquired, planes parallel to the collimator/crystal plane representing the object can be reconstructed by the computer. Milne et al.[33] reported on some preliminary clinical results using this system; no clear conclusions were reached, however, because of the incomplete nature of the software and limited clinical material.

Software for the bilateral two segment RSH collimator was developed and reported on by Lasher et al.[34] The software is capable of processing data from seven-pinhole as well as single or multiple projection RSH collimators. It reconstructs planes parallel to the camera's crystal. Weiland et al.[35] reported on the detection of coronary artery disease using this system in conjunction with ^{201}Tl myocardial perfusion imaging. They performed a prospective study for the detection of coronary artery disease (CAD) in 100 angiographically correlated patients. When compared to planar imaging, the tomographic method showed a significant improvement in both sensitivity and specificity for the overall and segmental detection of CAD. The system was used also to estimate relative changes in splenic volumes in response to epinephrine administration.[36]

In order to maximize the utilization of the crystal area of the scintillation camera for imaging a small object, a rotatable quadrant slant-hole collimator (QSH) was constructed by Chang et al.[18,27,37] This collimator (Figure 6) is equivalent to four smaller slant-hole collimators with each slanted section viewing the object from a different direction. It is constructed of four 90° pie-shaped segments with parallel channels angled such that two opposite quadrants are slanted toward each other. To obtain tomographic reconstructions, 2 successive 4-projection images are acquired, with a 45° rotation of the core of the collimator between the images. The computer then reconstructs planes parallel to the collimator using algebraic reconstruction techniques. The performance parameters of the QSH collimator system were compared to the seven-pinhole collimator system by Chang et al.[21,22] No extensive clinical experience with the QSH system has been reported. Some clinical work has, however, suggested its usefulness in ^{201}Tl myocardial perfusion imaging, gated blood-pool imaging, and cardiac chamber volume determination.[38,39]

A comparison of a RSH collimator system and rotating camera system for SPECT of the

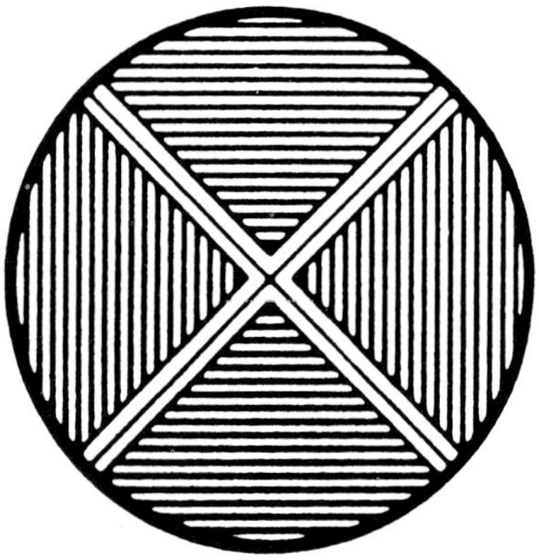

A

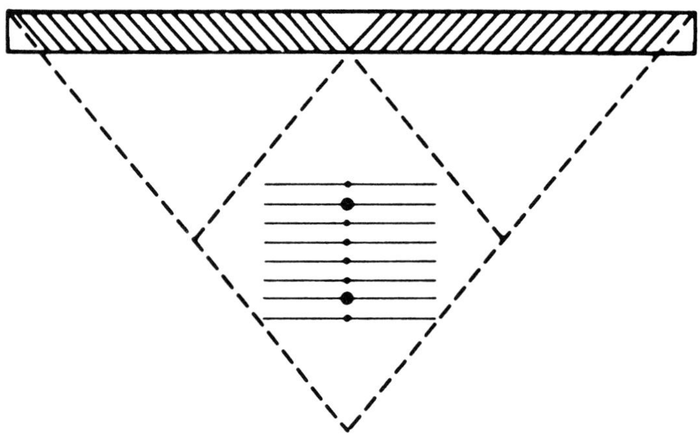

B

FIGURE 6. (A) Schematic drawing of the quadrant slant-hole collimator and (B) common volume generated by rotation of the collimator. (From Chang, W., Lin, S. L., and Henkin, R. E., *J. Nucl. Med.*, 23, 830, 1982.)

heart was reported on by Myers et al.[40] They made measurements of both systems using a standard heart phantom and ^{201}Tl. Although better intraplanar resolutions were obtained with the RSH system, the rotating camera was found to give superior definition of a defect and less propagation between reconstructed sections of the phantom.

III. BASIC DEFINITIONS FOR RSH TOMOGRAPHY

Common image space boundary (CIS) — The pixels in a projection selected for use during reconstruction. Each pixel of each projection in CIS must view at least one voxel common to all other projections (Figure 7A).

Common object space boundary (COS) — Common volume resulting from utilizing selected CIS (Figure 7B).

Common volume (CV) — The volume of space in which each voxel is seen in all projections (Figure 7C).

Slant angle — The angle of slant of the parallel collimator channels measured in degrees from the perpendicular to the crystal (Figure 7A).

Rotation angle — The angle of rotation of the collimator.

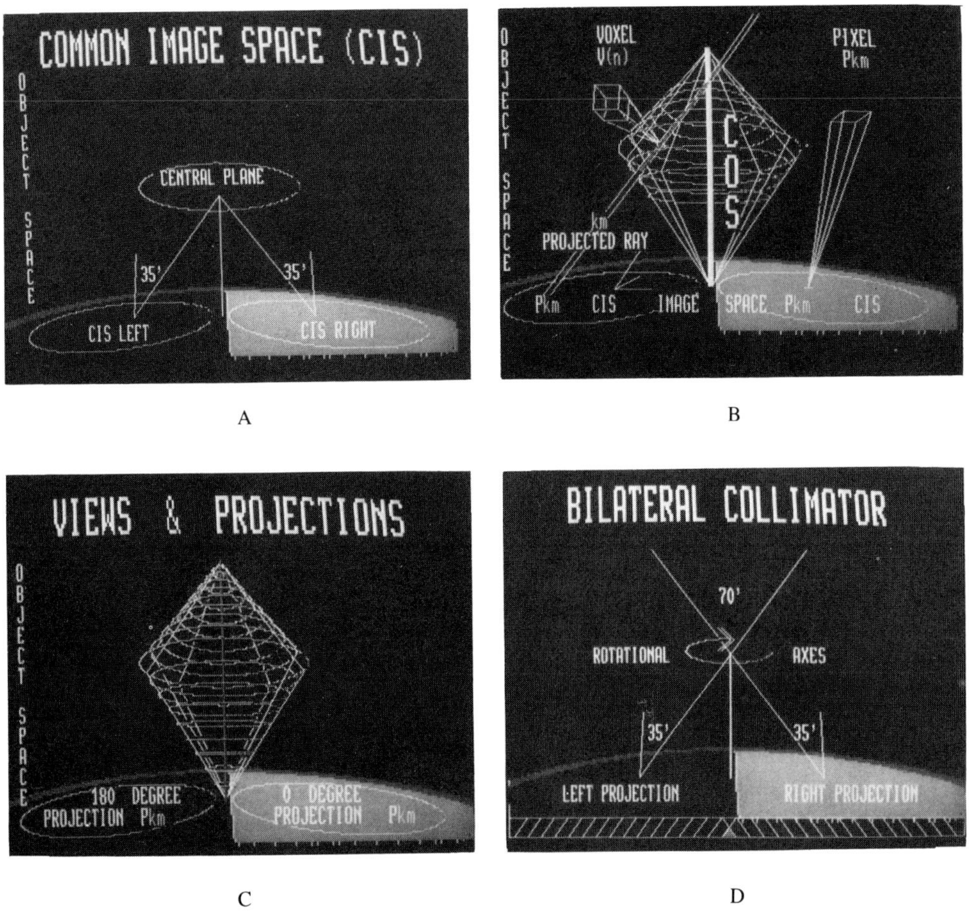

FIGURE 7. Illustrations used for definitions: (A) common image space, (B) common object space, voxel, and projected ray, (C) views and projections, and (D) bilateral collimator.

Tomographic angle — The angle between opposing projections (i.e., projections with rotation angles differing by 180°. The tomographic angle is 2× the slant angle (Figure 7D).

Central plane — Largest plane in the CV parallel to the crystal plane (Figure 7A).

IV. SPECIFIC ASPECTS OF SLANT-HOLE COLLIMATOR

Single slant-hole collimators have a useful field of view or CV that looks like a truncated cone which extends beyond the collimator face (Figure 3). The resulting CV is directly proportional to the cube of the crystal diameter and inversely proportional to the tangent of the slant angle.[9] The volume is calculated as follows:

$$V = pi * d^3/[24 * tan(a)]$$

a = Collimator slant angle

d = Diameter of CV at surface of collimator

V = Volume

Only points within this conical volume can be viewed by all projections. The diameter of the CV is always less than the diameter of the camera and depends on the distance from

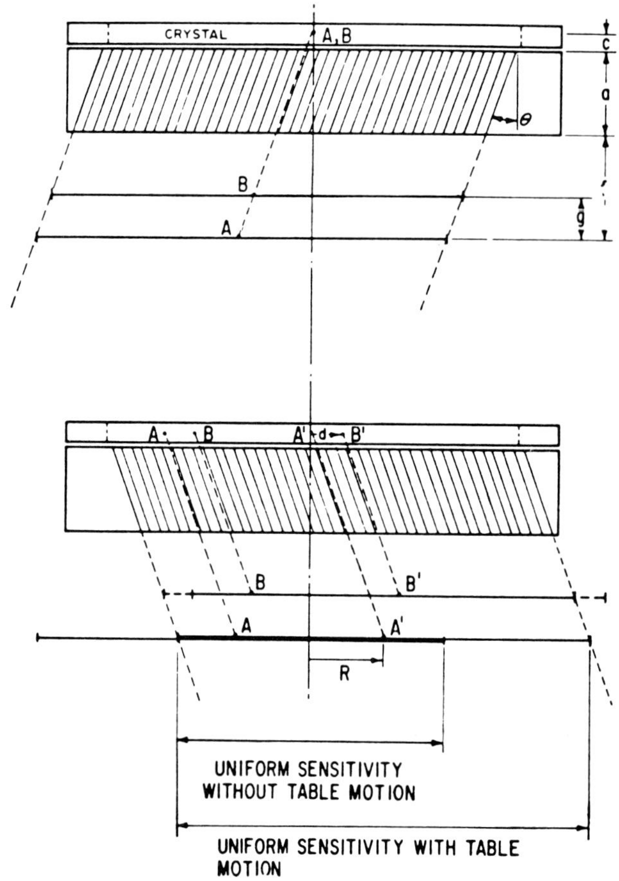

FIGURE 8. (Top) Sketch showing scintillation crystal, slanted-hole collimator, two sources A and B, and their images on the crystal. (Bottom) Same as (A) but collimator rotated 180° with table top stationary (source positions A and B) and table top moved (source positions A′ and B′).[5]

the collimator. At a distance of 10 cm from the collimator the CV diameter would be 13 cm for a 30° RSH collimator of 25-cm diameter. The equation for CV diameter as a function of distance from the collimator for a single-segment RSH collimator is as follows:

$$d' = d - 2 * z * \tan(a)$$

a = Collimator slant angle

d = Diameter of CV at surface of collimator

z = Distance from collimator to the plane

d′ = Diameter of CV at distance z from collimator surface

Various methods can be used to alter the cross-sectional area at increasing depths from a single slant-hole collimator's face.

Muehllehner's[5] method, using a moving table, can result in doubling the CV. This is accomplished by moving the patient in such a way that the volume to be imaged is kept within the field of view of the RSH collimator. To achieve this, a table with a movable top is rotated in a circular pattern in synchronization with the collimator's rotation (Figure 8).

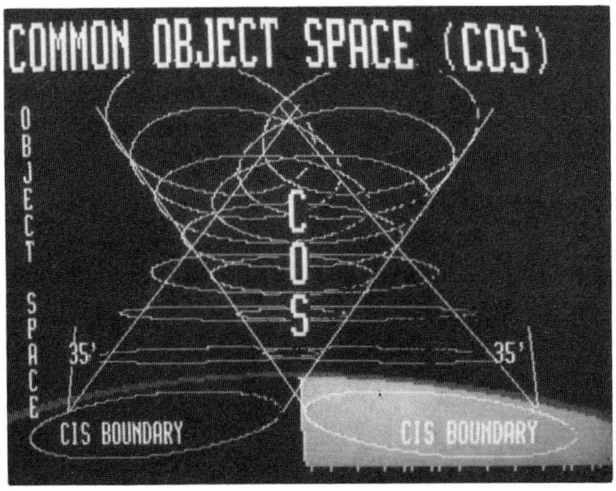

FIGURE 9. Common object space.

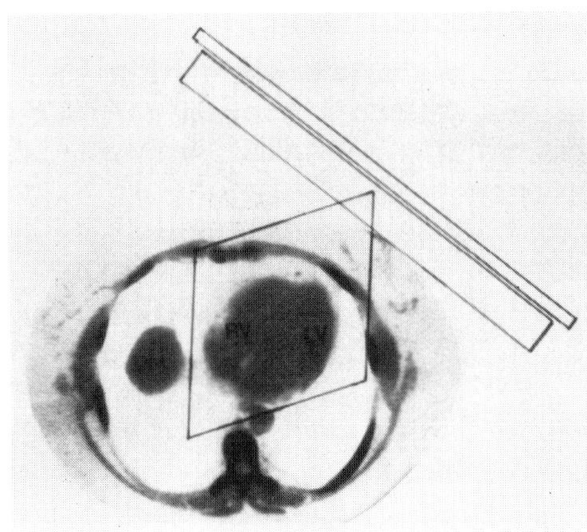

FIGURE 10. Common object boundary for 35° bilateral rotating slant-hole collimator for LFOV camera.

The image of point source A is stationary while the collimator rotates. Similarly, the image of all sources within the plane of A will be stationary on the crystal even though the collimator and camera rotate. Point source B, however, describes a circle on the crystal. Using this method, the useful area of uniform sensitivity for all sources in the plane of A can be equal to the useful area of the scintillation camera. The CV can be doubled when compared to Freedman's[9] method. This occurs when the CV takes on the form of two cones with a common base.

The two-segment or bilateral RSH collimator simultaneously collimates two spatially unique projections of the same object (Figure 9). The collimator is divided into opposite halves by a small triangular lead septum with its base parallel to the plane of the crystal. On each side of this septum, parallel channels slant toward each other at an angle measured perpendicular to the plane of the crystal. The collimator can be rotated parallel to the crystal's surface to form additional projections. The CV of the bilateral collimator can be thought of as two cones with a common base (Figure 7C). The common base or "central plane" has a diameter slightly less than one half the diameter of the crystal determined by the diameter of extracted circular projections. The common volumes for a large-field-of-view (LFOV) 35° bilateral collimator (Figure 10) and a standard-field-of-view (SFOV) 25° bilateral collimator (Figure 11) are illustrated by overlaying a common object space boundary on a transverse computed tomography (CT) section through the thorax. This large heart fits easily

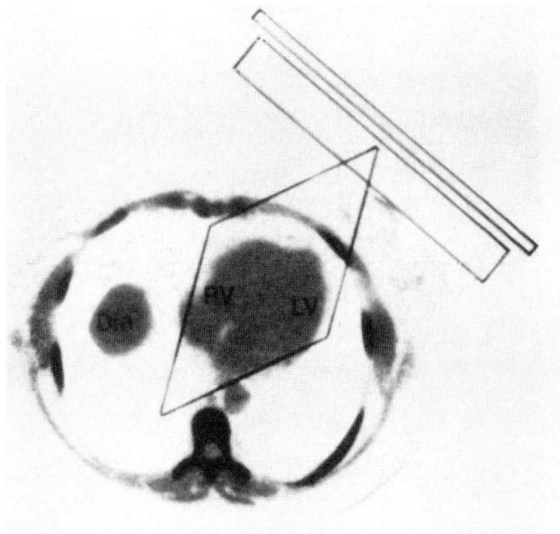

FIGURE 11. Common object boundary for 25° bilateral rotating slant-hole collimator for SFOV camera.

within the CV using a LFOV camera, but not as easily within the CV when a SFOV camera is used. If the primary interest is confined, however, to the left ventricle rather than the entire heart, the SFOV collimator may prove adequate for cardiac imaging even though its tomographic effect will not be as good as the LFOV.

The four-view or quadrant RSH collimator simultaneously views four spatially unique projections of the same object in space. Figure 6A illustrates the geometry of this CV. This collimator has generated interest because of its high imaging efficiency, large tomographic angle (40° on an LFOV), its potential for dynamic imaging, and the ease of positioning objects within CV.

Various single- and multiprojection slant-hole collimators have been constructed for both the LFOV and SFOV gamma cameras. The selection of the optimal collimator requires a knowledge of the intended use and considerations of the collimator design parameters. Parameters most important for collimator design in multisegment RSH collimators are calculated utilizing circular CIS boundaries as follows:

$Z_{v1} = [(D/2 - d') + s]/\tan(a)$	Z_{v1} = Distance from collimator to near vertex of CV
	d' = Diameter of extracted circles
	D = Collimator diameter
	s = Offset of center of extracted circle from center of segment
$z_{cp} = d'/\tan(a)$	Z_{cp} = Distance from collimator to the central plane
$V_{ms} = pi * d'^3/[12 * \tan(a)]$	V_{ms} = Volume of multisegment RSH collimator CIS

The collimator design should follow these guidelines:

1. Maximize the crystal size

2. Maximize the slant angle
3. Maximize the number of projections
4. Minimize the unusable crystal space

These guidelines are constrained by the following considerations:

1. Desired central plane height
2. Minimum required central plane width
3. Number of collimator segments
4. The camera to be used
5. Desired resolution
6. Desired sensitivity

The interactions of the various parameters and guidelines are complex and will not be elaborated on here. Table 1 lists specifications of various clinically useful collimators.

Experience with each of the three collimators described in Table 1 led to some conclusions. For routine imaging of left ventricular function and ^{201}Tl myocardial perfusion studies, the collimator and camera of choice is the high-sensitivity bilateral 35° RSH collimator on a LFOV gamma camera. This collimator has a desirable central plane height of approximately 14 cm. It is capable of imaging the largest of hearts with good imaging efficiency, excellent tomographic effect, and ease of positioning and repositioning.

A quadrant collimator on an LFOV gamma camera yields greater imaging efficiency when compared with the bilateral. There will be, however, some hearts that will not fit within its CV. The quadrant's CV is a subset of the bilateral's CV since increasing the number of projections has the effect of increasing the central plane height and decreasing the central plane width. The approximate relationship between volume for single, double, and quad-segment collimators is as follows:

$$V_{ss} = 4 * V_{ds} = 7.5 * V_{qs}$$

V_{ss} = Volume of single segment RSH collimator
V_{ds} = Volume of double segment RSH collimator
V_{qs} = Volume of quad segment RSH collimator

$$d_{ss} = 2 * d_{ds} = 2.47 d_{qs}$$

d_{ss} = Diameter of central plane for single segment RSH collimator
d_{ds} = Diameter of central plane for double segment RSH collimator
d_{qs} = Diameter of central plane for quad segment RSH collimator

ASSUMING
(1) Same crystal size.
(2) Same collimator slant angle.
(3) No dead space between segments.

The 25° bilateral collimator on a SFOV gamma camera is preferred over the single-slant collimator on a SFOV gamma camera. There will be, however, some hearts that will not fit within the bilateral's CV.

The rotating single-slant collimator offers the largest volume of reconstruction of all the

Table 1
RSH COLLIMATOR CHARACTERISTICS

Type collimator	Crystal diameter (cm)	Slant angle (degrees)	Central width (cm)	Plane height (cm)	CV (cm^3)
SFOV	25	25	25	0	4386
SFOV	25	30	25	0	3543
SFOV bilateral	25	25	12	13.9	970
SFOV bilateral	25	30	12	11.3	784
LFOV	38	30	38	0	12441
LFOV	38	35	38	0	10258
LFOV bilateral	38	30	18.5	16.9	2871
LFOV bilateral	38	35	18.5	13.9	2367
LFOV bilateral	38	40	18.5	11.6	1971
LFOV quadrilateral	38	38	14.4	15.1	1000

listed collimators. It does not, however, have the high imaging efficiency and ease of positioning that is inherent in multisegment collimators. Its CV is potentially four times as large as a bilateral's. This increase in CV is not clinically useful for left ventricular imaging since the left ventricle normally lies entirely within the portion of the CV that is common to both collimators.

V. RECONSTRUCTION THEORY AND METHODS

Due to the noise characteristics and lack of complete angular sampling with RSH collimators, tomographic reconstruction usually is accomplished utilizing iterative reconstruction techniques (IRTs).[34,41,42] The basic premise is to reconstruct a data set within the CV which appears to have the same characteristics as the original object when viewed from the various projections. This is achieved by comparing reprojections of successive estimates of the CV with the data projections acquired from the object. Because of incomplete angular sampling of the object, a unique solution for image reconstruction does not exist. A solution is sought, therefore, which is consistent with *a priori* knowledge of the object. Some *a priori* constraints utilized are (1) non-negative object, (2) entire object within CV, and (3) Poisson noise in the data projections.[16] It is, of course, not possible for all objects to reside totally within the CV. The CV constraint limits RSH tomography to relatively small objects surrounded by little or no other radioactivity.

The RSH algorithms to estimate a tomographic reconstruction fall into the general category of IRT. Two commonly utilized algorithms are simultaneous iterative reconstruction techniques (SIRT) and iterative least squares techniques (ILST). The SIRT forms successive approximations to the object voxels by altering a voxel value based on differences between observed and calculated sums of rays passing through the voxel independent of other voxel values. This operation is performed for each voxel with the result being the nth approximation of the object. After each iteration a new set of calculated projections (a new set of ray sums) is formed for use in the next iteration. SIRT corrections have been implemented in both an additive and a multiplicative algorithm.[41]

The ILST forms successive approximations to the object voxels by minimizing, in a *least-squares sense,* the relative error between observed and calculated ray sums for all rays passing through a voxel. ILST is similar to SIRT in this approach because both methods alter a voxel value based on all rays passing through the voxel independent of other voxels. The ILST forms successive approximations by adding a calculated correction factor to previous voxels. ILST utilizes the *a priori* constraints of Poisson statistics in calculation of the relative error where the error squared is divided by the variance and the variance is assumed to be equal to the observed count. Additionally, as discussed by Budinger and Gullberg,[41] a multiplicative damping factor (also calculated by least-squares methods) is employed to cause successive iterations to converge. Calculation of the damping factor is relatively complicated because it is intended to minimize simultaneously the relative errors between all observed and calculated ray sums.

An ILST for RSH tomography allowing single and multisegment collimators with varying numbers of views has been reported by Lasher et al.[34] A brief description of this ILST technique is given to illustrate the methodology.

Successive estimates to each voxel in common object space are formed by calculating V^{n+1} (i,j,k) as follows:

$V^{n+1}(i,j,k)$	$= V^n(i,j,k) + D^n * dV^n(i,j,k)$
$V^{n+1}(i,j,k)$	= n + 1th estimate of the voxel at row i, column j, and plane k
$V^{n+1}(i,j,k)$	= nth estimate of the voxel at row i, column j, and plane k
$dV^{n+1}(i,j,k)$	= Correction factor to be added for the nth estimate of the voxel at row i, column j, and plane k
D^n	= Damping factor to be used for the nth estimate

The correction factor dV^n (i,j,k) is calculated from all rays passing through the voxel i,j,k from the raw data projections (P) and the nth estimated projections (R^n). Letting P_1 and R^n_1 represent appropriate ray sums for the voxel (i,j,k), the correction factor is calculated by summing the relative error $(P_1 - R^n_1)/P_1$ over all projections and dividing by the sum of $1/P_1$ over all projections. To decrease processing time, an algorithm was designed to calculate the relative error for all voxels within the CV (or reconstruction volume) separately for each projection. Backprojection of all data can then be performed after relative errors for all projections have been determined. The final step is to backproject the reciprocal sum of $1/P_1$ into a separate volume and then multiply the volume of relative errors by the volume of reciprocal sums to get a volume of correction factors. The damping factor is calculated as outlined in the review article by Budinger and Gullberg.[41]

Lasher's software included seven distinct programs in a clinical package to enable users to acquire and process tomographic data with relative ease.

1. A program which determines the center of each projection, necessary for proper extraction and registration of all projections
2. A program which calculates pixels/mm, necessary for accurate plane spacing, image size, and reproducibility
3. A program to specify data acquisition parameters; acquisition information such as number of projections, pixel offset from center of projection, pixel size of projections, slant angle, and view angle are necessary for proper projection registration during reconstruction
4. A program to extract circular projections from the acquired views
5. A program to specify the reconstruction parameters such as plane separation, number of planes to reconstruct (1-16), starting plane (relative to central plane), and number of iterations
6. A program for reconstruction utilizing 1 to 5 above; typical reconstruction time employing three iterations was stated to be less than 90 s for 8 planes reconstructed from 8 projections

A 128 × 128 byte mode matrix was utilized for collimators with two or four segments. Data from each projection were extracted into 64 × 64 word mode matrices before reconstruction. Experience with this software has shown that three iterations are sufficient for clinical imaging.

VI. PERFORMANCE OF RSH SYSTEM

Since the slant-hole collimator is very similar to parallel-hole collimators its performance characteristics easily can be predicted.[5] The geometrical resolution of RSH collimators is determined from the following equation:

$$R = D(d + t + c)/t$$

R = Geometrical resolution distance
D = Diameter of collimator hole at collimator surface
d = Distance from collimator surface
t = Collimator thickness
c = Distance from collimator to crystal

Notes: 1. d,t,c are measured along a line perpendicular to the collimator surface.
2. D is not the diameter of the collimator channel. Diameter of collimator channel = D/cos(a) where a = slant angle.

This geometrical resolution distance is approximately equal to the full-width-at-half-maximum (FWHM) of the collimator line spread function[43] and is a measure of lateral resolution as a function of perpendicular distance from the collimator surface. The resolution for reconstructed tomography needs to be expressed for the three-dimensional space in which imaging occurs. Resolution from reconstructed data is generally reported as FWHM both laterally and longitudinally as a function of distance from the collimator along the axis of rotation. Resolution for a 30° bilateral RSH collimator is illustrated in Figure 12 as measured by Lasher and Kopp.[34] Longitudinal resolution of object distributions with large x and y dimensions is not possible with RSH systems because of the limited tomographic angle of the RSH collimator yielding insufficient angular sampling of the object longitudinally.[44]

The sensitivity of a RSH collimator is less than that of a standard parallel-channel collimator with the same resolution characteristics, due to the fact that the channels are longer and narrower for the RSH collimator, yielding poorer geometric efficiency. This disparity results from the fact that the actual distance from the object to the image for RSH collimators is greater than the collimator to object distance due to angulation of the collimator channels. Since RSH collimators can have more than one segment viewing the CV at one time, a gain in system sensitivity for tomographic imaging occurs. Assuming identical slant angles and collimator resolution and sensitivity, the sensitivity ratios for single, double, and quad RSH collimators are approximately 1:2:4. This increase in sensitivity is appreciated only for objects within the CV of all collimators. Measured sensitivity for two RSH collimators manufactured by Cardiac Medical Systems is given in Table 2.

Uniformity in the projections utilized in RSH tomography is a function of the gamma camera and collimator uniformity. Nonuniformity of the gamma camera (intrinsic) does not produce ring artifacts in RSH tomographic slices as has been reported for rotating camera tomography[45] because no location within the camera crystal is used repeatedly in the reconstruction of a single tomographic voxel. Gamma cameras without special uniformity correction have been used successfully for RSH tomography.[16,20,34] Collimator nonuniformity

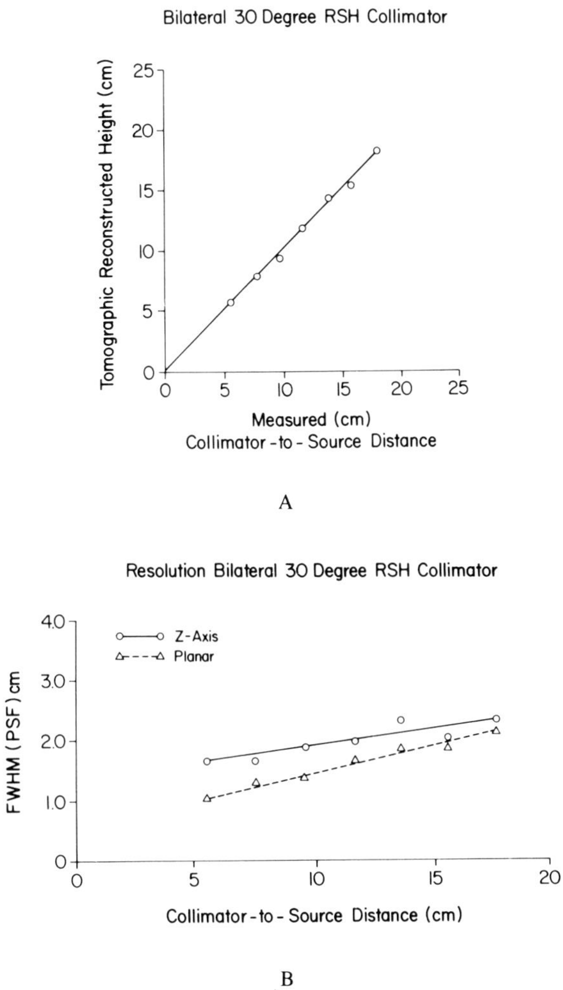

FIGURE 12. Bilateral 30° RSH collimator characteristics: (A) Reconstructed height vs. measured distance, (B) Resolution vs. distance.

Table 2
RSH COLLIMATOR SENSITIVITY

Collimator	Sensitivity[a]
Bilateral — 30° slant	1131 cpm/μCi
Quadrilateral — 38° slant	1895 cpm/μCi

[a] Determined with ^{57}Co point source at a distance of 10 cm from the collimator.

(extrinsic) is expected to have the greatest effect on reconstructed slices near the axis of rotation. The axis of rotation is the region of the CV which is viewed by the same collimator channels at all rotations during data acquisition. The collimator channels involved are those on a radial line which bisects the segment.

Because of the increased system sensitivity to objects within the CV when multisegment

RSH collimators are employed, a higher count rate will be experienced. The resolving time of the gamma camera should be sufficient to handle incident count rates of two times that expected for such studies.

VII. CLINICAL APPLICATIONS

Some of the initial clinical experience with a digital gamma camera tomographic system was described by Freedman in 1971 and 1973.[25,26] He felt that his method had been successful in demonstrating lesions not otherwise seen on conventional scans and was especially helpful in determining the depth and volume of these lesions. His final conclusion, however, was that tomographic evaluation by itself should not replace conventional studies nor would it be economically realistic to restudy all patients in the hope of locating the occasional lesion that could be picked up using this method. He did expect that future improvements of tomographic systems would justify their more widespread application. James et al.[28] and Goldsmith[29] reached similar conclusions about their general clinical experience in tomographic imaging with the Nuclear Chicago Tomocamera™, while Chamroenngan[7] was more positive about the application to brain imaging.

Myocardial infarct-sizing in dogs was reported by Lewis et al.[30] using several imaging systems. They felt that RSH tomography was superior to both multipinhole tomography and planar imaging for the detection of nontransmural infarction. Measurements of infarct size from RSH tomographic slices showed excellent correlation with infarct weight.

Ratib et al.[20] showed rotating single-slant tomography to be more sensitive than planar imaging in detecting simulated myocardial defects but indicated a potential limitation for the detection of perfusion abnormalities. This limitation is the appearance of decreased activity in a tomographic plane that may be secondary to the orientation of the camera to the long axis in the phantom or the left ventricle in patients. Chang et al.[46] pointed out in a letter to the editor that the tilt phenomenon observed by Ratib had already been described by them using seven-pinhole tomography,[38,47] and slant-hole tomography.[27] They found that there are ways to position seven-pinhole and multiview slant-hole collimators that usually will eliminate this problem.

Clinical applications of RSH tomography as applied to the cardiovascular system were reported by Herfkens et al.[31] They felt that RSH tomography of ^{99m}Tc-PYP myocardial perfusion imaging was useful in defining infarcted areas by separating rib uptake and blood-pool activity in the diffuse uptake pattern. The tomographic wall motion studies had been useful in defining chamber size and segmental motion abnormalities. RSH tomography was said to be useful in clearly defining ischemia and infarcted areas on ^{201}Tl myocardial perfusion imaging.

Weiland et al.[35] reported on the rotating two-view slant-hole (bilateral) tomographic system which was used for the detection of coronary artery disease using ^{201}Tl. They studied 100 angiographically correlated patients using a 30° bilateral LFOV tomographic system. The study compared the sensitivity and specificity of visual planar, visual tomographic, and quantitative tomographic methods for the detection of CAD on both a global and regional basis. They found that the visual methods of interpreting ^{201}Tl myocardial perfusion studies were inferior to the more objective quantitative means. It was felt, however, that the best clinical approach was to combine the visual planar and tomographic information with the quantitative information.

Rosen et al.[36] showed another use of the bilateral tomographic imaging system. They used the system to determine relative changes in splenic volume following administration of epinephrine. Their contention was that relative splenic volume changes would be less in patients with Hodgkin's disease involving the spleen than in patients with normal spleens. ^{99m}Tc-labeled heat-damaged red blood cells were used selectively to image the spleen.

Tomographic planes of the spleen were then acquired at several points in time, after which the relative splenic volume changes were determined by geometric counting of tomographic voxels on a study-by-study basis. The results showed that volume response to epinephrine appears to be significantly less in abnormal spleens and may serve to identify patients with unequivocally normal spleens prior to treatment.

Chang et al.[18,22,27] reported on the clinical use of a 25° SFOV rotating four-view slant-hole (quadrant) tomographic system and a 40° LFOV quadrant system. Their results with patients suggested that the CV of the 25° collimator was too small for routine cardiovascular imaging while the 40° LFOV collimator was optimal. As previously mentioned, artifacts were observed if the patient was improperly positioned, but this was felt not to be an insurmountable problem since mispositioning could be detected easily during the positioning stage.[27,46] Henkin et al.[38] reported on some preliminary results of gated blood-pool imaging of phantoms using the quadrant collimator.

There are several institutions using slant-hole collimators for clinical applications that do not involve tomographic imaging. Royal et al.[48] found the slant-hole collimator to be useful for several noncardiac, nontomographic applications. They felt that it permits the acquisition of views that would be physically impossible to obtain with a conventional collimator. In general, the slant-hole collimator is useful in obtaining cephalad and/or caudal angulation of the brain and oblique views of the chest and abdomen. Parker et al.[49] discussed the usefulness of a 30° slant-hole collimator during radionuclide ventriculography of the cardiac blood-pool to improve imaging of the heart in both the modified left anterior oblique and right anterior oblique views. Ohtake et al.[50] evaluated a nontomographic method of measuring the depth of internal mammary lymph nodes using the bilateral collimator which was originally designed for cardiac studies.

VIII. FUTURE OF SLANT-HOLE TOMOGRAPHY

Even though slant-hole collimator tomography was described in approximately 1969, it still has not gained widespread clinical acceptance. Most of the studies addressing specific applications, however, have been optimistic.

The question still remains as to whether RSH tomography would be worth pursuing if it were found to be beneficial to a group of patients representing only a small percentage of the total patient workload. The answer depends on several considerations such as the cost, operational ease, and ease of clinical interpretation. The cost is minimal since most systems today only require an RSH collimator ranging from $5000 to $7000 and software costing approximately $3000. Although most of the clinical trials have been limited, one of the more extensive studies[35] suggests that quantitative tomographic myocardial perfusion imaging using the bilateral RSH collimator represents an improvement over planar techniques and is easy both to perform and to interpret.

A comparison of RSH collimator tomographic techniques with those of the rotating gamma camera has recently been published by Myers et al.[40] Although better intraplanar resolutions were obtained with the RSH collimator, the rotating camera was found to give superior definition of a defect and less propagation between reconstructed sections of a phantom. In theory, there is little doubt that rotating gamma camera tomography is superior since it provides a complete set of information to define uniquely the distribution of activity.[37] This fact, however, does not prevent limited-angle tomography from contributing clinically significant information.

When applied to myocardial imaging, the unique geometry of the left ventricle and the symmetrical data sampling with respect to the long axis allow RSH tomography to define the distribution of activity quite well. It is also not clear whether the improved depth resolution offered by rotating camera tomography is necessary in the clinical situation. One possibility is that the contraction of the left ventricle might work against the gain in depth resolution. In the nonresearch situation an additional factor must be considered, that is, the cost-benefit ratio for myocardial imaging with the rotating camera as compared to the RSH collimator methods. The cost should include the time involved in data acquisition and processing as well as the cost of hardware and software. When applied to large organs, such as the liver, the RSH collimator methods probably have little clinical utility since there would be a great deal of activity outside the CV resulting in poor depth resolution and possible artifacts.

The future of RSH tomography may come from improved software algorithms; that is unlikely, however, to solve the limited angle sampling and attenuation problems.[51] Hybrid systems may be developed which exploit the desirable characteristics of both the RSH collimator and rotating camera methods. Koral et al.[42] simulated ECT of the left ventricle using a RSH collimator and two camera positions. This resulted in superior results when compared to the single camera position method, except when attenuation correction was attempted.

A statement from "Perspectives on Tomography" by John Keyes[52] is appropriate to RSH tomography: "SPECT is neither renaissance nor nonsense. It is a technique that will enhance many of the things that we do in nuclear medicine, but it is certainly not going to revolutionize the field in the same way that X-ray CT changed the field of radiography."

REFERENCES

1. **Andrews, J. R.,** Planigraphy. I. Introduction and history, *Am. J. Roentgenol.,* 36, 575, 1936.
2. **Kuhl, D. E. and Edwards, R. Q.,** Image separation radioisotope scanning, *Radiology,* 80, 653, 1963.
3. **Anger, H. O.,** Multiplane tomography gamma-ray scanner, in *Medical Radioisotope Scintigraphy,* Vol. 1, International Atomic Energy Agency, Vienna, 1969, 203.
4. **Freedman, G. S.,** Tomography with a gamma camera, *J. Nucl. Med.,* 11, 602, 1970.
5. **Muehllehner, G.,** A tomographic scintillation camera, *Phys. Med. Biol.,* 16, 87, 1971.
6. **Freedman, G. S.,** Gamma camera tomography — preliminary clinical experience, *Radiology,* 102, 365, 1972.
7. **Chamroenngan, S., Langan, J. K., Tratter, R. T., et al.,** Tomographic imaging with the scintillation camera in the detection and characterization of brain lesions, *Radiology,* 98, 445, 1971.
8. **Deland, F. H., James, E. A., Muehllenhner, G., et al.,** The value of tomography in liver scanning, *Radiology,* 102, 429, 1972.
9. **Freedman, G. S.,** Digital gamma camera tomography — theory, in *Tomographic Imaging in Nuclear Medicine,* Freedman, G. S., Ed., Society of Nuclear Medicine, New York, 1973, 68.
10. **Kuhl, D. E., Edwards, R. Q., Ricci, A. R., et al.,** The Mark IV system for radionuclide computed tomography of the brain, *Radiology,* 121, 405, 1976.
11. **Jaszczak, R. J., Murphy, P. H., Huard, D., et al.,** Radionuclide emission computed tomography of the head with Tc-99m and a scintillation camera, *J. Nucl. Med.,* 18, 373, 1977.
12. **Keyes, J. W., Orlandea, N., Heetderks, W. J., et al.,** The Humongotron-A scintillation camera transaxial tomography, *J. Nucl. Med.,* 18, 381, 1977.
13. **Vogel, R. A., Kirch, D., Lefree, M., et al.,** A new method of multiplanar tomography using a seven pinhole collimator and an Anger scintillation camera, *J. Nucl. Med.,* 19, 648, 1978.
14. **Vogel, R. A., Kirch, D. L., Lefree, M., et al.,** Thallium-201 myocardial perfusion scintigraphy: results of standard and multi-pinhole tomographic techniques, *Am. J. Cardiol.,* 43, 787, 1979.
15. **Rizi, H. R., Kline, R. C., Thrall, J. H., et al.,** Thallium-201 myocardial scintigraphy: a critical comparison of seven-pinhole tomography and conventional planar imaging, *J. Nucl. Med.,* 22, 493, 1981.
16. **Gottschalk, S. C., Smith, K. A., and Wake, R. H.,** Tomographic reconstructions with rotating slant-hole and seven-pinhole collimators on an Anger gamma camera phantom and clinical studies, in Emission Computed Tomography, No. 81-177, Paras, P. and Eikman, E., Eds., Food and Drug Administration, Rockville, MD, 1981, 105.
17. **Nalcioglu, O., Morton, M. E., and Milne, N.,** Computerized longitudinal tomography (CLT) with a bilateral collimator, *IEEE Trans. Nucl. Sci.,* NS-27, 430, 1980.

18. **Chang, W., Lin, S. L., and Kenkin, R. E.**, A rotatable quadrant slant-hole collimator for tomography (QSH), in *SPECT and Other Selected Computer Topics*, Sorenson, F. A., Ed., Society of Nuclear Medicine, New York, 1980, 81.
19. **Nalcioglu, O., Milne, N., and Morton, M. E.**, Performance of the BICLET system, in *Single Photon Emission Computed Tomography and Other Selected Computer Topics*, Sorenson, J. A., Ed., Society of Nuclear Medicine, New York, 1980, 73.
20. **Ratib, O., Henze, E., Hoffman, E., et al.**, Performance of the rotating slant-hole collimator for the detection of myocardial perfusion abnormalities, *J. Nucl. Med.*, 23, 34, 1982.
21. **Chang, W., Lin, S. L., and Henkin, R. E.**, Multisegmental collimator tomography: comparison of the system performance of the 7-pinhole and quadrant slant-hole collimators, in Emission Computed Tomography: The Single Photon Approach, Paras, P. and Eikman, E., Eds., No. 81-177, Food and Drug Administration, Rockville, MD, 1981, 65.
22. **Chang, W., Lin, S. L., and Henkin, R. E.**, A comparison of the performance parameters of the 7-pinhole collimator and the quadrant slant-hole collimator (QSH), in *SPECT and Other Selected Computer Topics*, Sorenson, F. A., Ed., Society of Nuclear Medicine, New York, 1980, 113.
23. **Freedman, G. S.**, Gamma camera tomography, *Radiology*, 102, 365, 1972.
24. **Muehllehner, G.**, Performance parameters for a tomographic scintillation camera, in *Tomographic Imaging in Nuclear Medicine*, Freedman, G. S., Ed., Society of Nuclear Medicine, New York, 1973, 76.
25. **Freedman, G. S.**, Clinical experience with a digital gamma camera tomography, in *Tomographic Imaging in Nuclear Medicine*, Freedman, G. S., Ed., Society of Nuclear Medicine, New York, 1973, 220.
26. **Freedman, G. S.**, Gamma camera tomography — preliminary clinical experience, *J. Nucl. Med.*, 12, 433, 1971.
27. **Chang, W., Lin, S. L., and Henkin, R. E.**, N-spot focal plane tomography in cardiac imaging, in *Functional Mapping of Organ Systems*, Esser, P. D., Ed., Society of Nuclear Medicine, New York, 1980, 185.
28. **James, A. E., Langan, J. K., Fisher, C. H., et al.**, Clinical experience in tomographic imaging with a tomocamera, in *Tomographic Imaging in Nuclear Medicine*, Freedman, G. S., Ed., Society of Nuclear Medicine, New York, 1973, 206.
29. **Goldsmith, S. J.**, Clinical artifacts encountered using circular tomography, in *Tomographic Imaging in Nuclear Medicine*, Freedman, G. S., Ed., Society of Nuclear Medicine, New York, 1973, 229.
30. **Lewis, S. E., Stokely, E. M., Devous, M. D., et al.**, Qualitation of experimental canine infarct size with multipinhole and rotating slanthole tomography, *J. Nucl. Med.*, 22, 1000, 1981.
31. **Herfkens, R. J., Shosa, D. W., Hattner, R. S., et al.**, Clinical applications of rotating slant-hole tomography to cardiovascular nuclear medicine, *J. Nucl. Med.*, 31(Abst.), 70, 1980.
32. **Shosa, D. W., O'Connell, J. W., and Hattner, R. S.**, Motivation for the rotating slant-hole approach to scintillation camera tomography, *J. Nucl. Med.*, 21(Abst.), 27, 1980.
33. **Milne, N., Nalcioglu, O., and Morton, M. E.**, BICLET: preliminary clinical results, in Emission Computed Tomography, Paras, P. and Eikman, E., Eds., No. 81-177, Food and Drug Administration, Rockville, MD, 1981, 105.
34. **Lasher, J. C., Blumhardt, R., Kopp, D. T., et al.**, Emission computed tomography: versatile limited angle software, in *Emission Computed Tomography: Current Trends*, Esser, P. D., Ed., Society of Nuclear Medicine, New York, 1983, 211.
35. **Weiland, F. L., Lasher, J. C., Uhl, G. S., et al.**, Bilateral emission scintislice tomography (BEST), in *Nuclear Medicine and Biology*, Proceedings of the Third World Congress of Nuclear Medicine and Biology, Paris, 1982, 3029.
36. **Rosen, P. R., Lasher, J. C., Weiland, F. L., et al.**, Predicting splenic abnormality in Hodgkin disease using volume response to epinephrine administration, *Radiology*, 143, 627, 1982.
37. **Chang, W., Lin, S. L., and Henkin, R. E.**, A new collimator for cardiac tomography: the quadrant slant-hole collimator, *J. Nucl. Med.*, 23, 830, 1982.
38. **Henkin, R. E., Chang, W., Salo, B. C., et al.**, Gamma camera tomography with multisegmental collimators: applications to Tl-201 and gated blood pool imaging, in Emission Computed Tomography: The Single Photon Approach, No. 81-177, Food and Drug Administration, Rockville, MD, 1981, 82.
39. **Chang, W., Henkin, R. E., Lin, S. L., et al.**, Chamber volume determination using a 4-quadrant slant-hole tomographic system, *J. Nucl. Med.*, 21(Abst.), 28, 1980.
40. **Myers, M. J., Sokole, E. B., and Bakker, J.**, A comparison of rotating slant-hole collimator and rotating camera for single photon emission tomography of the heart, *Phys. Med. Biol.*, 28, 581, 1983.
41. **Budinger, T. F. and Gullberg, G. T.**, Three-dimensional reconstruction in nuclear medicine emission imaging, *IEEE Trans. Nucl. Sci.*, NS-21, 2, 1974.
42. **Koral, K. F., Nolder, C., Ciliax, G., et al.**, Simulated ECT of the left ventricule using rotating slant-hole collimator and two camera positions, *J. Nucl. Med.*, 25, 343, 1984.
43. **Sorenson, J. A. and Phelps, M. E., Eds.**, *Physics in Nuclear Medicine*, Grune & Stratton, New York, 1980, 295.

44. **Chiu, M. Y., Barrett, H. H., Simpson, R. G., et al.,** Three-dimensional radiographic imaging with a restricted view angle, *J. Opt. Soc. Am.,* 69, 1323, 1979.
45. Tomography (ECT), in *Emission Computed Tomography: Current Trends,* Esser, P. D., Ed., Society of Nuclear Medicine, New York, 1983, 3.
46. **Chang, W. and Henkin, R. E.,** Performance of the rotating slant-hole collimator for the detection of myocardial perfusion abnormalities (letter), *J. Nucl. Med.,* 23(6), 547, 1982.
47. **Henkin, R. E., Hale, D. J., Salo, B. C., et al.,** Seven pinhole tomography: is it worth it?, *J. Nucl. Med.,* 21(Abst.), 69, 1980.
48. **Royal, H. D., Parker, A. J., and Kolodny, G. M.,** Noncardiac, nontomographic applications of the slant-hole collimator: concise communication, *J. Nucl. Med.,* 23, 786, 1982.
49. **Parker, J. A., Uren, R. F., Jones, A. G., et al.,** Radionuclide left ventriculography with the slant-hole collimator, *J. Nucl. Med.,* 18, 848, 1977.
50. **Ohtake, E., Ilo, M., Toyama, H., et al.,** Internal mammary lymphoscintigraphy using bilateral collimator: measurement of the depth of lymph node, *J. Nucl. Med.,* 21(Abst.), 82, 1980.
51. **Stokely, E. M., Parkey, R. W., Lewis, S. E., et al.,** Myocardial infarction imaging with single-photon emission computed tomography, in Emission Computed Tomography: The Single Photon Approach, No. 81-177, Food and Drug Administration, Rockville, MD, 1981, 53.
52. **Keyes, J. W.,** Perspectives on tomography, *J. Nucl. Med.,* 23, 633, 1982.

Chapter 9

SEVEN-PINHOLE TOMOGRAPHY IN NUCLEAR MEDICINE

U. Raff, D. L. Kirch, and W. R. Hendee

TABLE OF CONTENTS

I. INTRODUCTION

Among all tomographic techniques developed in the past decade, multiple-pinhole tomography using seven simultaneous views of the organ as separate images viewed from different angles has had the greatest clinical impact. This technique was initially designed for ^{201}Tl quantitation of myocardial perfusion and was restricted initially to applications in cardiovascular nuclear medicine. More recently, various noncardiac applications have emerged; however, their impact upon clinical nuclear medicine has been reduced by the introduction of rotating scintillation cameras, which offer more complete angular sampling. These commercially available single-photon emission computed tomography (SPECT) systems have facilitated extension of emission tomography to large organs. For small organ tomography, the seven-pinhole technique is still one of the more efficient tomographic procedures from technical, computational, and economic points of view.[1,2]

Seven-pinhole tomography has been commercially developed and widely used for myocardial perfusion and gated blood-pool studies. For satisfactory studies, careful clinical preparation of the patient is required. Various authors[3-7] have discussed the benefits and limitations of seven-pinhole systems.

A similar approach to SPECT using a four-pinhole collimator has been described by Stokely et al.[8] Lead separations were used in the same fashion as in seven-pinhole to provide nonmultiplexed data. An iterative deblurring algorithm based on work by Tomitani et al.[9] was applied to the backprojected reconstructions. An overview of the "physical attributes of single photon tomography" is available in Budinger's article.[10]

II. ASPECTS OF SEVEN-PINHOLE TOMOGRAPHY

A. Overview

Seven-pinhole tomography is the least complicated and least expensive approach to SPECT for evaluation of myocardial perfusion and left ventricular function. Static tomographic imaging and tomographic gated studies are easily performed.[11] Tomographic reconstructions from seven-pinhole images can be obtained with only the expense of a simple collimator and software accessories to any state of the art scintillation camera interfaced to a standard nuclear medicine computer. Hence the seven-pinhole approach provides an inexpensive alternative to the purchase of a rotating camera for smaller institutions desiring to add SPECT to their clinical capability.

Problems associated with ^{201}Tl uptake and washout[12] impose certain restrictions on myocardial planar imaging; for example, the required poststress imaging time of 30 to 40 min is a major limitation for optimal stress studies. The recommended injected activity of less than 3 mCi of ^{201}TlCl, and the low sensitivity of high resolution parallel-hole collimators, are the major reasons why 30 to 40 min are required for planar imaging. With the seven-pinhole approach, an interval of only 15 min is required for evaluation of ^{201}Tl myocardial perfusion.

The detection of ischemic areas in myocardial tissue using three to five planar views depends largely on the angle at which the views are obtained. Quantitative analysis of relative ^{201}Tl uptake in stress and redistribution phases requires a demanding computer analysis which is time consuming compared to the short processing times required by the seven-pinhole algorithm implemented by Stern[13] on most commercial nuclear medicine computers.

Dynamic flow and gated blood-pool acquisitions can be easily performed with the seven-pinhole technique, as long as sufficient computer memory is available for multiple 128 $\times$ 128-byte mode images. This amount of memory allows any view of the ventricle specified by the user to be reconstructed from a set of images acquired under a fixed left anterior oblique (LAO) position of the camera-collimator system. The advantages of seven-pinhole tomography for myocardial perfusion studies are accompanied by requirements for exacting technical control. These requirements have produced some reluctance to accept the diagnostic utility of the seven-pinhole approach to tomography.

Seven-pinhole imaging of the myocardium yields enhanced image contrast compared to planar imaging; this characteristic has caused some clinical researchers to regard the seven-pinhole approach as essentially an enhancement technique. On the other hand, the majority of clinical reports on seven-pinhole thallium imaging emphasize the benefits of reproducible quantitative information provided by this technique.

Two types of spatial distortion appear in the reconstructed images from the seven-pinhole, limited-angle, tomographic technique (54° between opposite pinhole views for cardiac-imaging collimators). In the first type of image distortion, the resolution within each transaxial slice varies from plane to plane at different depths. These resolution characteristics tend to overestimate activity toward the base of the myocardium; toward the apex, the resolution is better because the activity is closer to the pinhole collimator. In other words, tomographic sections far from the pinhole collimator show significant loss in spatial resolution. The second type of distortion is a longitudinal propagation of certain image details (e.g., ischemic areas) into planes above and below the one under consideration. The extent of this problem depends on the distance from the pinhole collimator and on the angle separating the outer views. Variation in magnification associated with pinhole images is a minor problem because the reconstruction software package can correct this effect (Figure 1).[12]

The success of seven-pinhole myocardial studies depends largely on patient preparation and on the protocol followed during the procedures.[14,15] Seven-pinhole tomography must be conducted with great care to ensure that no time is lost once the patient has been stressed and injected. Patient positioning must be done very carefully. This step is the most difficult and is often mentioned as one of the major technical demands of the seven-pinhole technique. Trained personnel can easily accommodate the challenge presented by the positioning procedure. Scheduling of patients should be done in advance to facilitate proper setup and calibration of the instrumentation (Figure 2).

The following aspects of patient preparation should be followed closely:

1. The breasts of female patients should be flattened against the chest with an elastic rib belt or bandage to minimize the amount of absorptive tissue.
2. To minimize stomach activity and gut uptake, the patient should have fasted for 2 h prior to injection.
3. The patient should be injected in an upright position to prevent lung uptake and be kept in this position until data acquisition is begun.
4. A total activity of 2 to 3 mCi $^{201}TlCl$ should be used to keep the imaging and positioning times as short as possible.
5. If clinically advisable, the patient should be removed from treatment with beta-blocking or vasodilating medications.

B. Stress ^{201}Tl Data Acquisition

Ischemic heart conditions are most easily detected under some form of exercise; hence, the patient should be adequately stressed just before imaging. The most common stress procedure is to use a graded treadmill device located close to the imaging room. The highest accuracy for detecting myocardial ischemia has been obtained by bringing the patient gradually to a state of physical exhaustion and/or typical pain symptoms under medical supervision. After injection of ^{201}Tl, the exercise procedure should be conducted for at least two additional minutes unless contraindicated by the patient's physical condition. Imaging should start within the next 10 min. A single 128 × 128 seven-pinhole image of 750,000 counts total is then acquired (Figure 2). Data acquisition is repeated approximately 2 to 4 h later

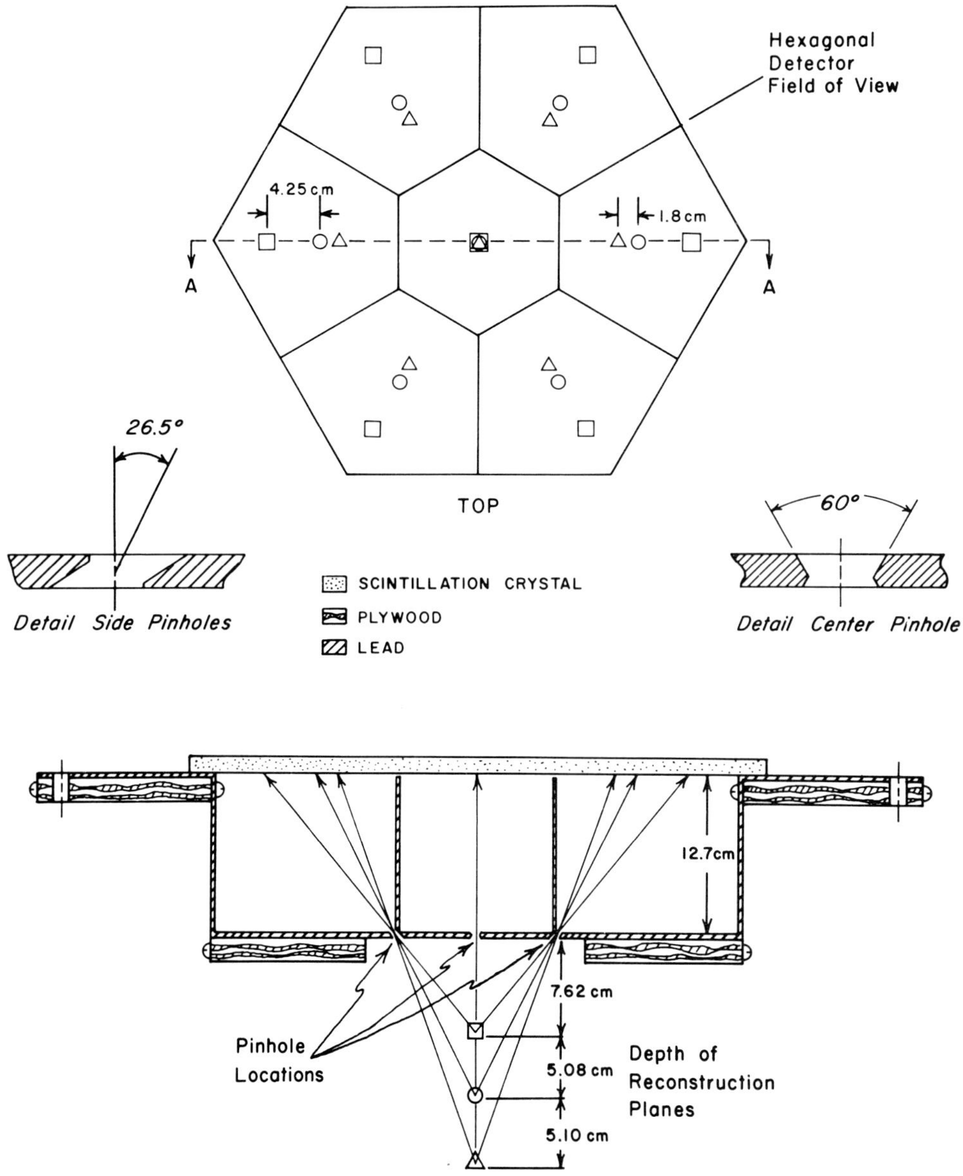

FIGURE 1. Seven-pinhole geometry; cross-sectional view through original large-field-of-view seven-pinhole collimator design.

at the stage of redistribution. The same data collection criteria are used for the redistribution image.

C. Seven-Pinhole Imaging Procedures

1. A solid ^{195}Au sheet source (half-life: 183 d; energies: 98.8 and 129.4 keV) is used to acquire the flood image and point-source calibration file. The camera is then repeaked for ^{201}Tl using a 40% asymmetric window over the 83 keV peak and a 15% window setting over the 167.4 keV peak. Peaking should be performed with the patient and the high-sensitivity seven-pinhole collimator in place.
2. The camera is placed initially in a 35% LAO orientation and the cephalad angulation

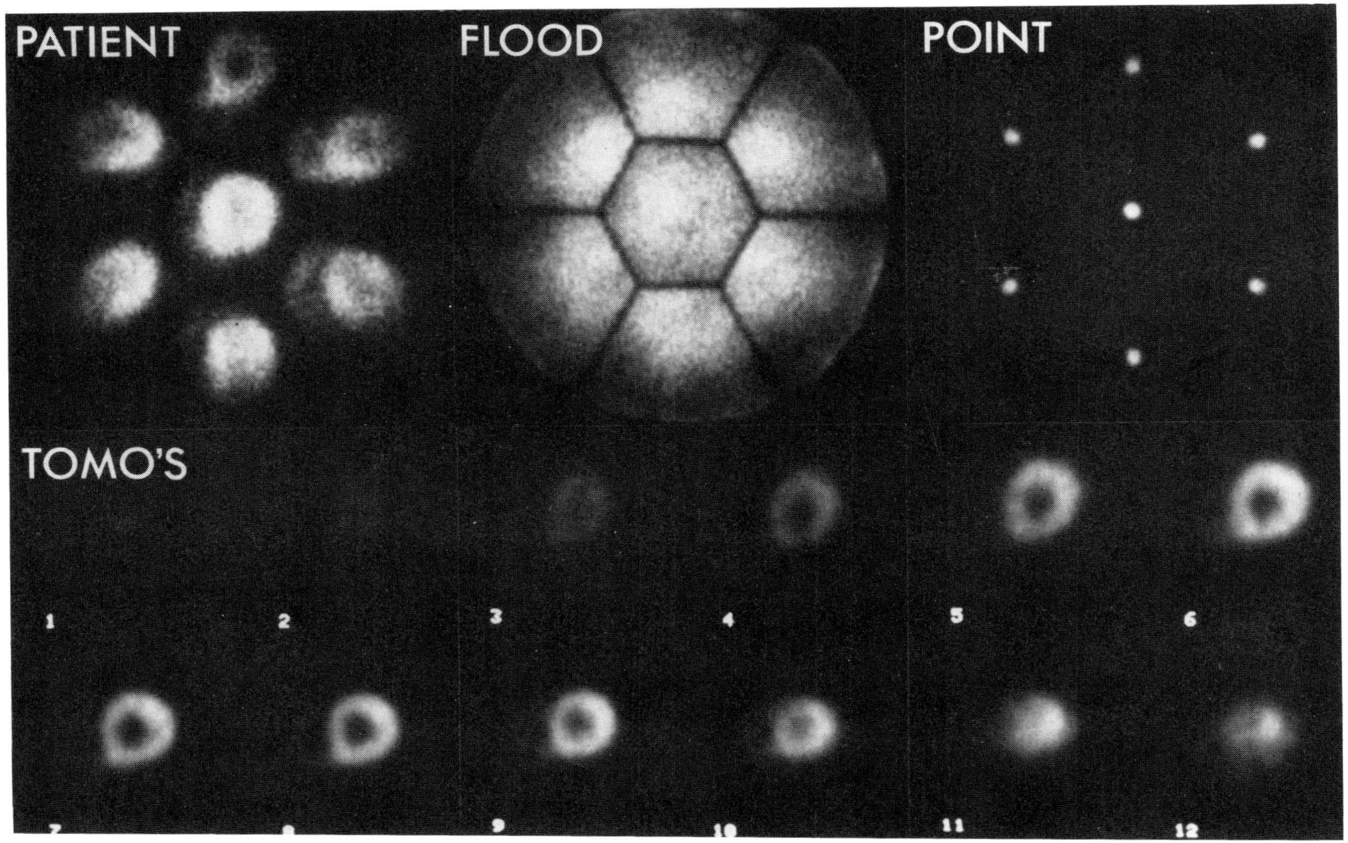

FIGURE 2. The top panel shows from left to right the original patient raw image, the calibration flood and point source images. The bottom panel shows 12 reconstructed tomographic slices perpendicular to the long axis of the left ventricle of a normal patient.

achieved by swinging the feet toward the camera stand, with the collimator as close as possible to the patient's chest. Special software can be used to monitor the positioning on the video display. The myocardium should be centered in the central view. The distance between the heart and the pinhole collimator is adjusted to center the outer six views in their respective sectors; this procedure will prevent clipping at the inner or outer sector margins.

3. After identifying the most circular view in the central sector (corresponding to alignment of the central pinhole with the longitudinal axis of the left ventricle (LV), the caudal patient angulation (foot swing) can also be adapted for individuals presenting cardiac anatomy that is oriented more vertically.
4. The patient file should be reviewed to verify proper positioning after collection of raw data. A positioning light source should be used to mark reference points on the patient's chest to facilitate positioning for the redistribution study. (Good vs. bad positioning, see Figures 3 and 4.)

D. Reconstruction Technique

A complete technical description of a seven-pinhole tomography system is available in Kirch et al.[16] The calibration flood and point-source data files are first processed by calibration software and are saved in mass storage for future use in the reconstruction of each individual patient study. Seven-pinhole data can be processed either by the simultaneous iterative reconstruction technique (SIRT)[17] to obtain multiple slices through the myocardium or by the minimum-impedance estimate first introduced by Kirch et al.[16] The latter algorithm computes first-estimate planes as an initial approximation of planes oriented parallel to the face of the camera at different depths. The first estimates are then modified by applying corrections from error planes obtained by comparing the ray-summed views to the original image data. Finally, tomographic planes are obtained corresponding to transaxial slices perpendicular to the longitudinal axis of the LV. The total depth of reconstruction ranges from 7 to 25 cm, and the slice thickness ranges from 0.75 to 2.5 cm. Examples of tomographic slices for stress and redistribution imaging are shown in Figure 5. With the impedance-estimator algorithm, processing time on a standard PDP11/34A minicomputer is less than 2 min for a complete set of tomographic sections.[13] The lead sectors of the seven-pinhole collimator prevent adjacent image projections from multiplexing (overlapping); hence, seven-pinhole projections are easier to process than are data acquired by other techniques. The processing time is significantly reduced compared to other coded aperture techniques where encoded multiplexed data must be decoded using time consuming algorithms.

Stress ^{201}Tl seven-pinhole tomography has been shown by Vogel et al.[18,19] to be a useful, noninvasive technique for detecting ischemic heart disease. In most reported studies, multipinhole tomography yields increased sensitivity for coronary artery disease (CAD) assessment with no loss in specificity compared to planar imaging. Resolution characteristics and weaknesses of the method are discussed by Williams et al.[4] In spite of its technical limitations, the seven-pinhole technique has several clinical advantages over other techniques. Besides the short imaging time (ideal for stress ^{201}Tl studies), qualitative visual interpretation and quantitative reproducibility of seven-pinhole myocardial tomograms are easily accomplished.

Because of improved contrast and reduced background activity, tomographic image interpretation is relatively easy compared to planar imaging. A relative lack of perfusion in ischemic areas is most likely to be detected when the collimator face is perpendicular to the long axis of the LV; otherwise, false positive perfusion defects may be observed. Insufficient LAO camera angulation results in decreased activity in the posterior wall in apical sections and in the anterior wall for most central and basal sections. Insufficient cephalad angulation produces decreased activity inferiorly in apical regions and superiorly in central and basal slices. The converse is observed for excessive LAO and cephalad angulation. In most

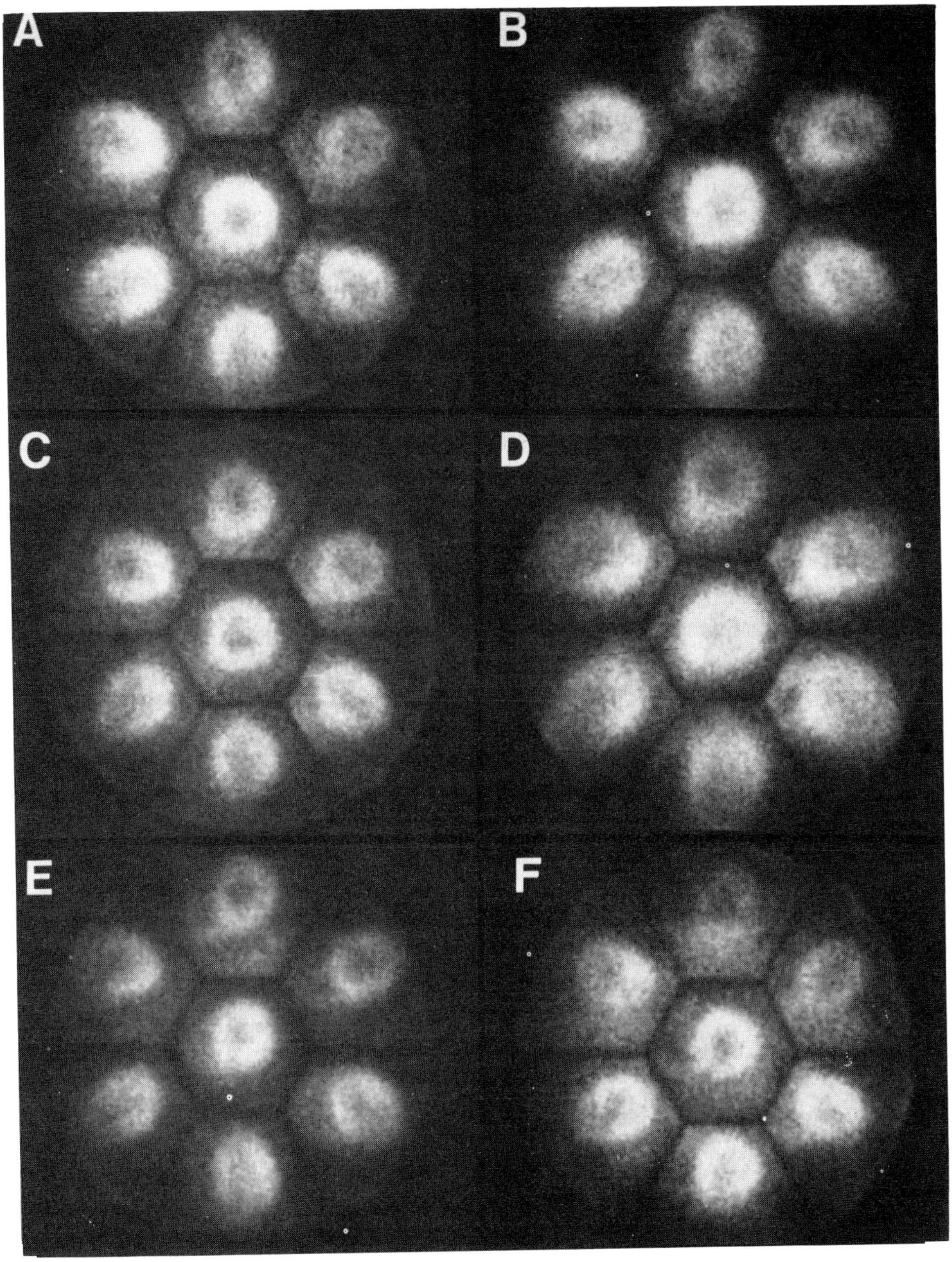

FIGURE 3. Acceptable seven-pinhole collimator positioning. (A) Excellent. (B) Excellent. (C) The patient is positioned slightly too far from the collimator, with the result that the outer cardiac views are positioned slightly centrally within their respective fields-of-view. (D) The patient is positioned slightly too close to the collimator, with the result that the outer cardiac views are positioned very near the periphery of their respective fields-of-view. (E) Two acceptable positioning variations are demonstrated by this scintigram. First, slightly too much caudal camera angulation is present, causing the upper cardiac image to be more annular in appearance than is the lower image. This is a common occurrence, especially in individuals with vertical hearts. Since the center cardiac image is the most annular of the seven, this scintigram is judged acceptable. Second, the patient is positioned slightly off center (high in the central and upper fields-of-view). (F) Somewhat excessive attenuation of the upper field-of-view is present. In this male patient, this is likely due to rib absorption. In female patients, the breast can cause similar problems and may necessitate retraction or compression. All of these seven-pinhole scintigrams will result in tomograms and quantitative data of high reliability and diagnostic certainty, despite their minor positioning imperfections. (Reprinted with permission from New England Nuclear and Picker Corp., A Pictorial Guide to Seven-Pinhole Tomographic Thallium-201 Scintigraphy, 1980.)

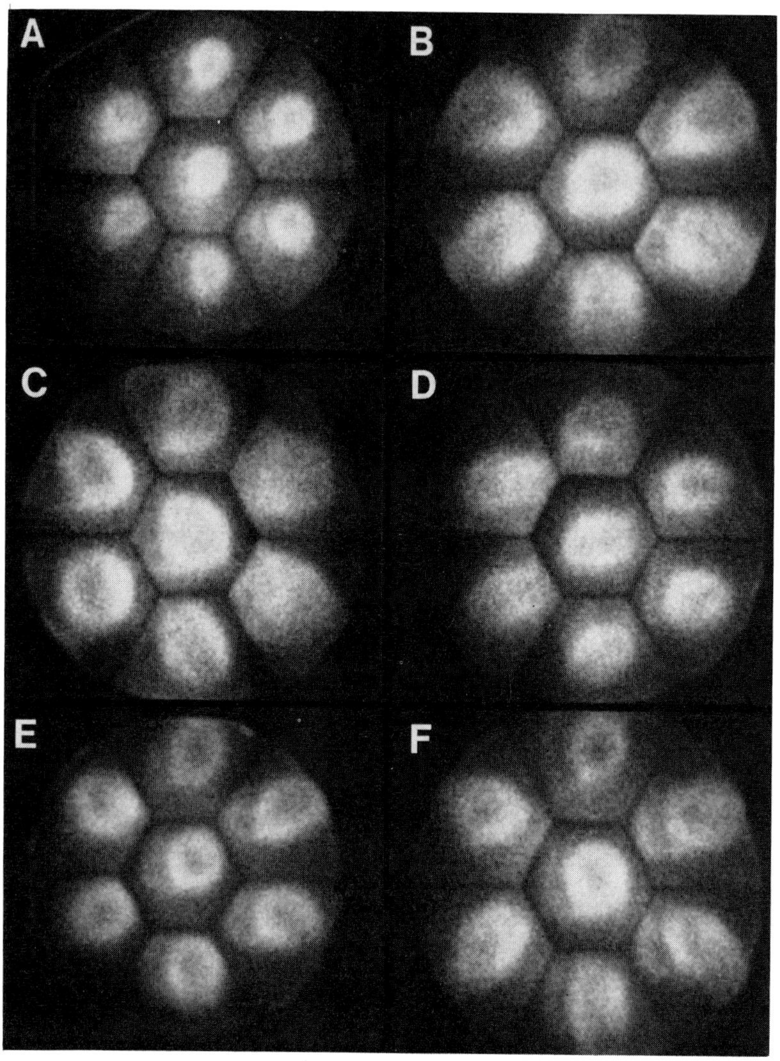

FIGURE 4. Unacceptable seven-pinhole collimator positioning. In each case, only the most predominate positioning fault is noted. (A) The patient is too far from the collimator, resulting in small, centrally positioned outer cardiac images. The patient needs to be moved closer to the collimator. (B) The patient is positioned too close to the collimator, resulting in large cardiac images which are cut off by the peripheral limits of the outer fields-of-view. The patient needs to be moved farther from the collimator. (C) The camera is angulated too anteriorly, resulting in maximum annularity of the two leftward cardiac images. The camera needs to be angulated more LAO, i.e., in a more lateral angle. (D) The camera is angulated too LAO, resulting in maximum annularity of the two rightward cardiac images. The camera needs to be angulated less LAO, i.e., more anteriorly. (E) The patient is positioned off center, resulting in a portion of the cardiac images being cut off by the edge of the fields-of-view. The patient needs to be positioned more centrally. (F) The camera was angulated too caudally, resulting in the upper cardiac images having the most annular appearance. The camera should be angulated more cephalad, i.e., aimed more upward toward the patient's head. In thin patients with vertical hearts, proper correction of this problem cannot always be achieved. For such cases, some degree of excessive caudal angulation can be tolerated if the consequences of a regional reduction in inferoapical activity are understood (see Figure 3). None of the above seven-pinhole scintigrams will yield reliable data. Repositioning should be undertaken as soon as these problems are discovered. (Reprinted with permission from New England Nuclear and Picker Corp., A Pictorial Guide to Seven-Pinhole Tomographic Thallium-201 Scintigraphy, 1980.)

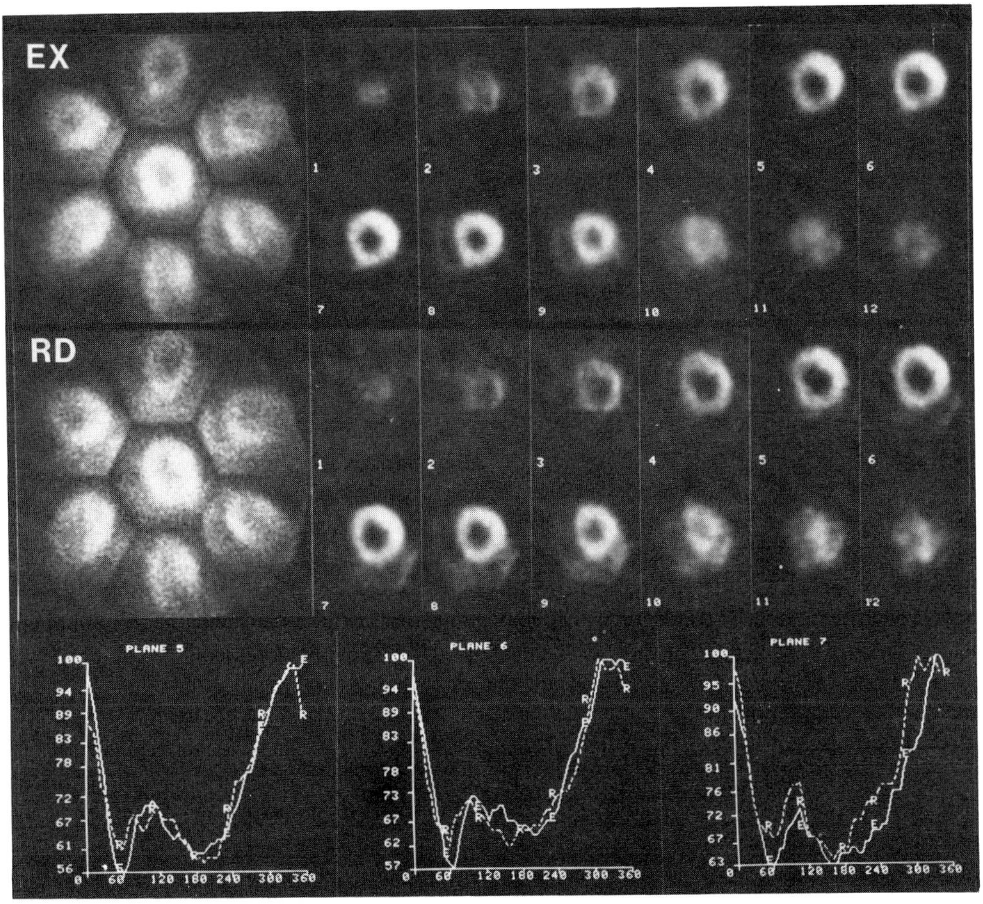

FIGURE 5. Positioning: The camera is angulated slightly too caudally, but acceptably. More caudal angulation is observed in the delayed study (RD). Central plane: 6. (Sections cutting through the cardiac cavity: 3—9.) Quantitative regional activity: Inferiorly and anteriorly, regional activity is at this institution's lower limits of normal. Redistribution: No significant redistribution seen. Pattern recognition: Normal pattern. Inferior regional (especially at the apex) activity is often reduced in circumstances of insufficient cephalad camera angulation; sometimes anteroseptal regional activity is also reduced. Impression: Normal. Certainty of impression: Low. (Reprinted with permission from New England Nuclear and Picker Corp., A Pictorial Guide to Seven-Pinhole Tomographic Thallium-201 Scintigraphy, 1980.)

transaxial sections of the normal LV, maximum activity is observed in the upperright quadrant corresponding to the posterior papillary muscle of the LV. In general, reduced activity in this region of the myocardium can be considered abnormal. In apical sections, decreased activity is observed in the inferior wall corresponding to the normal apical defect. In central sections the septum shows less activity than the free left ventricular wall, primarily because of differences in γ-ray absorption by left and right blood pools. Toward the base the interpretation of transaxial slices is difficult because of excessive blurring and because of the complex anatomy starting at the aortic valve plane. Motion is also a factor affecting interpretation of more apical planes. Normal and abnormal ^{201}Tl tomograms are shown in Figures 5 and 6, respectively.

Seven-pinhole tomography has succeeded mainly because of its ability to provide the clinician with an elegant approach to quantifying CAD in patients with myocardial ischemia or with a remote myocardial infarct. ^{201}Tl tomograms have been standardized by semiquantitative analysis in terms of relative activities circumferentially around the myocardial slices.[19]

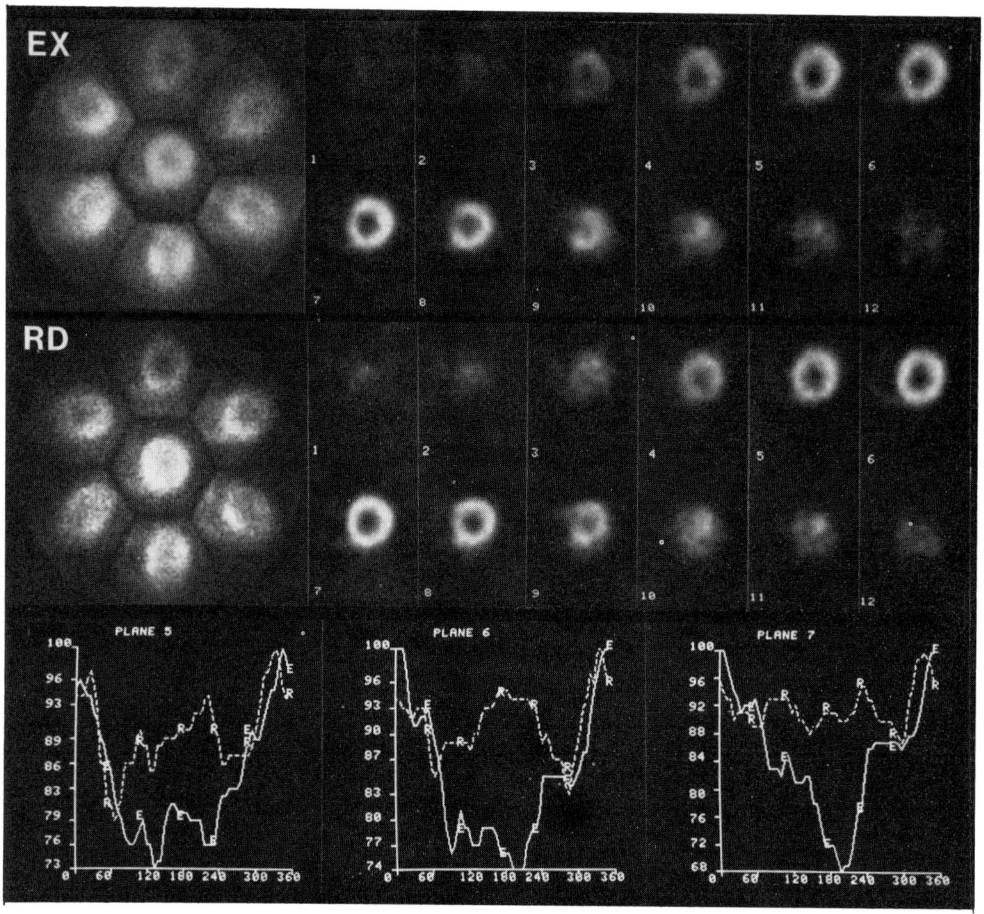

FIGURE 6. Positioning: Somewhat excessive attenuation is seen in the upper view; acceptable. Repositioning is very similar. Central plane: 6. Quantitative regional activity: All regions are well above the lower normal limit regional activity levels. Redistribution: Up to 23% increase in activity is seen during the redistributional period in the anterior region. Pattern recognition: Normal except for redistribution. Impression: Abnormal, anteroseptal regional ischemia. Certainty of impression: Moderate. (Reprinted with permission from New England Nuclear and Picker Corp., A Pictorial Guide to Seven-Pinhole Tomographic Thallium-201 Scintigraphy, 1980.)

The severity of cardiac disease can be evaluated by quantitative comparison of stress and redistribution patterns of regional perfusion. Visually detected inhomogeneities in the distribution of ^{201}Tl can be assessed in different ways. The most common technique is quantitation by circumferential profiles of maximum activities. This approach displays the maximum relative regional activity as a function of angular location. The circumferential profile technique, often described as "circle analysis", can be applied to any transaxial plane of the LV, as long as there is some annular myocardial activity detectable. By convention, the regional activity is plotted at 6° intervals in a clockwise fashion starting at a 3 o'clock position (Figure 7). Correspondence between the LV anatomy and the angle is given by:

0° or 360° = Posterolateral wall

90° = Inferior wall

180° = Anterior septal wall

270° = Superior wall

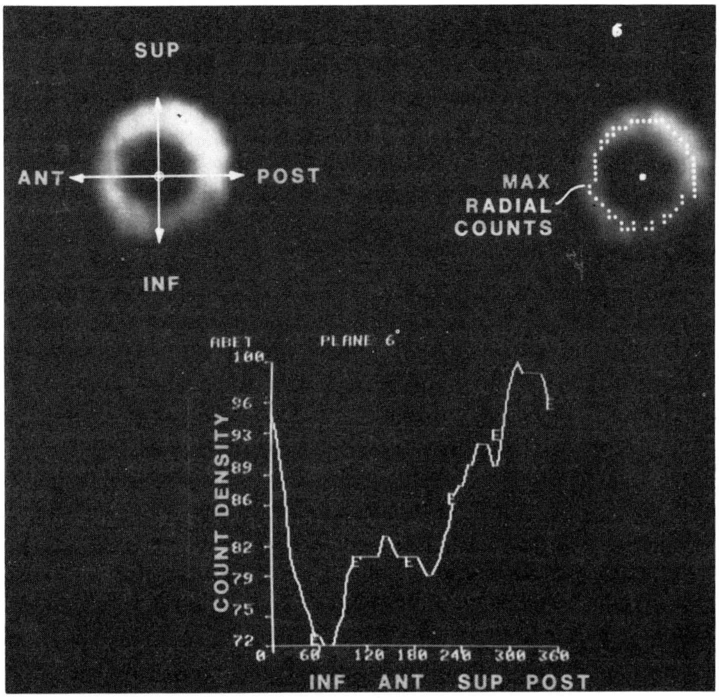

FIGURE 7. Upper left tomogram shows the location of superior (SUP), postero-lateral (POST), inferior (INF), and anterior (ANT) walls of the left ventricle. The upper right view displays the hottest pixels found in a radial search around the tomographic slice through the left ventricle. Lower panel shows the maximum relative regional activity as a function of angular location starting at a three o'clock position (0°). The curve corresponds to a clockwise rotation around the annular myocardial slice.

The regional activity curve obtained from the highest pixel values in this radial search is plotted in either absolute values or after normalization where the highest pixel value is set to 100%. So long as the absolute uptake of radiotracer is not of importance, the latter method is advantageous because it allows the generation of quantitative ranges for normal patients from both stress and redistribution patterns. In general, the three to eight most centrally located slices through the LV are used. One major difficulty is the large amount of data generated for each patient when eight sections are included in the studies. Circumferential analysis makes it difficult to integrate all of the available information and, therefore, sometimes complicates the diagnostic interpretation.

The concentric polar profile plot (CPP plot) has been introduced to overcome problems with circle analysis. According to Johnson et al.,[20] plotting the regional activity as a Cartesian function of angle does not help ease the correlation of the curves with the anatomy of the myocardium, because the observer has to associate the displayed curves mentally with the myocardial sections. In the CPP approach, up to eight circumferential profiles are assembled to facilitate diagnostic interpretation. The plot consists of a set of concentric rings in which the information from circle analysis, as described earlier, is mapped onto polar coordinates. Each data point to be plotted is labeled with a number corresponding to the myocardial section (depth information) and the angle at which the regional activity was measured. Temporal relations for tomographic ^{201}Tl stress and redistribution studies are very important. Profiles are generated for exercise (E) and redistribution (R) counts, and the ratios R/E for corresponding locations are plotted for a single tomographic plane as shown in Figure 8A. Individual rings in the CPP plot are scaled arbitrarily from an inner boundary of 0.6 to an

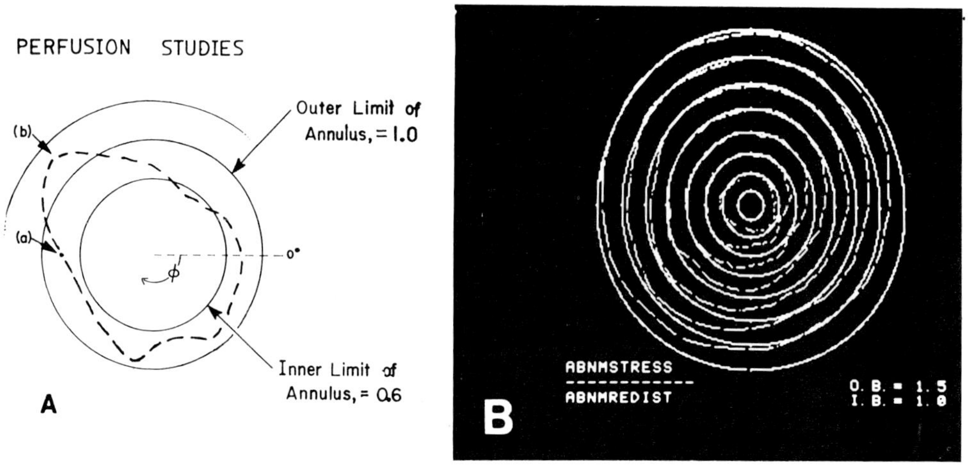

FIGURE 8. Regional redistribution changes of ^{201}Tl uptake. Changes in redistribution are generated with profile arrays for exercise (E) and redistribution (R) studies determining the ratios of counts for corresponding points. Figure 8A shows the ratio (R/E) for a single tomographic slice. The radial position at which a given ratio is plotted is determined by scaling the ring width linearly from an inner boundary of 0.6 to an outer boundary of 2.0 for the display of (R/E) curves. Figure 8B shows the ratios (E/R) (abnormal stress/abnormal redistribution) for eight consecutive slices through the left ventricle. Note that in this case inner boundary (I.B.) and outer boundary (O.B.) are arbitrarily set to 1.0 and 1.5, respectively. Regions of significant redistribution associated with ischemic tissue are indicated by inward bulges on the curve. Patient had abnormal tomograms. Posterolateral-inferior ischemia can be observed.

outer boundary of 1.0, as shown in Figure 8A, or from an inner boundary of 1.0 to an outer boundary of 1.5 for the ratio E/R. A single CPP plot displays a set of curves describing the relative changes of radiotracer concentration between R and E for up to eight myocardial sections. If a region has experienced significant redistribution associated with ischemia, the ratios R/E greater than or equal to 1 will appear as inward sags of the curve, as shown in Figure 8A. Visual and quantitative tomographic analysis is performed in three steps:

1. Normalized poststress regional activity in comparison with group standard lower limits of normal
2. Normalized redistribution regional activity in comparison with poststress results
3. Pattern recognition

Vogel et al.[18] have found that the minimum normal lower limit values for different normalized regional activities are approximately:

1. Inferior region 50 to 55%
2. Anterior region 55 to 60%
3. Superior region 65 to 75%
4. Posterior region 65 to 75%

These lower normal limits may vary considerably, however, from one institution to another, depending primarily on the population and to a lesser extent on the equipment used to determine the values. Lower normal limit profiles of the apical, central, and basal sections are generated from a known normal population. CAD is assessed at the University of Colorado Health Sciences Center (UCHSC) by comparing normalized values to those obtained from a population of 140 normal individuals taken from a multicenter study.

E. Normalized Regional Activity

A normalized regional increase of approximately 20% from immediate poststress to a 4-h delayed curve is diagnostically positive for regional ischemia, even in the presence of a stress regional activity curve falling within normal limits. Stationary ischemia is indicative of infarction alone. An increase in regional activity less than that mentioned above is indicative of partial regional ischemia. Pattern recognition is very important in these cases. Absolutely correct positioning and repositioning has to be checked. Some variations in the redistribution pattern can be expected in the 4-h poststress study.

F. Pattern Recognition

There is a qualitative recognition of characteristic patterns in a set of slices transaxial to the long axis of the LV. The decreased normalized activity of the inferior wall usually increases from apex to base. This kind of pattern, typical for regional ischemia or even infarction, should be examined for borderline cases. Missing apical activity cannot easily be quantified and must be recognized visually from a set of displayed sections. Recognition of characteristic seven-pinhole patterns, together with stress and redistribution data, is very helpful in borderline cases of ischemia. Normal and abnormal stress and redistribution patterns, together with corresponding normalized quantitative results, are shown in Figure 5 and 6, respectively.[13] A single composite image display has been developed by Klingensmith et al.[21] to visualize the shape, size, and extent of myocardial lesions involving multiple sections. The normalized quantitative information obtained from the tomograms of the LV described above is used to generate an "en face" gray-scale image of the superior, inferior, anteroseptal, and posterolateral LV surfaces (Figure 9). These four surfaces are displayed with their apices touching so that the LV appears open in a fashion similar to a peeled banana (Figure 10). The apical parts are obtained by extrapolation since circle analysis cannot be performed on these sections. A small exclusive apical defect will still be missed by this method, emphasizing the importance of pattern recognition as discussed above. First, two composite images for stress and rest are generated and displayed (Figure 11). A gray-scale composite image of the myocardium with greater perfusion at redistribution is generated by subtracting the "stress" composite image from the "rest" composite image. A second composite image is then obtained for abnormal decreased perfusion at rest by subtracting the rest composite image from the left lower normal limit image. Finally, a composite image is created where normal areas of the myocardium, with significant improvement in perfusion at rest, and areas of irreversible ischemia are coded into three different gray levels, as shown in Figure 11. Displaying the different composite images in the same gray scale as in the original images is essential so that small differences in activity will not appear significant by changes in gray level. This display method has the advantage of being applicable to any tomographic method (seven-pinhole, slant-hole, or rotating-camera).

Quantitation of an exercise ^{201}Tl study is displayed in the "bull's eye"[22] functional image shown in Figure 12. The apex is at the center and is shown without activity because of the lack of quantitation discussed previously. The activity of each successive transaxial slice is displayed as a new ring of increasing radius from the apex to the base located at the periphery. Myocardial activity is distributed according to the degree of perfusion. The "bull's eye" display can be used to generate the same type of quantitative information as that available in the single composite image; the method of choice is a matter of personal preference. Quantitation schemes such as those presented here are especially useful in following the progress of pharmacological interventions, percutaneous transluminal coronary angioplasty, and coronary artery bypass grafting.

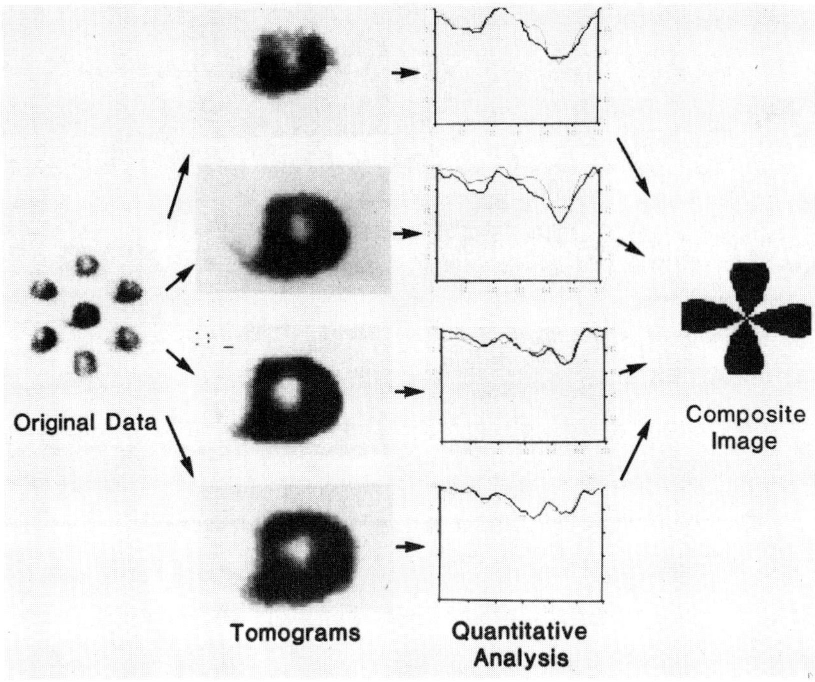

FIGURE 9. The composite image of left ventricular perfusion is constructed by (a) acquiring left ventricular images in multiple projections with a seven-pinhole collimator (original data), (b) reconstructing the seven nontomographic images into a series of tomographic images along the long axis of the left ventricle (tomograms), (c) quantitatively analyzing each tomogram with a circle program (the results of both stress and rest studies are shown (quantitative analysis), and (d) combining the three-dimensional quantitative perfusion information into a single composite gray-scale display (composite image). In this last display, the left ventricle is segmented along four lines extending from the apex to the base and displayed as four surfaces with the apical part of each surface joined at the center of the image. The superior surface of the left ventricle extends upward, the inferior surface downward, the anteroseptal surface to the left, and the posterolateral surface to the right. This patient had had a documented anterior myocardial infarct. (Reprinted with permission from Klingensmith, W. C., III, Stern, D., and Spitzer, V. M., *Radiology*, 141, 242, 1981.)

III. MYOCARDIAL IMAGING

A. Diagnostic Accuracy

Results of seven-pinhole tomography applied to myocardial perfusion studies show an overall increase of 5 to 10% in sensitivity with unchanged specificity, compared to standard planar imaging. Variations in diagnostic accuracy reported for seven-pinhole tomography are due largely to many factors associated with multicenter studies, including:

1. Differences in instrumentation
2. Selection and preparation of patients and sequence of imaging
3. Interpretive methods used for an objective intercomparative study
4. Methods used to display images (BW, color, Polaroid®, etc.)

For example, selection of a large number of patients with prior myocardial infarction (MI) will substantially increase diagnostic sensitivity. Exercise protocols vary from institution to institution, as does the total number of counts acquired (at least 750,000 cts/raw data file should be used). Redistribution imaging can be altered by factors during the delay such as

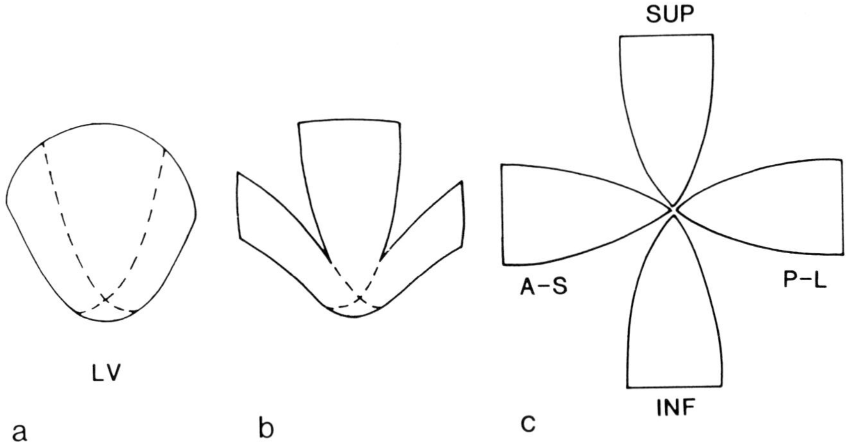

FIGURE 10. Segmentation and flattening of the three-dimensional left ventricle into two dimensions is depicted diagrammatically. The left ventricle is segmented along four lines which run from the apex to the base at equally spaced distances around the ventricular cross-section (a). The segments are then ''peeled'' forward so that the ventricle will occupy only two dimensions (b). The segmentation results in superior (SUP), inferior (INF), anteroseptal (A-S), and posterolateral (P-L) segments or surfaces. (Reprinted with permission from Klingensmith, W. C., III, Stern, D., and Spitzer, V. M., *Radiology,* 141, 242, 1981.)

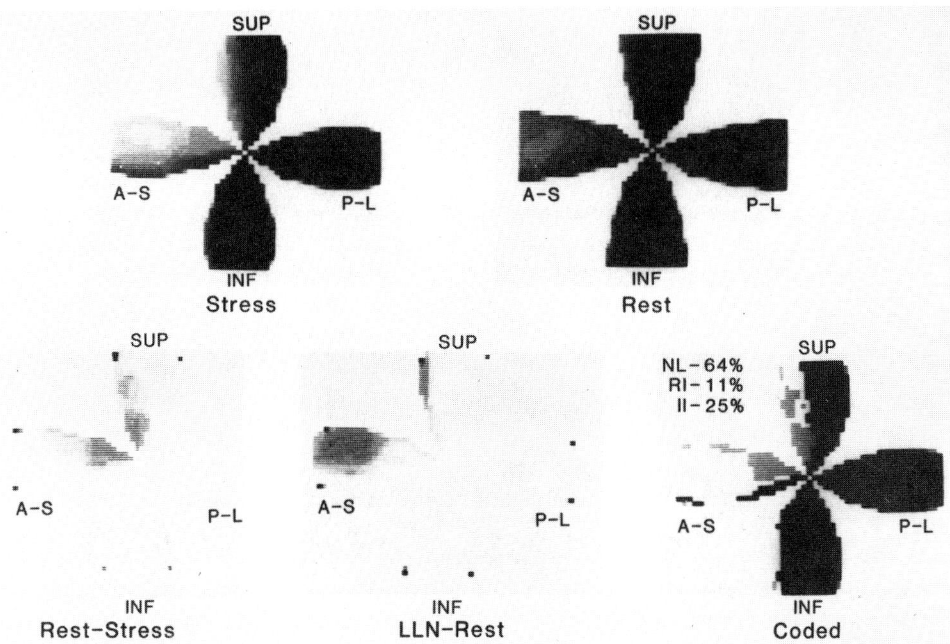

FIGURE 11. Quantitative information from tomographic sections constructed with a seven-pinhole tomographic system is used to construct composite images of relative perfusion at stress (exercise) and rest (redistribution). A composite gray-scale image of myocardium with greater perfusion at rest is created by subtracting the composite stress image from the composite rest image from the LLN composite image. Finally, a coded composite image is created in which normal myocardium is displayed as black, areas of myocardium with significant improvement in perfusion from stress to rest are displayed as medium gray, and areas of irreversible ischemia are displayed as light gray. The percentage of myocardium in each of the three categories is calculated and displayed along with the coded image. SUP = superior, INF = inferior, A-S = anteroseptal, and P-L = posterolateral images. (Reprinted with permission from Klingensmith, W. C., III, Stern, D., and Spitzer, V. M., *Radiology,* 141, 242, 1981.)

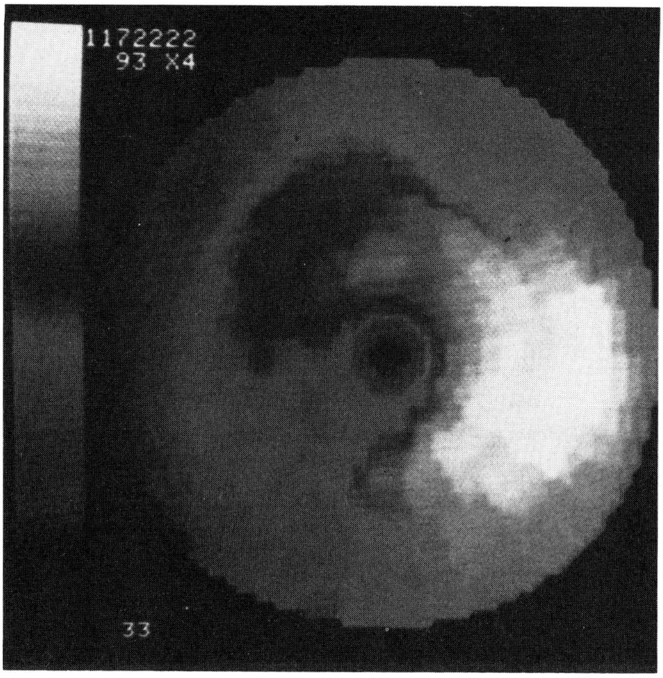

FIGURE 12. "Bull's-eye" display for exercise ^{201}Tl single-photon emission computed tomogram (SPECT) in short axis. The apex is at the center and the base is at the periphery. There is a large defect extending from the base to apex in the septum and a portion of the anterior wall. Color coding can also be useful to display areas of normal perfusion and areas of ischemia or infarction.

food consumption, alcohol, cigarettes, etc. Gastric and lung uptake can alter background activity over the redistribution waiting period. Differences also exist among various commercially available software routines for reconstruction imaging and quantitative analysis.

For comparative studies, planar imaging and seven-pinhole tomography should not be randomly executed in time. Instead, the stress seven-pinhole acquisition should always precede planar imaging, since the data-collection time is shorter.

B. Review of Clinical Studies

After introduction of the seven-pinhole technique for myocardial imaging by Vogel and Kirch[2,3,16] in the late 1970s, a large number of investigators reported on the clinical efficacy of the new technique compared with planar imaging[23-29] and other techniques,[30] and the first multi-institutional studies appeared.[31] Preliminary results for noncardiac applications were also reported.[32,33] Qualitative and quantitative improvement were quoted for assessment of single- and multi-vessel CAD. The first clinical results from Vogel et al.[19] described two groups of patients: the first group included 65 patients (23 without and 42 with angiographically suspected CAD; i.e., more than 70% luminal stenosis). These patients underwent stress seven-pinhole and planar imaging. A second group was composed of 7 normal patients and 32 patients with documented CAD. The patients from this group underwent seven-pinhole stress and redistribution imaging. Comparison of planar images to seven-pinhole tomograms showed that 31 of 42 patients had an abnormal planar study, while 40 of the 42 patients with stenosis were identified correctly with the seven-pinhole technique. In the second group, none of the normal patients had an abnormal tomogram, while 31 of 32 patients with CAD had abnormal tomographic study. Left-ventricular disease was defined by an ejection fraction below 55%; the LV was considered normal for an ejection fraction above 55%. With these criteria, the seven-pinhole approach improved the sensitivity by about 20% when compared to planar imaging.

Ritchie et al.[34] examined patients with prior MI. Thirty-six patients with prior MI, and 14 without, had myocardial ^{201}Tl imaging at rest using the planar and seven-pinhole techniques. Sensitivities for planar imaging were based on qualitative visual diagnosis, a Polaroid® output video display format, and semiquantitative analysis. These techniques yielded sensitivity scores of 69, 80, and 75%, respectively. Quoted specificities were 100, 93, and 71%. Seven-pinhole procedures had a sensitivity of 83% by qualitative (visual) inspection and 86% by semiquantitative analysis. Specificities for the tomographic technique were 71% (visual) and 57% (semiquantitative). Although the seven-pinhole approach improved the visual sensitivity by 14% and the semiquantitative sensitivity by 11%, the authors concluded that the gain in sensitivity was not statistically significant and that the seven-pinhole technique had no distinct advantages over planar imaging. They drew the same conclusion for specificity, although it was lower by 20% for seven-pinhole. The specificity was evaluated with a small group of only 12 patients, leaving the statistical significance of the specificity conclusion to be somewhat of an open issue.

A third major comparison of seven-pinhole tomography with planar imaging has been reported by Rizi et al.[35] Results are reported for 63 patients, with 52 of them showing a luminal stenosis ≥70% after angiography. The authors emphasize the critical point of patient positioning and thoroughly discuss important factors such as collimator-subject orientation, collimator centering, and collimator-object distance. Only 11 patients without CAD were examined. Preliminary results for detection of CAD using seven-pinhole tomography were sensitivity 94%, specificity 91%, and accuracy 94%. The authors point out that specificity for both the planar and tomographic techniques depends largely on patient selection, since abnormal ^{201}Tl uptake is observed in various cardiac diseases including valvular heart disease and cardiomyopathy. Inter- and intraobserver agreement had different outcomes for planar and tomographic imaging. With or without additional computer analysis of the data, the superiority of the tomographic analysis was apparent in this study. Sensitivity is very high in both planar and tomographic images for patients with prior myocardial infarction. In patients without prior myocardial infarction, however, the tomographic approach yielded better results than did planar imaging. Only 3 patients of 52 with significant CAD had false negative results by analysis of tomograms; in all three cases, the planar images also were normal. The difficulty of positioning every patient ideally with the seven-pinhole technique was emphasized as an inherent, unalterable limitation of that tomographic approach.

Bateman et al.[36] evaluated seven-pinhole tomography for detection and localization of CAD in terms of major coronary arteries and compared the results to quantitative planar imaging. Seven-pinhole tomography and planar scintigraphy were performed under stress and redistribution conditions for 40 patients (23 with angiographically documented CAD, 8 normals, and 9 with a likelihood ≤1% for CAD). The same quantitation procedures were applied for ^{201}Tl distribution and washout. Seven-pinhole tomography did not significantly improve the outcome of these studies. In the study of 31 patients with coronary angiography, 23 were found to have stenosis ≥50% in one or more major vessels. Eight patients had normal coronary arteries. Two-vessel disease (stenosis of LAD and/or LCx or RCA) was revealed in 12 patients and 6 showed single-vessel disease. Identification of CAD was accomplished by quantitative ^{201}Tl stress and redistribution analysis using software based on bilinear interpolative background subtraction[37] and nine-point smoothing. For the planar imaging studies, 21 of 23 patients were correctly identified with CAD (sensitivity of 91%) and 16 of 17 showed absence of disease (specificity of 94%). The tomographic results showed a slightly higher sensitivity of 96% (22 of 23 patients) and a slightly lower specificity of 88%. With regard to identification of the diseased vessel, the seven-pinhole technique identified 44 of 51 cases correctly (sensitivity 86%) and the absence of disease in 57 of 69 vessels (specificity 83%). Planar scintigraphy had a lower sensitivity (71%) and a comparable specificity (87%). Similar results have been reported by the authors for multivessel CAD identification. The seven-pinhole technique showed an overall improvement of 10% in sensitivity with no change in specificity; however, tomography yielded a 14% (85 vs. 71%) improvement in sensitivity for detection of CAD, mainly due to a 27% increase in sensitivity for detection of LCx artery stenosis. The gain in sensitivity seems to be accompanied by a loss in specificity. The conclusion of the authors was that seven-pinhole tomography is a cost effective alternative to evaluation of CAD compared to planar scintigraphy.

Recently Tamaki et al.,[38] using a rotating scintillation camera, have compared myocardial ^{201}Tl emission tomography to seven-pinhole tomography and planar imaging. Cardiac phantom studies and clinical studies performed on 47 patients with MI are reported. The results show that tomograms obtained with a rotating camera yield higher contrast images than those obtained with the seven-pinhole approach. The propagation of image details through nearby planes with seven-pinhole approach is similar to that reported by Williams et al.[4] The sensitivity obtained with the seven-pinhole system (93%) was comparable to that obtained with the rotating camera (96%). Poor specificity is reported for the seven-pinhole technique (68%) compared to the rotating SPECT system (89%), while planar imaging provided 95% sensitivity and 89% specificity. The rotating camera tomograms allow reliable reconstruction of coronal and sagittal planes without significant loss of resolution. However, the data acquisition time with the rotating camera is 50% greater than that required with the seven-pinhole system, leading to some concern associated with ^{201}Tl redistribution studies. Although the rotating SPECT system seems conceptually superior, its cost is significantly greater than the seven-pinhole system. A teaching editorial by Mullani et al.[39] reveals a marginal superiority of rotating SPECT cameras over seven-pinhole systems. Mullani et al. also concluded that neither of the two tomographic modalities show a dramatic improvement over planar imaging for detection of cardiac lesions. According to them, both tomographic methods should be considered as an improvement over planar scintigraphy in terms of diagnostic technique. Additional comparative studies are needed to determine the absolute clinical utility of both tomographic techniques.

C. Quantitation of Dynamic Myocardial Perfusion

Massie et al.[40] recently developed a quantitative scintigraphic index of myocardial ischemia using the seven-pinhole technique. ^{201}Tl scintigrams were acquired immediately poststress, followed by redistribution 3 h later in 15 normal patients. The same protocol was applied to 55 catheterized patients with typical chest pain. A 3-h clearance curve was generated using circumferential type analysis for three sections through the LV. A "scintigraphic ischemic score" (SIS) was defined by summing the area between stress and the 3-h delay curves for 3 transaxial sections, together with the area for which the clearance curve fell below the lower limit defined by normal subjects. The SIS that combines quantitative redistribution and clearance abnormalities to the stress level yielded the best sensitivity for diagnostic purposes, the best separation of patients with multivessel disease from those with zero or one vessel involvement, and the best correlation with a coronary arteriography score (CAS) and a treadmill exercise score.

Brady et al.[41] reported the use of seven-pinhole tomography to assess regional ^{201}Tl kinetics for detection of patients with CAD. Twelve dogs were used for the study: 6 of them had a temporary occlusion (average 15 min) of LAD and 6 had a temporary occlusion of LCx. Serial seven-pinhole images were acquired during occlusion and reflow (175 min). The central pinhole image and reconstructed tomograms were used to analyze the time activity distributions by looking at region of interests (ROI) in normal and ischemic myocardial tissue. The same data were reanalyzed by circle analysis. In addition, the ^{201}Tl activity was recorded directly with a Cd-Te radiation probe sutured within the posterior wall of the myocardium. Poor correlation was found between direct counting in the posterior wall and the time activity change using ROI and circumferential analysis. Nevertheless, Brady et al. concluded that the seven-pinhole technique is very sensitive for detection of myocardial ischemia.

Sklar et al.[42] used the seven-pinhole technique to determine myocardial clearance of thallium by extension of the quantitative seven-pinhole method to follow the dynamics of ^{201}Tl redistribution after stress. Slow ^{201}Tl clearance appears to be characteristic of myocardial tissue supplied by stenosed coronary arteries. Seven-pinhole tomograms, circumferential count profiles, and blood samples for thallium concentration obtained 2 and 4 h after stress were studied for 28 patients. The thallium clearance from the blood (TCB) was compared to the thallium clearance from each myocardial segment (TCM) between 2 and 4 h. In 17 of 20 cases found with CAD, at least one lesion yielded a TCM less than the TCB. Of 8 normal patients 7 had TCM greater than TCB. Of 13 patients with multi-vessel CAD, 11 had multiple lesions with TCM less than TCB. Using this approach, the authors identified 31 of 39 obstructive coronary arteries. The observation of slow myocardial clearance may improve diagnostic sensitivity for the detection of multivessel CAD. Examples of normal and abnormal late clearance analysis are shown in Figures 13 and 14, respectively.

Another clinical application of seven-pinhole tomography with ^{201}Tl has been reported by Schuler et al.[43] to assess intracoronary fibrinolysis in MI using streptokinase. In 16 patients, recanalization was achieved within approximately 4 h after acute MI. Cross-section through the LV of the myocardium were obtained from seven-pinhole data to assess the ^{201}Tl perfusion defect and to express it as a percentage of the left-ventricular circumference activity. Intracoronary fibrinolysis may reduce thallium perfusion defects in patients with acute MI. The validity of the seven-pinhole technique is also discussed by Schuler et al.[43] However, since each patient was used to assess the success of fibrinolysis in acute MI using streptokinase, and since the reproducibility of the seven-pinhole tomography is adequate, technical limitations should not affect the clinical results. By analyzing reperfusion 4 h after the onset of acute myocardial infarction, the presence of residual coronary flow due to extensive collaterals or to subtotal stenosis of the affected main arteries can be detected.

Although largely displaced by rotating scintillation cameras, seven-pinhole tomography remains a valuable research tool for myocardial perfusion studies and can still be considered as a viable approach for detection of remote MI and reversible states of ischemia.[44,45]

Bizais et al.[46] have reported another use of the seven-pinhole technique for emission tomography. Two orthogonal sets of projections obtained with seven-pinhole collimators (dual seven-pinhole tomography) are used for tomographic studies. The acquisition system, reconstruction algorithm, and results based on the liver phantom study are presented. Advantages and disadvantages over the standard conventional seven-pinhole technique are also discussed. Improved sensitivity and resolution are reported. The resolution variation within the reconstruction volume can be neglected.

IV. NONCARDIAC APPLICATIONS OF SEVEN-PINHOLE TOMOGRAPHY

Very few noncardiac applications of seven-pinhole tomography have been reported.

Because of its small size, the thyroid is the most tomographically examined organ with the exception of the myocardium. Detection and localization of cold thyroid nodules are greatly enhanced by the seven-pinhole technique. Although nodules in the central seven-pinhole image appear equivalent to those in a planar image, contrast is generally poor. A normal thyroid study is shown in Figure 15. Better delineation of hot and cold nodules by seven-pinhole tomography is illustrated in Figure 16. Telepak et al.[47] have published results of seven-pinhole tomography for noncardiac clinical applications and have shown that this

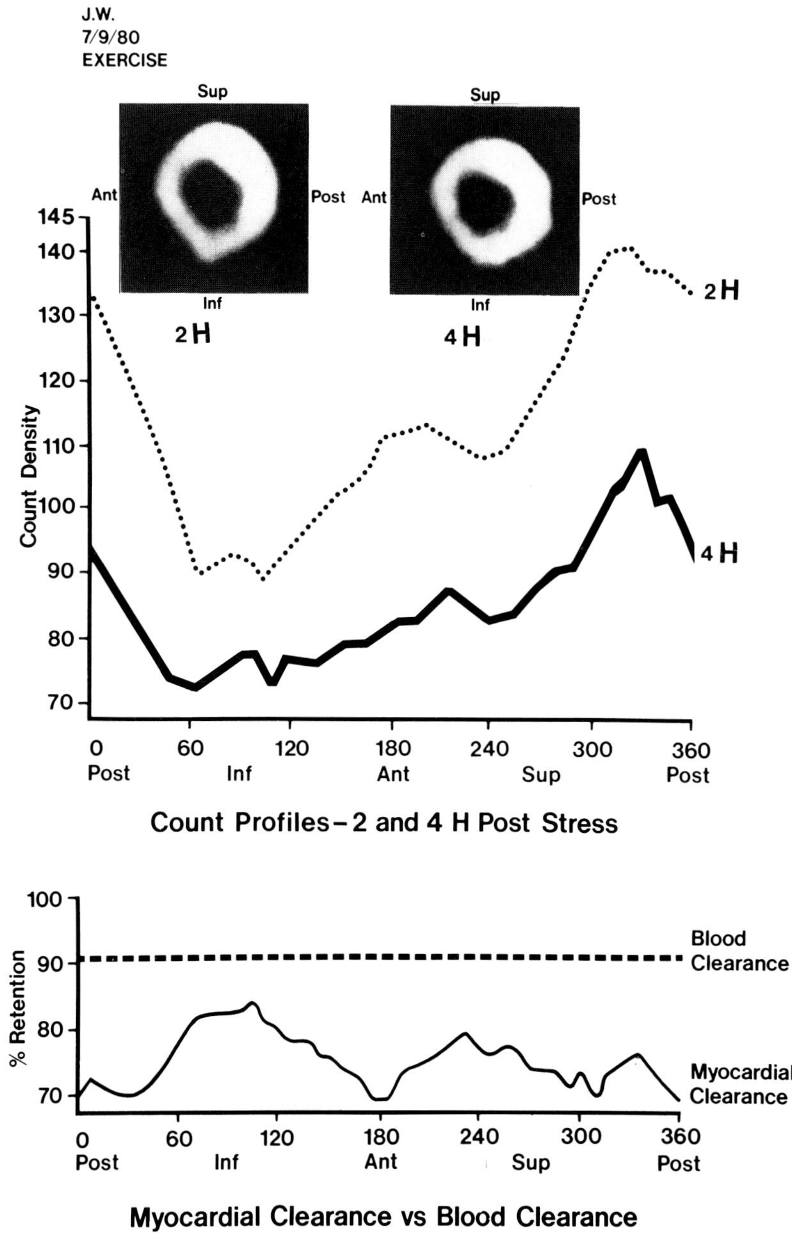

FIGURE 13. A normal late clearance analysis. On top are the midventricular tomographic planes from the 2- and 4-h thallium scintigrams. The upper section shows the absolute circumferential count profiles derived from those planes. The lower section shows the blood clearance rate (expressed as percent retention) and the myocardial clearance profile (expressed as percent retention of counts) between 2 and 4 h. The myocardial clearance curve is lower than the blood clearance line throughout; thus, thallium washed out of all regions of myocardium faster than it cleared from the blood. (Reprinted with permission from Sklar, J., Kirch, D., Johnson, T., et al., *Circulation,* 65, 1504, 1982.)

approach to emission tomography is an excellent complement to standard planar scintigraphy. The major advantages of seven-pinhole tomography are increased lesion detectability through improved contrast and low cost associated with the instrumentation. Among the major drawbacks mentioned in the work by Telepak et al.[47] are the stringent positioning requirements for the patient and the nonuniform plane spacing resulting in degradation of resolution

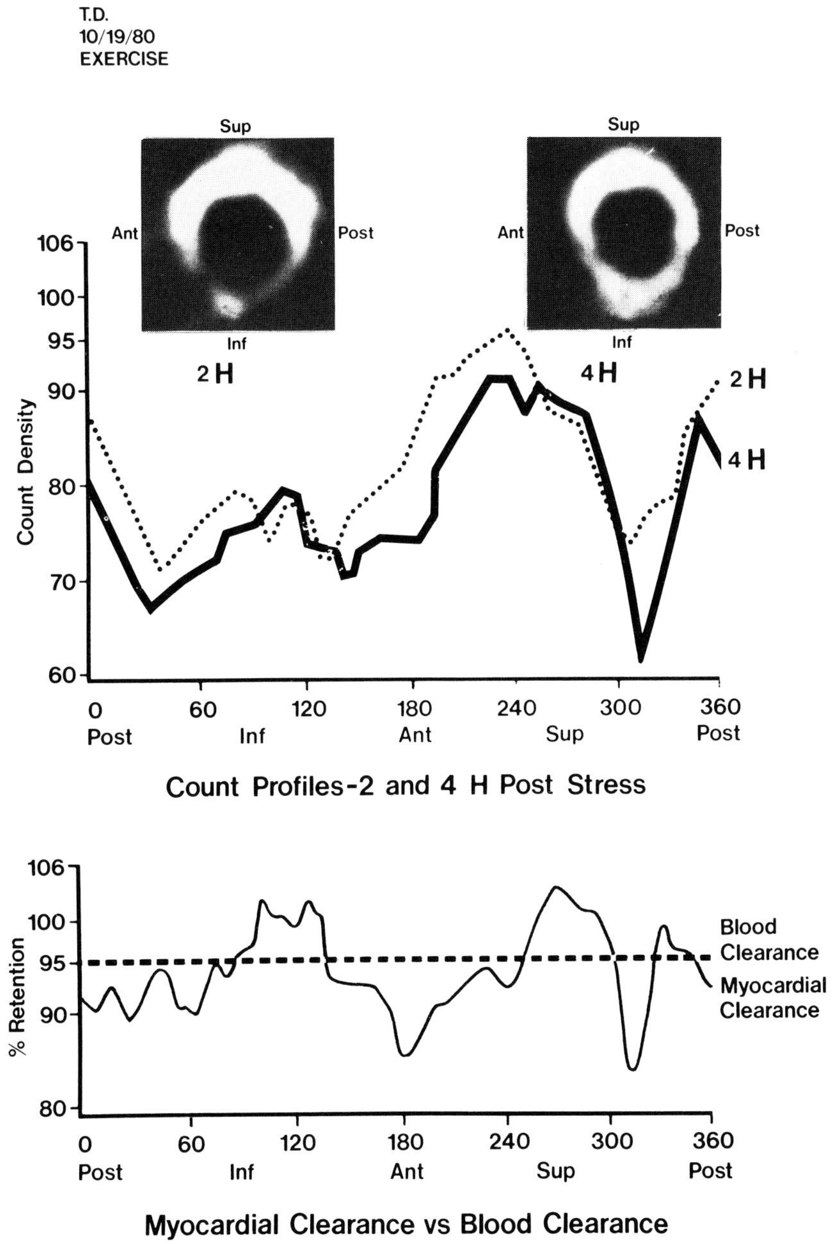

FIGURE 14. An abnormal late clearance analysis; same format as Figure 13. The myocardial clearance curve is higher than the blood clearance line in two (possibly three) locations; thus, in these locations, thallium cleared from myocardium slower than it cleared from blood. This correctly suggests multivessel coronary artery disease involving the right (inferior), left anterior descending or diagonal (anterosuperior), and possibly circumflex (superoposterior) coronary arteries in this patient. (Reprinted with permission from Sklar, J., Kirch, D., Johnson, T., et al., *Circulation,* 65, 1504, 1982.)

with depth. A commercial seven-pinhole collimator was used with two different aperture sizes: larger pinholes (6 mm) were used for positioning the patient, and smaller pinholes (4 mm) were used for data acquisition. ^{99m}Tc-radiopharmaceuticals were used with standard dosages. In addition to the tomographic data, planar scintigraphic images were also acquired. The time to position the patient was about 5 min. Since noncardiac applications utilize

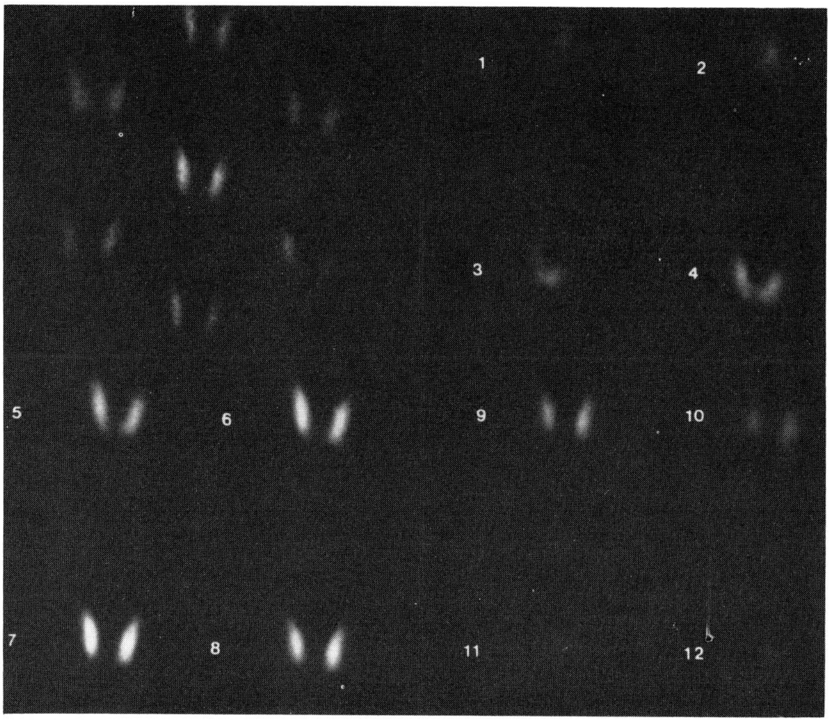

FIGURE 15. Normal seven-pinhole thyroid study. Upper left image shows raw images. Tomographic slices obtained through the thyroid (anterior to posterior) are displayed in the upper right.

radiotracers other than ^{201}Tl problems associated with redistribution and washout are not present.

Other applications of the seven-pinhole technique (bone scans of the posterior pelvis and scans of patients with Wagner hip prostheses) are described by Telepak et al.[47] Good results have been achieved for lesions in glucoheptonate renal cortical scans. Unfortunately, there are no specific guidelines for noncardiac applications similar to those for cardiac scans with an optimized software for thallium myocardial imaging. In another paper, Telepak et al.[48] discussed nontomographic uses of seven-pinhole collimators for thyroid imaging with both ^{99m}Tc-pertechnetate and ^{123}I-sodium iodide. Imaging was performed with a modified pinhole plate (pinhole sizes 2 and 3 mm) to increase resolution.

Single-pinhole thyroid scans are known to be the most accurate approach to detection of thyroid lesions. The standard single-pinhole views are anterior, left anterior oblique, and right anterior oblique for planar imaging. The low sensitivity, however, associated with the single-pinhole technique increases considerably the imaging time. The time factor becomes a significant drawback if multiple views are needed. The advantage of thyroid imaging with a seven-pinhole collimator becomes obvious; besides the standard anterior view, multiple oblique views are produced simultaneously. The seven-pinhole image can be computer-stored for later processing if the results of planar scintigraphy are insufficient for diagnosis. Imaging thyroid phantoms with a seven-pinhole collimator with known lesion sizes helps to identify abnormal thyroid scans.

Hips and kidneys are also suited for seven-pinhole tomography because of their relatively small size. Brain and liver seven-pinhole tomography requires a special seven-pinhole plate, and these organs were seldom imaged with the seven-pinhole approach. Results of seven-pinhole brain studies are shown in Figures 17 and 18.

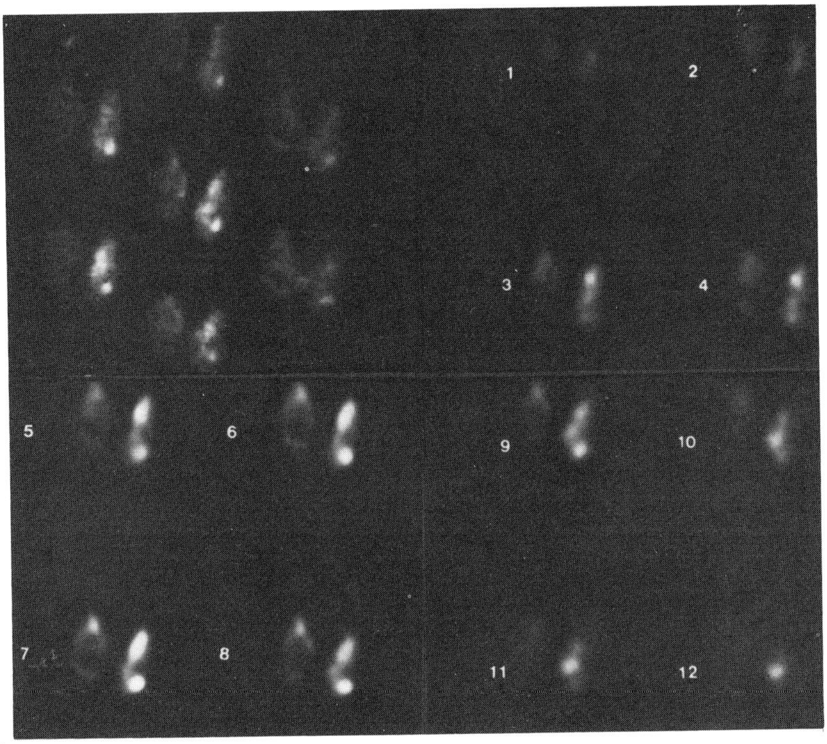

FIGURE 16. Abnormal seven-pinhole thyroid study. Upper left image shows the seven pinhole patient image. Planar central pinhole view and oblique views show cold and hot nodules. Reconstructed tomographic slices through the thyroid show clearly the size and depth of cold and hot nodules.

The seven-pinhole technique has also been applied to gated emission computed tomography, yielding the possibility of a three-dimensional representation of myocardial wall motion. Results of gated acquisition studies are displayed with the ''bird cage'' technique and are shown in Figure 19.

The seven-pinhole technique can be considered clinically as a useful add-on to planar imaging to assess diagnostic procedures, especially in small institutions. As other techniques for emission tomography come into prominence, it becomes apparent that the technical stringencies necessary to make them reliable may be equal to or greater than these for seven-pinhole. All in all, it is also becoming apparent that the real value of these techniques is in improved lesion contrast and relative quantification.

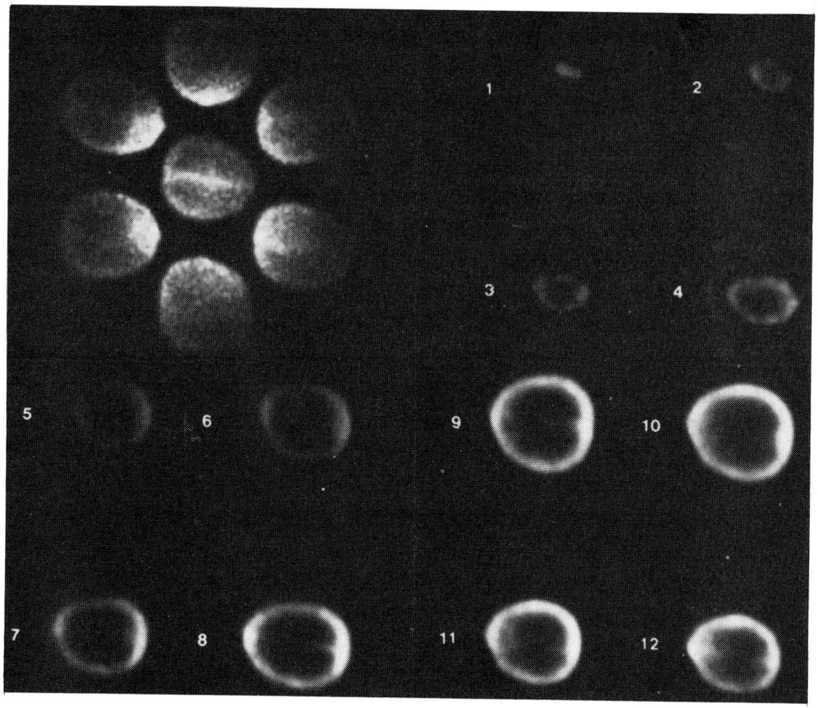

FIGURE 17. Normal seven-pinhole brain study. Upper left image shows the raw image. Twelve tomographic slices through the brain (cephalad to caudal) are displayed starting in the upper right. Plane #3, thickness 0.84 cm — starts at a depth of 10.78 cm and plane #10 — thickness 4.15 cm ends at a depth of 23.83 cm.

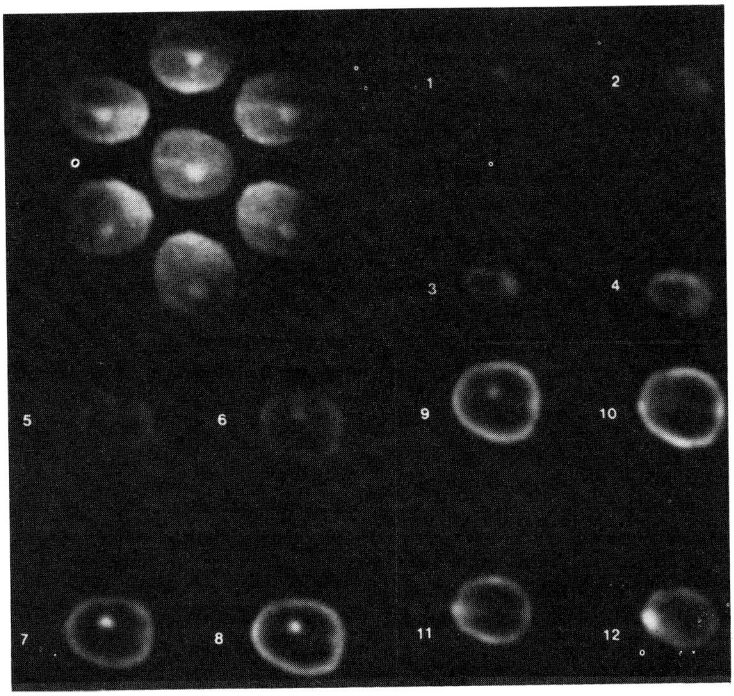

FIGURE 18. Abnormal seven-pinhole brain study. Upper left shows the seven-pinhole acquisition image. Raw data shows abnormal radiotracer concentration in the brain parenchyma. Reconstructed tomographic slices show clearly the size and location of a meningioma confirmed by CT scan. Tomographic sections are the same thickness and start at the same depth as those displayed in Figure 17.

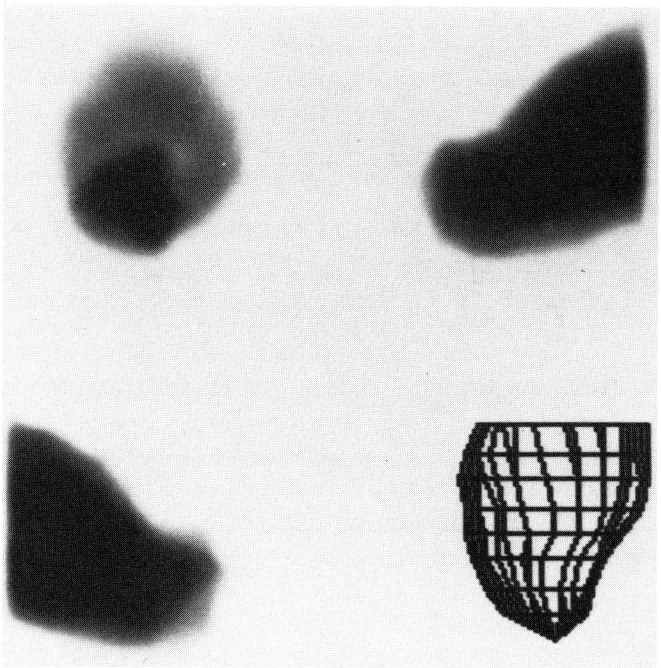

FIGURE 19. Gated myocardial seven-pinhole study. From left to right, top to bottom: LAO view, LPO view, RAO view, and "bird cage" in anterior view. Acquisition (LAO, LPO, RAO, and ANT) uses eight frames for display in cine mode. "Bird cage" can be displayed for all cases to simulate three-dimensional display. A large apical aneurysm can be observed. (Courtesy of Eisenhower Hospital, Colorado Springs, CO.)

REFERENCES

1. **Vogel, R. A., Kirch, D. L., and LeFree, M. T.,** A new method of emission tomography using compound collimation, in *The Proceedings of the 5th International Conference on Information Processing in Medical Imaging,* ORNL/BCTIC-1, Biomedical Computing Technology Information Center, Oak Ridge, 1977, 636.
2. **Vogel, R. A., Kirch, D. L., LeFree, M. T., and Steele, P. P.,** A new method of multiplanar emission tomography using a seven pinhole collimator and an Anger scintillation camera, *J. Nucl. Med.,* 19, 649, 1978.
3. **LeFree, M. T., Vogel, R. A., Kirch, D. L., and Steele, P. P.,** Seven-pinhole tomography — a technical description, *J. Nucl. Med.,* 22, 48, 1981.
4. **Williams, D. L., Ritchie, J. L., Harp, G. D., Caldwell, J. H., and Hamilton, G. W.,** *In vivo* simulation of thallium-201 myocardial scintigraphy by seven-pinhole emission tomography, *J. Nucl. Med.,* 21, 821, 1980.
5. **Brookeman, V. A. and Maisey, M. N.,** Performance characteristics of seven-pinhole tomography, *Br. J. Radiol.,* 55, 229, 1982.
6. **Brookeman, V. A.,** Performance characteristics of seven-pinhole tomography, *J. Nucl. Med.,* 21, 28, 1980.
7. **Rollo, F. D. and Patton, J. A.,** Perspectives of seven pinhole tomography, *J. Nucl. Med.,* 21, 888, 1980.
8. **Stokely, E. M., Tipton, D. M., Buja, L., Lewis, S. E., DeVous, M. D., Bonte, F. J., Parkey, R. W., and Willerson, J. T.,** Quantitation of experimental canine infarct site using multipinhole single-photon tomography, *J. Nucl. Med.,* 2, 55, 1981.
9. **Tomitani, T. and Tanaka, E.,** Three-dimensional reconstruction in longitudinal tomography by means of iterative approximation, in *Proceedings of the 5th International Conference on Information Processing in Medical Imaging,* ORNL-BCTIC-2, Biomedical Computing Technology Information Center, Oak Ridge, 1977, 174.

10. **Budinger, T. F.,** Physical attributes of single-photon tomography, *J. Nucl. Med.*, 21, 579, 1980.
11. **Chang, W. and Henkin, R. E.,** Seven pinhole multigated tomography and its application to blood-pool imaging: technical parameters, *J. Nucl. Med.*, 21, 682, 1981.
12. **McKillop, J. J.,** Is ^{201}thallium imaging clinically valuable in coronary artery disease?, *Diagnostic Imaging*, 18, 167, 1981.
13. **Stern, D. M.,** Research Systems, Inc., 2021 Albion Street, Denver, Colorado, 80207, personal communication.
14. **Kirch, D. L., Vogel, R. A., and LeFree, M. T.,** An Operational Guide to Performing Seven-Pinhole Tomographic Myocardial Perfusion Studies, The Denver Veterans Administration Medical Center and the University of Colorado Health Sciences Center, Denver, 1980.
15. **Vogel, R. A., and LeFree, M. T.,** A Pictorial Guide to Seven-Pinhole Tomographic thallium-201 Scintigraphy, Research pamphlet, Denver Veterans Administration Medical Center and the University of Colorado Health Sciences Center, Denver, 1980.
16. **Kirch, D. L., Vogel, R. A., LeFree, M. T., Sklar, J., Hasegawa, B. H., and Steele, P. P.,** An Anger/camera computer system for myocardial perfusion tomography using a seven pinhole collimator, *IEEE Trans. Nucl. Sci.*, NS-27, 412, 1980.
17. **Lakshminarayanan, A. V. and Lent, A.,** The simultaneous iterative reconstruction technique as a least-squares method, *SPIE Opt. Instr. V*, 96, 108, 1976.
18. **Vogel, R. A., Kirch, D. L., LeFree, M. T., and Steele, P. P.,** Improved Diagnostic Results of Myocardial Perfusion Scintigraphy by Large-Field Anger Camera, Veterans Administration Hospital, Department of Cardiology, 1979.
19. **Vogel, R. A., Kirch, D. L., LeFree, M. T., Rainwater, J. O., Jensen, D. P., and Steele, P. P.,** Thallium-201 myocardial perfusion scintigraphy: results of standard and multi-pinhole tomographic techniques. *Am. J. Cardiol.*, 43, 787, 1979.
20. **Johnson, T., Kirch, D., Hasegawa, B., Sklar, J., and Steele, P. P.,** A concentric polar plotting technique for analysis of emission cardiac tomography, *J. Nucl. Med.*, 22, 21, 1981.
21. **Klingensmith, W. C., Stern, D., and Spitzer, V. M.,** Single-composite image display of information from tomographic myocardial perfusion studies, *Radiology*, 141, 242, 1981.
22. **Berger, H. J., McClees, E. C., Eisner, R., Malko, J., and Fajman, W. A.,** New advances in tomographic cardiac imaging. Current concepts, *Diagn. Nucl. Imaging*, 1, 10, 1984.
23. **Yonekura, Y., Ishii, Y., Yamamoto, K., Muaki, T., Fujita, T., Minato, K., and Torizuka, K.,** Clinical efficacy of myocardial perfusion tomography with 7-pinhole collimator, *J. Nucl. Med.*, 21, 71, 1980.
24. **Green, A., Berman, D., Caldwell, J., Thrall, J., and Vogel, R.,** A multicenter comparison of standard 7 pinhole tomographic myocardial perfusion imaging: rock analysis of qualitative visual interpretation, *J. Nucl. Med.*, 21, 70, 1980.
25. **Berman, D., Freeman, M., Garcia, E., Staniloff, H., Pantaleo, N., Maddahi, J., Forrester, J. Swan, H. J. C., and Waxman, A.,** Clinical comparison of multiple pinhole tomography with planar imaging for thallium-201 stress myocardial scintigraphy, *J. Nucl. Med.*, 21, 70, 1980.
26. **Thrall, J. H., Besozzi, M., Kline, R., Brady, T., Rogers, L., Keyes, J., and Pitt, B.,** Thallium-201 imaging for detection of coronary artery disease: comparison of planar and seven-pinhole tomographic techniques, *J. Nucl. Med.*, 21, 71, 1980.
27. **Henkin, R. E., Hale, D. J., Salo, B. C., Rao, A., and Chang, W.,** 7-Pinhole tomography. Is it worth it?, *J. Nucl. Med.*, 21, 69, 1980.
28. **Myers, R. W., Bails, R. P., Reed, V. R. et al.,** Tomographic radionuclide angiography, *J. Nucl. Med.*, 21, 70, 1980.
29. **Wainwright, R. J., Brookeman, V. A., Brennand-Roper, D. A., Arocha, J., Hilson, A. J. W., Sowton, E., and Maisey, M. N.,** Comparison of seven-pinhole computed tomograms and planar scintigrams in thallium-201 myocardial imaging, *Nucl. Med. Commun.*, 1, 334, 1980.
30. **Smith, K. A. and Wake, R. H.,** Comparison of seven pinhole and rotating slant tomography of a cardiac phantom, *J. Nucl. Med.*, 21, 27, 1980.
31. **Vogel, R., Alderson, P., Berman, D., Caldwell, J., Thrall, J., van Aswegan, A., Becker, L., Brady, T., Freeman, M., Kirch, D., LeFree, M., Links, J., Pantaleo, N., Ritchie, J., Staniloff, H., Hamilton, G., and Pitt, B.,** A multicenter comparison of standard and seven pinhole tomographic Tl-201 scintigraphy: results of quantitative interpretation of tomograms, *J. Nucl. Med.*, 21, 70, 1980.
32. **Grove, R. B., Rodewald, A., Bell, R. L., and DeBlanc, H. J.,** Application of multiple pinhole emission radionuclide tomography to imaging of the brain and thyroid, *J. Nucl. Med.*, 21, 87, 1980.
33. **DeLand, F. H., Kim, E. E., Domstad, P. A., and Magoun, S. L.,** Contributions of the seven pinhole collimation to cisternography, *J. Nucl. Med.*, 21, 88, 1980.
34. **Ritchie, J. L., Williams, D. L., Caldwell, J. H., Stratton, J. R., Harp, G. D., Vogel, R. A., and Hamilton, G. W.,** Seven-pinhole emission tomography with thallium-201 in patients with prior myocardial infarction, *J. Nucl. Med.*, 22, 107, 1980.

35. **Rizi, H. R., Kline, R. C., Thrall, H. H., Besozzi, M. C., Keyes, J. W., Jr., Rogers, W. L., Clare, J., and Pitt, B.**, Thallium-201 myocardial scintigraphy: a critical comparison of seven-pinhole tomography and conventional planar imaging, *J. Nucl. Med.*, 22, 493, 1981.
36. **Bateman, T., Garcia, E., Maddahi, J., Rozanski, A., Pantaleo, N., Staniloff, H., Freeman, M., Waxman, A., and Berman, D.**, Clinical evaluation of seven-pinhole tomography for the detection and localization of coronary artery disease: comparison with planar imaging using quantitative analysis of myocardial thallium-201 distribution and washout after exercise, *Am. Heart J.*, 106, 263, 1983.
37. **Goris, M. L., Daspit, S. G., McLaughlin, P., and Kriss, J. P.**, Interpolative background subtraction, *J. Nucl. Med.*, 17, 744, 1976.
38. **Tamaki, N., Mukai, T., Ishii, Y., Yonekura, Y., Kambara, H., Kawai, C., and Torizuka, K.**, Clinical evaluation of thallium-201 emission myocardial tomography using a rotating gamma camera: comparison with seven-pinhole tomography, *J. Nucl. Med.*, 22, 849, 1981.
39. **Mullani, N. A., Gould, K. L., and Gaeta, J. M.**, Tomographic imaging of the heart with thallium-201: seven-pinhole or rotating gamma camera?, *J. Nucl. Med.*, 22, 925, 1981.
40. **Massie, B. M., Hollenberg, M., Wisneski, J. A., Go, R., Gertz, E. W., and Henderson, S.**, Scintigraphic quantification of myocardial ischemia: a new approach, *Circulation*, 68, 747, 1983.
41. **Brady, T. J., O'Keefe, D. D., Okada, R. D., Jacocks, M. A., Johnson, R. G., Geffin, G. A., Merril, D., Strauss, H. W., Daggett, W. M., and Pohost, G. M.**, Inability of seven-pinhole myocardial tomography to obtain accurate 201-Tl kinetic data, *Eur. J. Nucl. Med.*, 8, 425, 1983.
42. **Sklar, J., Kirch, D., Johnson, T., Hasegawa, B., Peck, S., and Steele, P. P.**, Slow late myocardial clearance of thallium: a characteristic phenomenon in coronary artery disease, *Circulation*, 65, 1504, 1982.
43. **Schuler, G., Schwarz, F., Hofmann, M., Mehmel, H., Manthey, J., Maurer, W., Rauch, B., Herrman, H. J., and Kubler, W.**, Thrombolysis in acute myocardial infarction using intracoronary streptokinase: assessment by thallium-201 scintigraphy, *Circulation*, 66, 658, 1982.
44. **Massie, B., Wisneski, J., Hollenberg, M., Gertz, E., Go, R., and Henderson, S.**, Scintigraphic quantitation of myocardial ischemia, *J. Nucl. Med.*, 24, 19, 1983.
45. **Massie, B., Wisneski, J., Inouye, I. K., Hollenberg, M., Gertz, S., and Henderson, S.**, Detection and quantitation of remote myocardial infarction by tomographic exercise-redistribution Tl-201 scintigraphy, *J. Nucl. Med.*, 24, 36, 1983.
46. **Bizais, Y., Zubak, I. G., Rowe, R. W., Bennett, G. W., and Brill, A. B.**, Dual seven pinhole tomography, *IEEE Trans. Nucl. Sci.*, NS-30, 703, 1983.
47. **Telepak, R. J. and Wood, E. L.**, Noncardiac clinical applications of seven-pinhole tomography, *Clin. Nucl. Med.*, 6, 344, 1981.
48. **Telepak, R. J., Bunker, S. R., Lancaster, J. L., Hartshorne, M. F., and Blumhardt, R.**, Another use for the seven-pinhole collimator routine nontomographic imaging of the thyroid, *Clin. Nucl. Med.*, 8, 163, 1983.

Chapter 10

SEVEN-PINHOLE TOMOGRAPHIC RECONSTRUCTION ALGORITHM

B. H. Hasegawa

TABLE OF CONTENTS

I. SEVEN-PINHOLE TOMOGRAPHIC RECONSTRUCTION TECHNIQUE

A. Introduction

This section outlines the reconstruction algorithm used in 7-pinhole (7PH) tomography. Much of the information is derived from the description by LeFree et al.[1] and the reader is referred to that work. In this discussion, the acquired image and the reconstructed tomographic planes are represented as continuous functions of the continuous spatial variables x and y, which is done primarily to simplify notation. In practice, the reconstruction algorithm is implemented in a digital format with discrete functions of discrete spatial variables. We will describe some of the digital aspects of the images but will leave it to the reader to translate the discussion of the reconstruction algorithm from the analog into the digital realm.

B. Description of Data Acquisition

The tomographic algorithm requires three images all acquired with the 7PH collimator: (1) the flood (or uniformity calibration) image, (2) the point source (or reference point projection) image, and (3) the patient image. The flood image provides a uniformity correction of the patient data. It can be shown that the projected count density from a uniform sheet of radioactivity viewed through a pinhole falls off as the cosine cubed of the angle measured from the axis normal to the sheet source through the pinhole. This geometric nonuniformity as well as inherent camera nonuniformities are corrected by dividing the patient image by the flood image on a pixel-by-pixel basis. The depth calibration (distance from the pinhole collimator endplate) is provided by an image of a simple point source held at a known distance along the central normal axis of the collimator. In the reconstruction algorithm, tomographic planes are reconstructed by combining the simultaneously acquired views obtained with the 7PH collimator. The views are shifted relative to the projected coordinates of the point source to reconstruct planes at different depths.

As Shabason et al.[2] point out, the recorded positions of events vary as a function of photon energy and the incident angle of the photons with the detector. For this reason, it is important that the flood and point source images be acquired with the same photon energy used in the patient image. Typically we use ^{99m}Tc calibration images for gated blood-pool studies while ^{195}Au is used to acquire the calibration images for thallium perfusion studies.

All images are acquired as 128 $\times$ 128 matrices. The flood and point source images have approximately 2.5 million and 40 thousand total counts, respectively. The ^{201}Tl patient images are acquired with 5.5-mm pinholes in approximately 10 min with a 1.5 to 2.0 mCi patient dose and contain approximately 750,000 total counts. Of course, larger pinholes can be used to increase sensitivity and decrease imaging time with a corresponding loss of spatial resolution. Improved resolution can be obtained with smaller pinholes and with sensitivity loss.

C. Overview of the Reconstruction Algorithm

Figure 1 provides a simplified description of the 7PH tomographic reconstruction algorithm. By way of definition, the term ''view'' will denote a projection image as seen by the detector while the term ''plane'' will denote a tomographic reconstruction image representing radioactivity distributions in the object. The reader should differentiate the terms ''original views'', ''estimate views'', ''error views'', ''estimate planes'', ''error planes'', and ''final planes'' and correlate the following description of the algorithm with Figure 1.

In this diagram, the N-pinhole collimator views radioactive objects (denoted 0 and X) placed at two different distances from the pinhole endplate. Following uniformity correction with the flood image, the simultaneously acquired images (original views) of the object are separated. For the central view, the two objects placed along the central collimator axis are superimposed. In comparison, for the outer views, superficial objects (denoted by ''X'' in

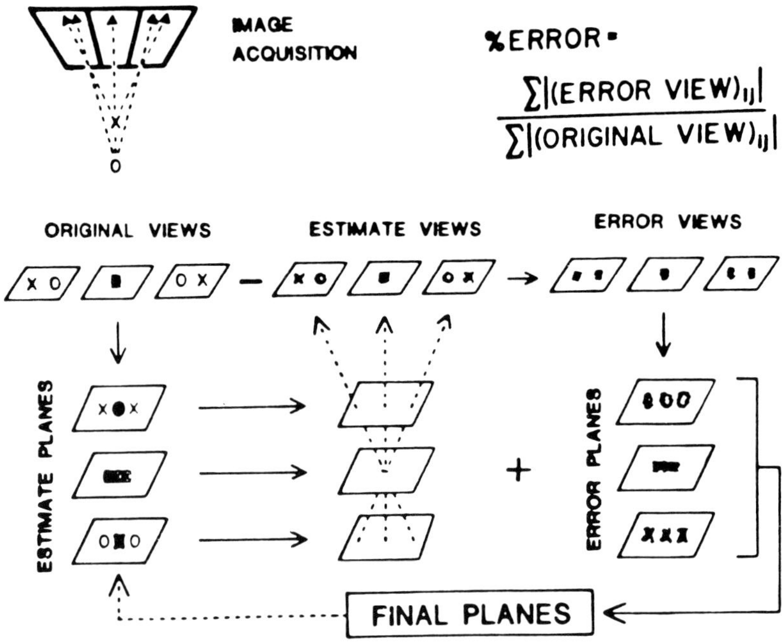

FIGURE 1. Diagram of N-pinhole tomographic reconstruction algorithm.

Figure 1) are projected to the periphery while distal objects (denoted by 0 in Figure 1) are projected more centrally. Tomographic planes are reconstructed by superimposing and shifting the acquired views and combining them. With the central view stationary, shifting the outer views toward the center first superimposes distal objects with additional shifts providing estimate planes of more superficial objects. The resulting estimate planes then are reprojected (simulating the image acquisition process) to provide estimate views. These estimate views represent the images that would have been acquired if the estimate planes had accurately represented the radioactivity distribution in the object. The difference between the original views and the estimate views form the error views which contain the errors in the reconstructed (estimate) views relative to the original views. The error views then are backprojected to form tomographic error planes. The error planes distribute the errors in the estimate views to the depth of the corresponding estimate planes and are added to the estimate planes forming the final planes. The tomographic algorithm can be continued iteratively by using the final planes as the estimate planes in a second reconstruction cycle. In practice, the reconstruction algorithm converges within acceptable tolerances in one iteration and additional iterations are generally unnecessary.[1,3]

II. SEVEN-PINHOLE TOMOGRAPHIC ALGORITHM

The previous section presented a conceptual overview of the 7PH tomographic algorithm. In this section we will build on this conceptual framework and present a detailed description of the 7PH algorithm.

A. Data Preparation

The first stage of the reconstruction algorithm prepares the three images (point source, flood, and patient) for processing. The point source image supplies the projected coordinates in each view of a point source placed at a known distance from the pinhole endplate. These coordinates are determined by a simple search algorithm. The approximate position of the point source coordinates are known from prior acquisitions. Only a small region around the historically known point source coordinates, therefore, are searched for maxima to reduce computation time; the entire image need not be searched for these maxima. The point source coordinates are saved for each view and are used, as described later, to superpose mathematically the different views of the patient radionuclide distribution in forming the tomographic planes.

The flood image is used for two purposes. The first is to provide a uniformity calibration of the patient image. The patient image is divided pixel-by-pixel by the flood image smoothed by convolution with a 3 × 3 equally weighted kernel. As previously described, this corrects for both geometric and intrinsic nonuniformities of the patient image. Second, the flood image provides information to separate the different views of the patient image. One-bit images, called masks, are constructed to delineate the image area comprising each view. The masks can be obtained in a number of ways. One can search radially outward from the coordinates of the point source projection in the central view to locate its borders and then search along the edge of the central view to find the peripheral septa outlining the outer views. The region contained within contiguous collimator septa is filled with 1's while surrounding areas are filled with 0's. Each of the seven resulting masks are used in a logical operation with the patient image resulting in seven separate images, each containing only one view of the patient data. After masking, each view is extracted and placed within a 64 × 64 matrix centered on the coordinates of the projected point source image corresponding to that view.

B. Background Correction

At this point, the data consists of the seven masked, flood-corrected views of the patient radionuclide distribution. Each view is contained within a 64 × 64 matrix and is centered on the coordinates corresponding to the projected point source image for that particular view. (Superposition of the centers of the views will allow reconstruction of the tomographic plane at the depth of the calibration point source.) Before the tomographic planes are reconstructed, each view is corrected for background. The view is searched for its maximum pixel count. The values of all pixels having values less than 50% of this maximum count are replaced with the average value of these pixels. There are two motivations for this background correction. First, as explained in the following section, the impedance estimator used to reconstruct the first estimate planes requires nonzero background values. Second, a value of 50% of the maximum pixel count is used as a criterion for background rather than a smaller value, due to a large fraction of counts contributed from radioactivity in the blood pool. The replacement of low-count pixels with a constant value provides a zero-frequency subtraction of the input data for the reconstruction algorithm. This partially accounts for edge enhancement[4,5] attributed to the 7PH reconstruction algorithm when applied to non-anatomic radionuclide distributions such as cubes and spheres. These reports are discussed further in the last segment of this section.

C. Reconstruction of the First Estimate Planes

Iterative tomographic reconstruction algorithms typically begin with a uniform distribution of pixel values in the first estimate tomographic planes.[6] One unique feature of the 7PH tomographic reconstruction algorithm is use of the Impedance Estimator (IE) to generate the first estimate planes.[1,7] This formula combines the acquired views by adding the reciprocals of pixel values from mathematically superposed views and then taking the reciprocal of the resulting sum. Different tomographic planes are obtained by shifting the views relative to their centers (defined by the projection of the point source image) before the impedance estimator is applied.

Table 1
UNIT SHIFT VECTORS FOR THE 7-PINHOLE COLLIMATOR

View no. (i)	Orientation angle θ	Shift vector (r(i),s(i))
0	Central view	(0, 0)
1	90	(0, 1)
2	30	$(^1/_2\sqrt{3},\ ^1/_2)$
3	330	$(^1/_2\sqrt{3},\ -^1/_2)$
4	270	(0, −1)
5	210	$(-^1/_2\sqrt{3},-^1/_2)$
6	150	$(-^1/_2\sqrt{3},\ ^1/_2)$

Note: Presented are the unit shift vectors (r(i),s(i)) for the 7-pinhole collimator used in Equations 1, 2, and 4. The central view corresponds to i = 0 while the outer views are numbered i = 1 to i = 6 in a clockwise direction starting from the view normally presented in the uppermost position of the image. The orientation angle θ is measured with respect to the positive x-axis and points from the origin of the coordinate system to the center of the view. The observant reader will note that for the outer views having an orientation angle of θ the unit shift vector has coordinates (cos θ, sin θ).

In the following discussion, tomographic planes will be indicated by P_n^k with the superscript k indicating the iteration index and the subscript n indicating the plane number (different values of n indicate different depths in the reconstruction volume). The views will be indicated by V_i^k with the superscript k again indicating the iteration index (where k = 0 for the original views) and the subscript i indicating the view number (i = 0, 1, ... , 6 with i = 0 for the central view). The first estimate tomographic plane P_n^1 at depth n is given by

$$P_n^1(x,y) = \left(\sum_{i=0}^{6} V_i^o[x + n \cdot r(i),\quad y + n \cdot s(i)]^{-1}\right)^{-1} \tag{1}$$

When n equals 0, the plane at the depth of the calibration point source is reconstructed. Negative values of n yield more distal planes and positive values of n yield more superficial planes. The shift vectors (r(i),s(i)) are unit vectors originating at the center of central view and pointing toward the point source projection for the ith view. Typical values are given in Table 1 for a 7PH collimator.

The resulting tomographic planes are normalized so that the total number of counts in all of the reconstructed planes equals the total number of counts in the original background-corrected views. This is performed by multiplying each pixel value in all of the planes by a constant equal to the total number of counts in the views divided by the total number of counts in the planes.

The motivation for a nonzero background correction of the acquired views also can be identified. Since the impedance estimator (Equation 1) inverts the pixel values, zero pixel values would lead to indeterminant results. This is avoided by forcing nonzero background values before the impedance estimator is applied to the input data.

D. Formation of the Estimate Views

The estimate planes P_n^k obtained with Equation 1 are not exact representations of the three-dimensional radionuclide distribution. The tomographic process accounts for errors by re-projecting the estimate planes to form estimate views which are compared against the original views. In the kth iteration, the ith view V_i^k is given by

$$V_i^k(x,y) = \sum_n a_n \, P_n^k[x - n \cdot r(i), \quad y - n \cdot s(i)] \tag{2}$$

in which a_n is an attenuation correction constant which is multiplicatively applied to each plane P_n^k. The summation extends over all tomographic planes obtained in Equation 1 and is repeated for each view. If the estimate planes were exact representations of the radionuclide distribution, then the estimate views obtained from Equation 2 would equal the original views. In general, this is not the case and a correction to the estimate planes must be applied, as explained below.

E. Formation of the Final Planes

Following formation of the estimate views, the error views (ΔV_i^k) are formed as the difference between the original views (V_i^o) and the estimate views (V_i^k) in the kth iteration

$$\Delta V_i^k(x,y) = V_i^o(x,y) - V_i^k(x,y) \tag{3}$$

The error views contain information in projection form about the errors distributed in the estimate planes. The estimate views are smoothed with a 3×3 equally weighted convolution kernel before the error views are formed. This produces an unsharp masking of data in the original views and results in edge enhancement in both the error planes and the final planes to improve delineation of perfusion defects. Simple backprojection of the error views to form error planes (ΔP_n^k)

$$\Delta P_n^k(x,y) = \sum_{i=0}^{6} \Delta V_i^k[x + n \cdot r(i), \quad y + n \cdot s(i)] \tag{4}$$

distributes these errors into the corresponding tomographic planes. Full application of the error plane to the estimate plane often causes oscillations in the iterative process.[1] The error planes are, therefore, multiplied by a damping factor q (typically equal to 0.25) before the error planes are added to the estimate planes. The final planes P_n^{k+1} are formed by adding the damped error planes to the estimate planes

$$P_n^{k+1}(x,y) = P_n^k(x,y) + q \cdot \Delta P_n^k(x,y) \tag{5}$$

The final planes can be used as the estimate planes in another iterative cycle by using them to recalculate new estimate planes (step 4). As previously stated, the algorithm converges satisfactorily after one iteration so that additional reconstruction cycles generally are unnecessary.

III. DISCUSSION

A. Comparison of First Estimate Reconstruction Techniques

The original motivation for the impedance estimator (Equation 1) was to reconstruct accurately regions of low radioactivity in ^{201}Tl myocardial perfusion studies in the first estimate planes. Other first estimate algorithms are possible.[8] The most obvious is simple backprojection in which the views are shifted and added to reconstruct the tomographic planes. For myocardial perfusion studies, this approach dulls perfusion defects with counts from over- and underlying structures. Multiplicative estimation reconstructs tomographic planes by multiplying, rather than adding, the shifted views. As in impedance estimation, multiplicative estimation maintains perfusion defects and can be implemented with logarithmically transformed data using digital look-up tables. When applied to point sources and myocardial phantoms, simple backprojection produces tomograms with poorer spatial resolution in the z-direction and with less accuracy of the known activity distributions in comparison to impedance estimation and multiplicative estimation. Due to these errors, simple backprojection requires multiple iterations to produce acceptable final planes. The differences between multiplicative estimation and impedance estimation were less dramatic, although multiplicative estimation produces tomograms with slightly better spatial resolution but slightly more noise than impedance estimation.

B. Edge Enhancement in the Reconstructed Planes

The 7PH tomographic algorithm was designed for studies of myocardial perfusion with ^{201}Tl. Edge enhancement improves delineation of perfusion defects and minimizes contamination of the lesion with activity from the blood pool. Edge enhancement is produced both from the method of background subtraction and by smoothing the estimate views before the error views are formed. These operations account for edge enhancement reported when the 7PH algorithm is applied to cylindrical or cubical activity distributions,[4,5] but do not indicate a fundamental property of the 7PH technique. Rather, they are a manifestation of characteristics which act to improve the reconstruction accuracy of radioactivity from the myocardial wall when surrounded by a large background contribution. One can improve the quantitative accuracy of reconstructions of cylindrical or cubical source distributions by removing edge enhancement in the reconstruction algorithm, should one wish to do so.

C. Spacing of the Tomographic Planes

The spacing of the tomographic planes is determined by the values of n in Equations 1, 2, and 4. The relationship between the value of n and the depth of the reconstructed plane is nonlinear and uniformly spaced values of n in Equations 1, 2, and 4 result in unequally spaced tomographic planes. Alternatively, one can select unequally spaced values of n to obtain equally spaced tomographic planes. The exact relationship between n and the depth of the tomographic plane can be derived from simple geometrical considerations and is left as an exercise for the reader.

D. Fractional Pixel Shifting

Pixel shifting in Equations 1, 2, and 4 is determined by the value of the vector $(n \cdot r(i), n \cdot s(i))$ which may have nonintegral pixel coordinates. In the 7PH tomographic algorithm, the shift vector coordinates generally are rounded to integral pixel values before the shifting is performed. This is not possible in 12-pinhole tomography[9] since a unit shift in the inner views corresponds to a 3-unit shift in the outer views. It is mandatory that the inner views be shifted fractional pixels to provide sufficient numbers of planes in the reconstruction volume. Fractional-pixel shifting can be performed with a convolution of the image data as described in the Appendix of Reference 9. It is possible to perform pixel shifting in the 7PH algorithm without rounding the components of the shift vector, by applying the same fractional-pixel shifting operation. Since the shifted views are more accurately placed before they are combined, the fractional-pixel shifting routine improves spatial resolution at the cost of increased processing time. Fractional-pixel shifting has not been included in any of the commercially available 7PH tomographic algorithms and probably is a second-order improvement in the algorithm. This is not the case in the 12-pinhole tomographic algorithm where fractional-pixel shifting is a necessity unless higher matrix dimensions (256×256 or 512×512) are used in acquisition and processing of the image data.

REFERENCES

1. **LeFree, M. T., Vogel, R. A., Kirch, D. L., and Steele, P. P.,** Seven-pinhole tomography — a technical description, *J. Nucl. Med.,* 22, 48, 1981.
2. **Shabason, L., LeFree, M. T., Kirch, D. L., and Hasegawa, B. H.,** Energy and angular dependent distortions in Anger camera images, *J. Nucl. Med.,* 21 (Abstr.), 81, 1980.
3. **Kirch, D. L., Vogel, R. A., LeFree, M. T., Sklar, J., Hasegawa, B. H., Steele, P. P.,** An Anger camera-computer system for myocardial perfusion tomography using a 7-pinhole collimator, *IEEE Trans. Nucl. Sci.,* NS-27, 412, 1980.
4. **Patton, J., Price, R., Bowen, R., Pickens, D., Touya, J. J., and Rollo, F. D.,** A comparison of PHO/CON and 7-pinhole collimator computerized reconstruction imaging with Tl-201, in *Single Photon Emission Computed Tomography and Other Selected Computer Topics,* Sorenson, J. A., Ed., Society of Nuclear Medicine, New York, 1980, 127.
5. **Brookeman, V. A.,** Performance characteristics of seven-pinhole tomography, *J. Nucl. Med.,* 21 (Abstr.), 28, 1980.
6. **Brooks, R. A. and DiChiro, G. A.,** Principles of computer assisted tomography (CAT) in radiographic and radioisotopic imaging, *Phys. Med. Biol.,* 21, 689, 1976.
7. **Vogel, R. A., Kirch, D. L., LeFree, M. T., Rainwater, J. O., Jensen, D. P., and Steele, P. P.,** Thallium-201 myocardial perfusion scintigraphy: results of standard and multi-pinhole tomographic techniques, *Am. J. Cardiol.,* 43, 787, 1979.
8. **Hasegawa, B. H., Kirch, D. L., and Steele, P. P.,** First estimate reconstruction techniques for N-pinhole radionuclide tomography, *Med. Phys.,* 8 (Abstr.), 567, 1981.
9. **Hasegawa, B. H., Kirch, D. L., Stern, D. M., Adams, M., Sklar, J., Johnson, T. K., and Steele, P. P.,** Single-photon emission tomography with a 12-pinhole collimator, *J. Nucl. Med.,* 23, 606, 1982.

Chapter 11

CODED APERTURE TOMOGRAPHY

U. Raff, R. E. Hendrick, and W. R. Hendee

TABLE OF CONTENTS

I. INTRODUCTION AND PHYSICAL PRINCIPLES

Coded apertures were originally developed to improve the collection efficiencies of imaging systems in X-ray astronomy. In 1961, Mertz and Young[1] developed a Fresnel zone-plate aperture, a series of concentric transparent and opaque rings of equal areas, as shown in Figure 1. In 1968, Dicke[2] and Ables[3] independently proposed the use of arrays consisting of pinholes randomly distributed on an opaque background plane, as shown in Figure 2. Both Fresnel zone-plates and random pinhole arrays are roughly 50% transparent to X-rays and both coded apertures generate their own decoding matrices. Unfortunately, neither array design permits encoding and decoding without some residual ghosting. In 1971, Golay[4] proposed a coded aperture design, the nonredundant pinhole array, that eliminated severe ghosting but at the expense of transparency. The best nonredundant pinhole arrays have a limited number of pinholes and low transmission of photons. In 1978, Fenimore and Cannon[5-7] developed a class of arrays called uniformly redundant arrays that are 50% transmitting and, in principle, eliminate the ghosting problem. Examples of two types of uniformly redundant arrays are shown in Figure 3.

It was recognized early that the improved photon collection efficiencies of coded apertures might be used to advantage in nuclear medicine emission imaging. Beginning in 1972, Barrett and co-workers[8-10] applied Fresnel zone-plates to nuclear medicine. In 1975, Koral et al.[11] reported on the use of time-varying multipinhole apertures for clinical imaging, and Simpson and Barrett[12,13] investigated the use of annuli in nuclear medicine. Rotating-slit coded apertures were suggested by Tanaka and Iinuma[14] in 1975 and later were investigated in detail by Barrett and co-workers at the University of Arizona.[15] Uniformly redundant arrays are currently under investigation for use in nuclear medicine imaging by investigators at the University of Arizona[16,17] and the University of Colorado.[18]

Coded aperture imaging consists of two basic steps. The first step is encoding or multiplexing. To encode an image, a coded aperture is placed between the photon-emitting object and the image receptor, as shown in Figure 4. Multiple pinholes in the array cast a number of overlapping pinhole images of the emitting object on the image receptor. The second step in coded aperture imaging is to decode or de-multiplex the overlapping images to reconstruct one or more planar images of the object.

In nuclear medicine the object of interest is the radioactive distribution within the patient. The image receptor is a film or, more often, a scintillation camera with the collimator removed. Decoding of the overlapping images cast by the aperture is usually done with the aid of a high-speed computer.

Coded aperture imaging can be interpreted as simply another approach to emission computed tomography. Tomography with coded apertures is sometimes referred to as longitudinal tomography, since the coded aperture approach reconstructs a set of planes parallel to the aperture plane.

In principle, coded aperture data can be either multiplexed or unmultiplexed. The conventional approach to coded aperture imaging has been to cast overlapping images onto the detector to improve the photon collection efficiency. On the other hand, an approach such as seven-pinhole tomography[19] that does not produce overlapping images is also a form of coded aperture imaging. Each pinhole records data on a distinct area of the scintillation crystal surface so that the data are "unmultiplexed", or nonoverlapping, and no decoding algorithm is needed to obtain tomographic sections. High contrast images and short computing times provided by the impedance estimator algorithm developed by Kirch,[20] as well as the low cost of this tomographic approach, account for the success of the seven-pinhole approach to tomographic imaging in nuclear medicine. This review concentrates on the clinical viability of multiplexed data collection using coded apertures.

The primary motivation for replacing parallel multihole collimators or single-pinhole

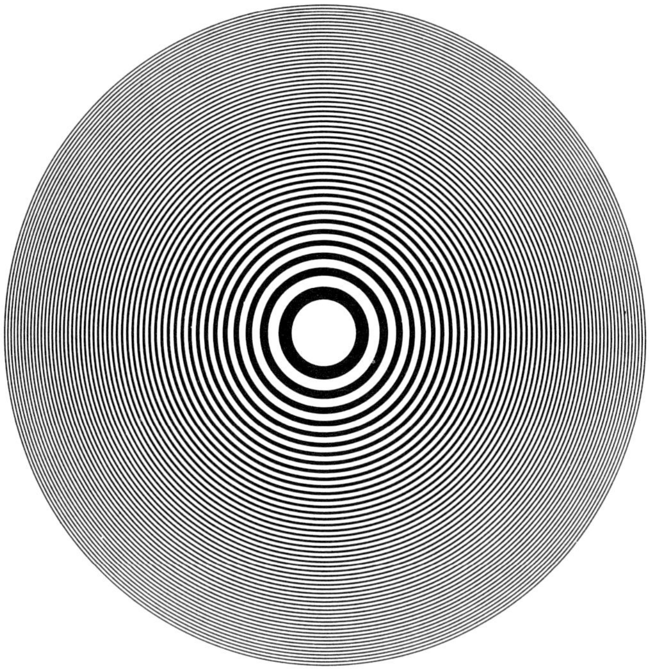

FIGURE 1. A Fresnel-zone plate. (From Barrett, H. H. and Swindell, W., *Radiological Imaging,* Academic Press, New York, 1981. With permission.)

FIGURE 2. A random array. (From Cannon, T. M. and Fenimore, E. E., *Appl. Opt.,* 18, 1052, 1979. With permission.)

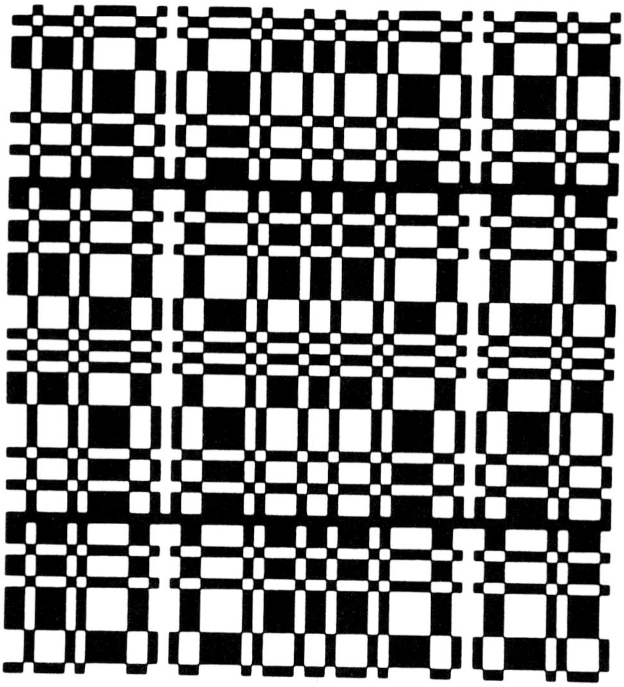

A

B

FIGURE 3. (A) Uniformly redundant array based on quadratic residues. (B) A uniformly redundant array based on m sequences. (From Cannon, T. M. and Fenimore, E. E., *Appl. Opt.*, 18, 1052, 1979. With permission.)

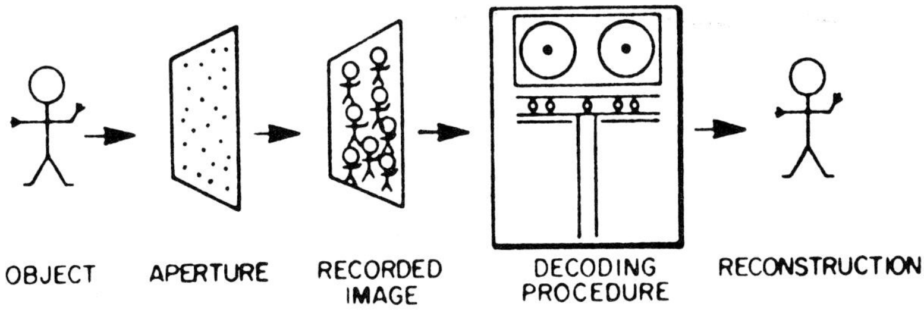

FIGURE 4. The basic steps in encoding and decoding an image acquired using coded apertures. (From Fenimore, E. E. and Cannon, T. M., *Appl. Opt.*, 17, 337, 1978. With permission.)

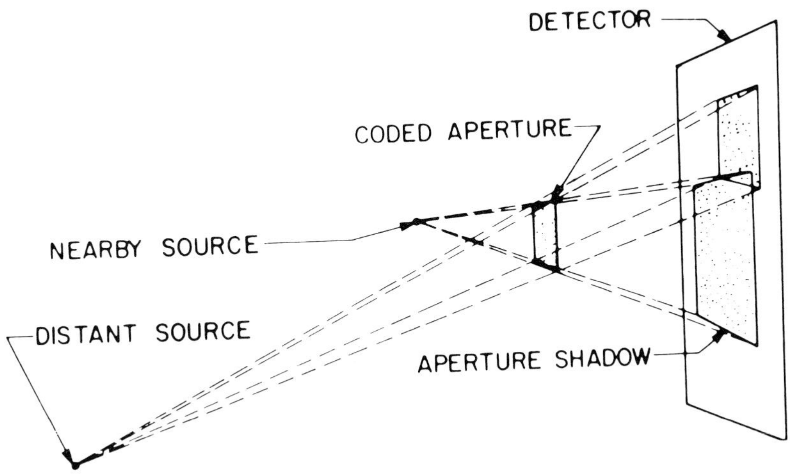

FIGURE 5. The method used by coded aperture systems for obtaining depth information is shown. Distant sources cast smaller aperture shadows than closer sources. By correlating the encoded image with decoding patterns of different sizes, images of the source distribution at different depths can be retrieved. (From Cannon, T. M. and Fenimore, E. E., *Appl. Opt.*, 18, 1052, 1979. With permission.)

apertures with coded apertures in nuclear medicine is to improve the photon collection efficiency of the imaging system. Single-pinhole apertures and parallel multihole collimators used with scintillation cameras typically have collection efficiencies of 10^{-4} or less. The replacement of these collimators with coded apertures increases the collection efficiency by a factor of 100 to 1000. If collection efficiency were the only factor of importance in nuclear medicine imaging, coded apertures would permit substantial reductions in injected activity, imaging time, or both.

A second potential advantage of coded apertures is their potential for tomographic imaging. In principle, a single image acquisition contains all the information needed to reconstruct parallel planar images at any depth in the reconstructed object. Depth information is reflected in the size of the shadow cast by the coded aperture on the image receptor, as shown in Figure 5. A plane at a chosen depth may be reconstructed by using a decoding matrix of the appropriate size. All planes other than the plane at the in-focus depth are blurred and superimposed on the plane of interest, much like the blurring of out-of-focus planes on a conventional tomographic transmission image.

Collection efficiency is not the only characteristic of interest in a nuclear medicine imaging system. The signal to noise ratio (SNR) of the system is another important descriptor of the system's ability to detect low-contrast objects in the presence of a noisy background. Both theoretical[21] and experimental studies[18] of coded aperture imaging systems indicate that the SNR is excellent for point-like objects but decreases quickly with increasing object size. To understand this observation, consider an extended object as a collection of point sources. Each point in the object casts a different shadow of the coded aperture on the image receptor. In the multiplexing scheme, photons striking a particular resolution element on the image receptor may have originated from any of a number of points in the object and may have passed through any of a number of pinholes in the aperture. With an extended object, the signal (i.e., unattenuated photons) emitted by one point in the object adds noise to the signal emitted by another point in the object. As the object size is increased, more noise is added to the signal cast by each point in the object, and the SNR is reduced.

As might be expected, the reduction in SNR is more dramatic in coded apertures with higher transmission ratios resulting from a greater density of pinholes or more open area. A filled array (i.e., a 50% transmitting aperture) will have a substantially lower SNR than a parallel-multihole collimator registering the same number of counts from an extended object.

In addition to the reduction in SNR caused by multiplexing signals from an extended object, conventional coded apertures provide a limited angular view of the radioactive distribution being imaged. In the conventional imaging geometry for coded apertures illustrated in Figure 5, the object, aperture, and detector are fixed in a single orientation during data collection. It has been pointed out in recent work[22-24] that a single limited angle view of an object restricts the collected data so that full tomographic reconstruction of the object is impossible. This difficulty has stimulated the use of multiple views for data collection with coded apertures.[17]

A complete review of the physical and mathematical properties of coded apertures is available in *Radiological Imaging, The Theory of Image Formation, Detection and Processing* by Barrett and Swindell.[25] The present review stresses the clinical applications and viability of coded aperture systems.

II. FRESNEL ZONE-PLATE CODED APERTURES IN NUCLEAR MEDICINE

The first coded aperture used in nuclear medicine imaging was the Fresnel zone-plate aperture. This pattern consists of alternate concentric rings of opaque (lead) and transparent (Lucite) material, with each ring having the same area. The transmission factor through the plate is therefore roughly 50% regardless of the number of rings employed. Figure 6 shows a positive (transparent central zone) and negative (opaque central zone) plate, each with 32 rings, used at the University of Colorado. The number of rings was chosen to resolve the two outermost transparent rings when point sources were imaged in a 128 × 128 matrix on a large-field-of-view (LFOV) GE-400AT camera with an intrinsic resolution of 3.3 mm.

The use of Fresnel zone-plates in light optics to produce an incoherent hologram of a light source distribution is well known. A coherent light source (laser) allows the reconstruction or decoding of the diffraction pattern to recover the initial structure of the object. The potential advantages of Fresnel zone-plates in nuclear medicine imaging are obvious: the amount of radiotracer activity can be reduced considerably, while the imaging time can be decreased compared to imaging methods with pinhole collimators. A review of theoretical aspects and physical properties of zone-plate imaging can be found in various textbooks or original articles.[25-27] Applications to γ-ray imaging have been published by Barrett and Horrigan[9] and Barrett and Swindell.[25]

Simple applications of Fresnel zone plates to nuclear medicine have been reported by several authors.[8,28-33] The source of radiation (i.e., the patient) is placed in front of the zone plate and the encoded information is captured on transparency film. Images representing

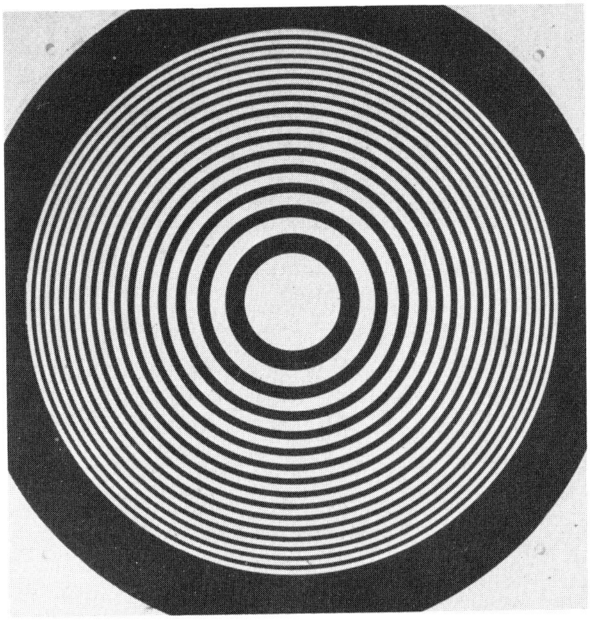

A

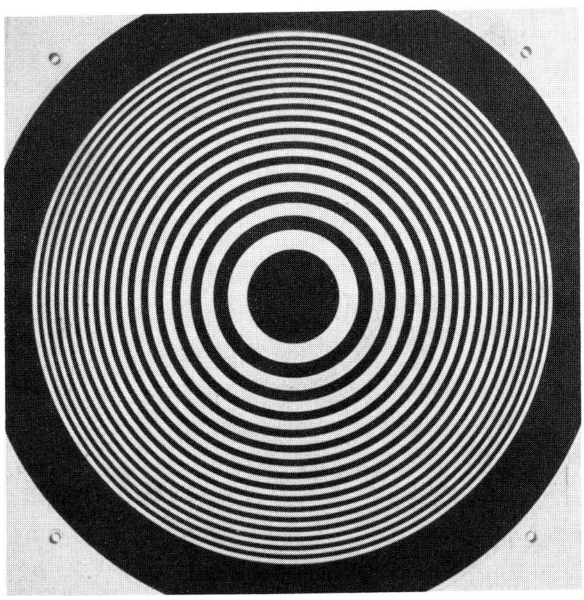

B

FIGURE 6. Positive (A) and negative (B) 32-ring Fresnel-zone plates. (Unpublished work of U. Raff, University of Colorado Health Sciences Center, Denver.)

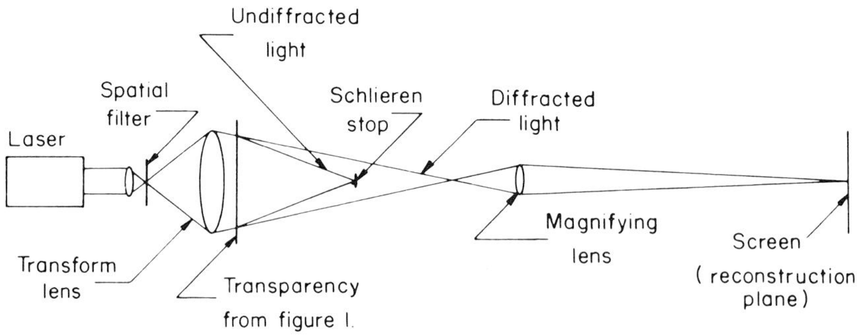

FIGURE 7. Reconstruction system for decoding images obtained with a zone plate camera. (From Barrett, H. H., *J. Nucl. Med.*, 13, 382, 1971. With permission.)

planes through the source distribution are reconstructed by transmitting coherent light through the transparency. Images are reconstructed in three dimensions, as in standard holography. This analog tomographic approach offers two major advantages: (1) the photon collection efficiency is a factor of approximately 100 greater than the efficiency of usual collimators and (2) the spatial resolution is improved beyond that obtained with conventional devices.

There are, however, some major shortcomings to the analog method of zone-plate imaging. The recording medium must have an extremely wide dynamic range, and noise from the film may be a limiting factor. In addition, the transmitted plane waves through the zone plate produce a high background and a superimposed virtual image. It has been shown by Leith et al.[34] that the signal amplitude in holograms decreases as 1/N, where N is the total number of point source holograms that contribute incoherently to the encoded information. As a consequence, extended objects yield poorer contrast. Furthermore, extended objects require larger recording media. The recording medium can be decreased in size by reducing the diameter of the zone plate. In this case, however, the density of multiplexed shadows increases on the recording medium and the amplitude of the signal is decreased. The background arising from undiffracted plane waves and defocused virtual images can be reduced by special filtering and off-axis techniques.[34] This approach has been described in the early work of Barrett.[8,29] The reconstruction system used for decoding the image in shown in Figure 7. First results, imaging a thyroid phantom loaded with 10 μCi of ^{131}I using an on-axis zone plate can be seen in Figure 8.

The use of zone plates for clinical studies with scintillation cameras has been characterized as promising, even for large objects. Tipton et al.[30] analyzed the feasibility of imaging extended γ-ray distributions as large as 20 cm by using a dark-centered negative zone plate. As the object size increases, the image contrast decreases and finally reaches zero. Further enlargements in the object size increase the DC term (background) and reduce the image intensity by destructive interference. An interesting effect is that the contrast eventually reverses so that high contrast images are obtained in a negative sense.

In the optical analog approach to zone-plate imaging described above, tomographic imaging is implemented visually by means of a fast Fourier transform (FFT) to obtain the tomographic in-focus plane. An interesting approach to zone-plate tomography has been described by Macdonald et al.[35] and Budinger et al.,[36] in which the decoding of the image is performed digitally with a computer. The large DC term appearing in the digitized hologram can be eliminated by a method that does not require an off-axis zone plate: the shadowgram obtained with a negative zone plate is subtracted from the one obtained with a positive zone plate.[36] A similar method has been applied to random-pinhole apertures.[37] If all the point sources are within one plane, excellent results can be obtained; however, heavy blurring of sources from out-of-focus planes is superimposed on the in-focus plane. For isolated point

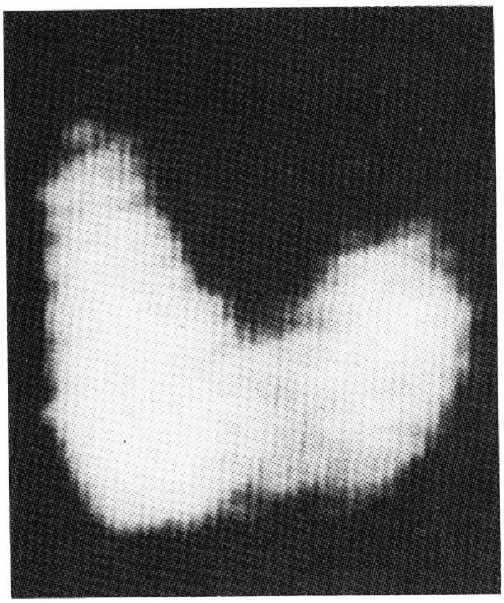

FIGURE 8. Reconstructed image of a 10-μCi thyroid phantom taken with lead zone plate (on-axis) and Anger camera. (From Barrett, H. H., *J. Nucl. Med.*, 13, 382, 1971. With permission.)

sources in a plane, the SNR from zone-plate imaging is far superior to that from pinhole imaging. With increasing object size, however, the noise increases with the number of object points (or resolution areas) with a faster increase for zone plates than for pinhole imaging. This characteristic sharply reduces the advantage of the high collection efficiency of the zone plate.

Optical analog decoding has been compared to digital reconstruction methods by Dance et al.[38] using the autocorrelation approach. These investigators evaluated the response function and the SNR for a single point source using zone plates with varying numbers of zones. Their results are summarized in Figure 9. The autocorrelation technique was found to be superior to the optical technique, yielding a 50% greater SNR. The resolution, however, of the autocorrelation approach was inferior to that of optical processing because with the optical technique, the number of zones can be increased without sacrificing SNR. In the digital method, a compromise between SNR and spatial resolution must be identified based on a choice of the number of zones in the plate. Digital decoding of data recorded with a scintillation camera has been explored by Wilson et al.[39] with computer simulations to obtain insight into noise effects, solid-angle variations, shape of detector, and detector resolution. Tomographic results are provided for line sources and for a standard thyroid phantom loaded with ^{99m}Tc. Geometrical efficiency and SNR are compared for camera zone plates and high-resolution parallel-hole collimators. The SNR for the collimator can be taken as $\sqrt{\text{counts}}$ per pixel in the image. The SNR depends on the spatial resolution but is relatively independent of the object-collimator distance. For an equal number of total counts in the image, the ratio

$$R = \text{SNR (zone plate)/SNR (collimator)}$$

is always less than 1 and thus does not favor the use of the coded aperture. This result, however, ignores the fact that the count rate is much higher (20 to 100 times) for the zone plate than for the parallel-hole collimator. For equal counting times, the ratio R depends on the source to camera distance and may be greater than 1. For example, a line source imaged

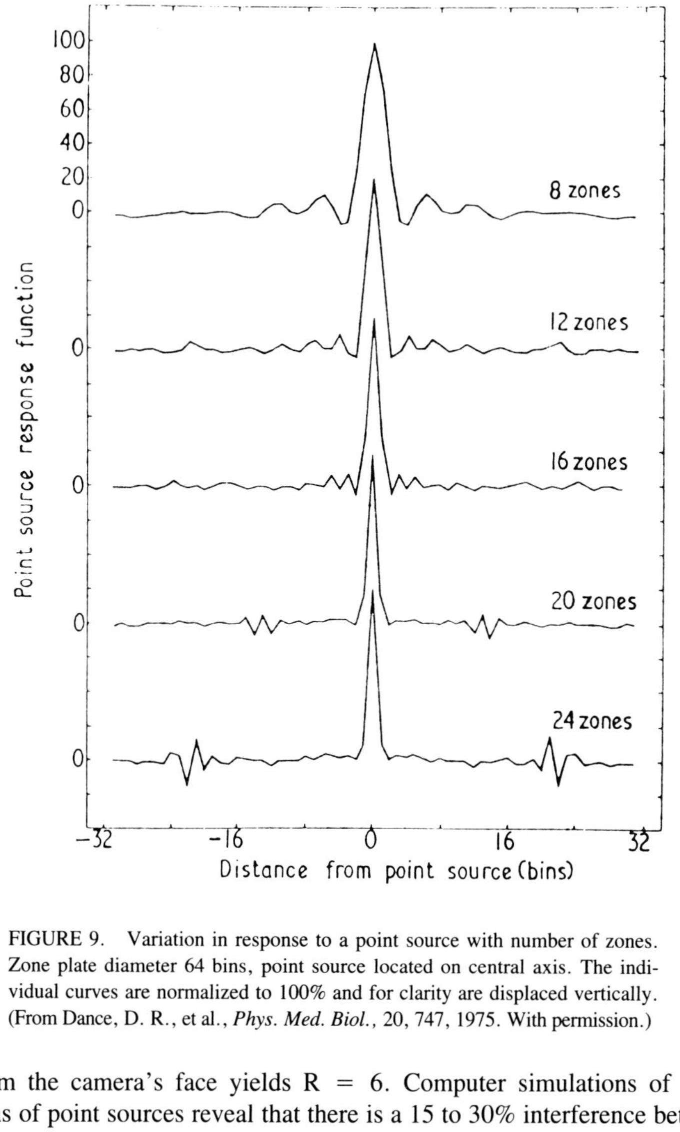

FIGURE 9. Variation in response to a point source with number of zones. Zone plate diameter 64 bins, point source located on central axis. The individual curves are normalized to 100% and for clarity are displaced vertically. (From Dance, D. R., et al., *Phys. Med. Biol.*, 20, 747, 1975. With permission.)

at 15 cm from the camera's face yields R = 6. Computer simulations of tomographic reconstructions of point sources reveal that there is a 15 to 30% interference between planes 10% apart. The interference was smallest for points located at the center of the object matrix and largest for points at the edges of the object matrix.

Singleton et al.[40] have reviewed optical and digital tomographic reconstruction techniques for Fresnel zone plates. Digital reconstruction is achieved by decoding using direct deconvolution. Off-axis Fresnel zone-plate apertures (Figure 10) requiring a "half-tone" (bar pattern) screen to collect the data are compared to on-axis zone-plate apertures. The advantage of the off-axis zone plate is that multiply diffracted waves are spatially separated, thereby avoiding interference with other waves. However, an on-axis zone plate cannot simply be replaced by an off-axis plate because the off-axis plate produces encoded images with very low contrast. Practically no light can be diffracted through the photoreduced transparency by decoding this type of image. Interposing a bar pattern screen between a radioactive organ and an off-axis zone plate introduces artificial high-frequency components in the encoded image. When the modulating bar pattern satisfies the Nyquist criterion, however, no information is lost in collecting the encoded image.

For scintillation camera imaging, the spatial resolution in the decoded image is approximately three times poorer in the off-axis case.[25] This behavior explains why off-axis zone

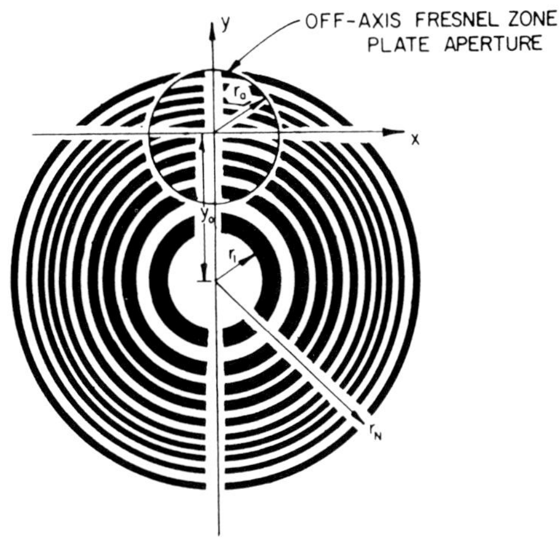

A

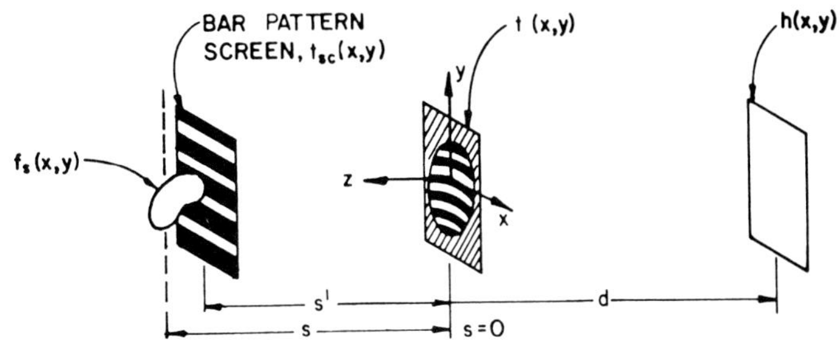

B

FIGURE 10. (A) Transmittance of the off-axis FZP aperture, where r_a is the aperture radius, y_o is the shift from the center, and r_N is the total zone plate radius. (B) Arrangement using an off-axis FZP aperture and a bar pattern screen to obtain a recording which yields a separated image. (From Singleton, R. M., et al., *IEEE Trans. Biomed. Eng.*, BME-23, 239, 1976. With permission.)

plates have found very little applicability with scintillation cameras. A solution to this dilemma has been found by using a combination of multiple on-axis zone plates, an approach used successfully to image flat objects such as the thyroid phantom shown in Figure 11. This image was obtained with three on-axis zone plates.

Recently, Budinger[41] reviewed the physical properties of emission computed tomography, including multiple-pinhole arrays, stochastic apertures, and Fresnel zone plates. The effects of limited angular sampling in reconstructions are examined when prior information is known about object shape, geometry of the imaging system, and noise characteristics. A major benefit of coded aperture tomography may be the ability to perform dynamic SPECT studies.

Until now, the clinical use of Fresnel zone-plate tomography has been a practical failure, due primarily to problems arising from the limited-angle image acquisition. So far, only a few clinical trials have been attempted. Farmelant et al.[42] studied a series of patients who were given ^{123}I and were imaged with both a rectilinear scanner and a zone-plate aperture. Tomographic decoding was done optically. Normal and abnormal (multinodular goiter) thyroid tomographic studies are shown in Figure 12. Using this approach for large objects (e.g., lungs), the amount of out-of-focus data is generally greater than the data used to reconstruct the in-focus tomogram, and a diagnostic interpretation is impossible.

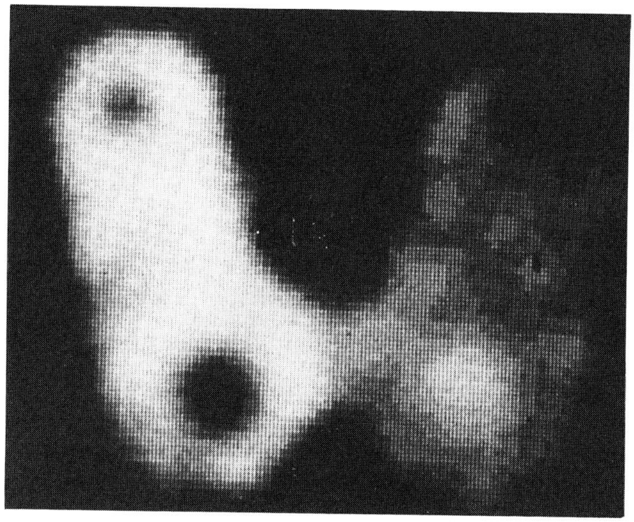

FIGURE 11. Image of the Picker thyroid phantom with a Picker Dynacamera 4/15. Obtained with three on-axis zone plates. Total exposure time was the same as with standard parallel-hole collimator. (Unpublished work of Reinhardt, E. R., Laub, G., and Bloss, W. H., University of Stuttgart, and Feine, U. and Müller-Schauenburg, University of Tübingen. Reprinted with permission from Barrett, H. H. and Swindell, W., *Radiological Imaging*, Academic Press, New York, 1981.)

Probably the most successful clinical attempt of tomography with a Fresnel zone-plate aperture has been described by Holman et al.,[43] who assessed regional myocardial perfusion using an animal model. Optical reconstruction of the hologram provided tomographic sections of the heart. Planar scintigraphy was also performed and compared to the tomographic results. Myocardial perfusion was studied by injecting 100,000 microspheres (20 to 40 μm) labeled with 20 mCi of ^{99m}Tc directly into the left main coronary artery. Ischemia was generated by coronary artery occlusion obtained by embolization via a catheter guidewire system. The camera zone-plate system used is shown in Figure 13. Gamma rays passing through the aperture are encoded directly on X-ray film. Reconstruction of this multiplexed information (''unscrambling of data'') was performed with coherent laser light that passed through the minified (1:100) version of the recorded hologram of the heart. By moving a lens in the laser system, different in-focus planes could be obtained and recorded photographically while over- and underlying structures were blurred. The coded aperture system consisted of an off-axis zone plate and a half-tone screen combination. Imaging of the dog's heart was accomplished in a 45° left anterior oblique (LAO) and right anterior oblique (RAO) position and, when possible, in a right and left lateral position. Five 1-m exposures were performed for each view. Because of the poor sensitivity of the detector used, the sensitivity of the ''Fresnel zone camera'' was quoted as low as no better than 5% of the scintillation camera. The extent of perfusion defects obtained from the Fresnel zone image was compared to the reduction in perfusion measured by *in vitro* assays using gamma well-counters. Tomographic zone-plate sections were obtained in $^1/_2$-in. increments from 2 to 4 in. from the aperture plane. Normal tomographic sections are shown in Figure 14 and myocardial perfusion images following occlusion of the LAD artery are shown in Figure 15. Contrast was satisfactory and was superior to that obtained in planar imaging. As soon as the radiotracer was distributed around the organ to be imaged, artifacts from other structures became a major disadvantage. The poor sensitivity of the Fresnel zone camera used by Holman et al.[43] was due primarily to the lack of an adequate film-screen combination for the 140 keV

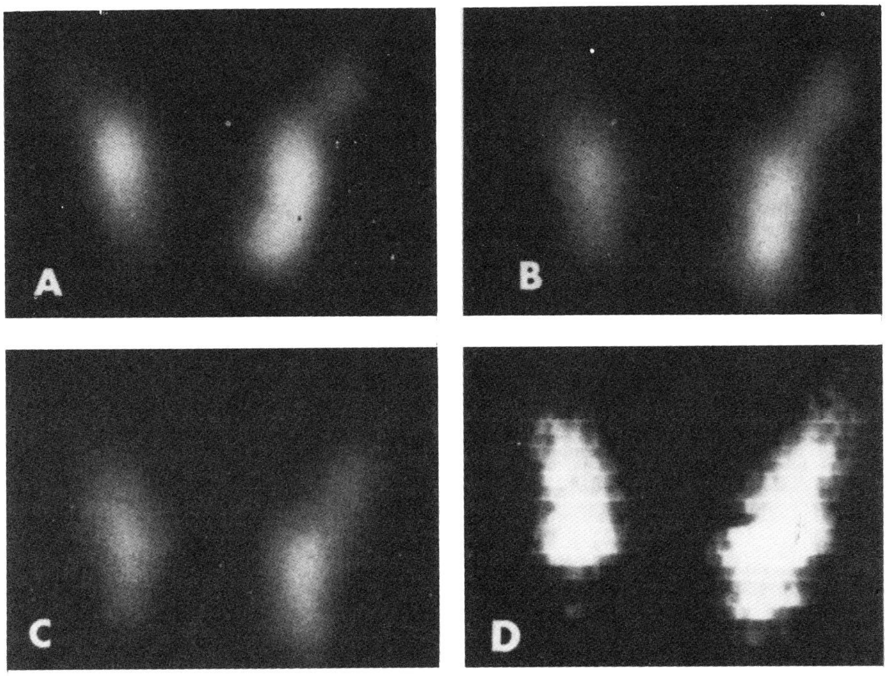

a

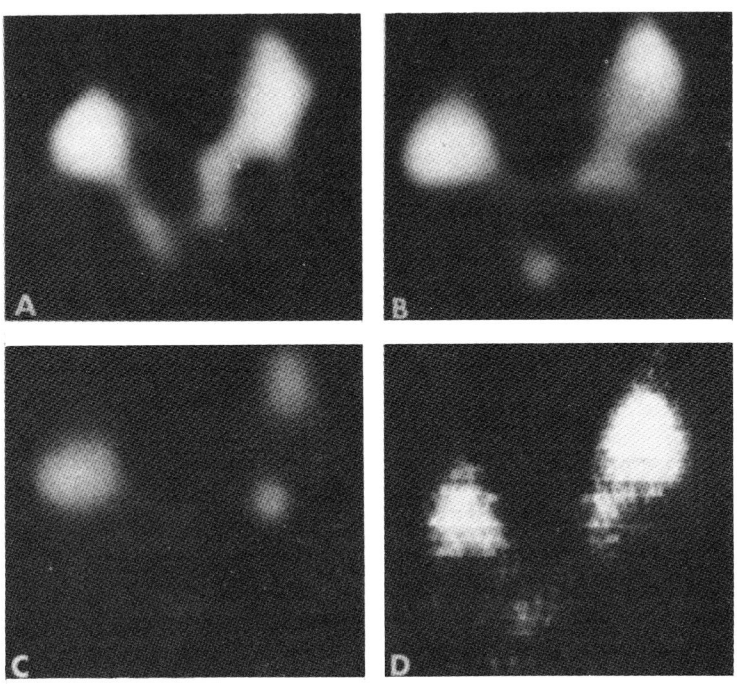

b

FIGURE 12. (a) Comparison of zone-plate and rectilinear normal thyroidal images. (A to C) are "cuts" from front, middle, and rear of the reconstruction encompassing less than 2 cm in total thickness (^{123}I). Band-like area of reduced uptake in left upper lobe appears as narrowing when viewed on television monitor without discontinuities of reproductions. (b) Large multinodular nontoxic goiter (^{123}I). Zone-plate series at 1.2-cm intervals (A to C). Whereas rectilinear scan (D) is diagnostic, zone-plate series more clearly define nodules. (From Farmelant, M. H., et al., *J. Nucl. Med.*, 16, 183, 1975. With permission.)

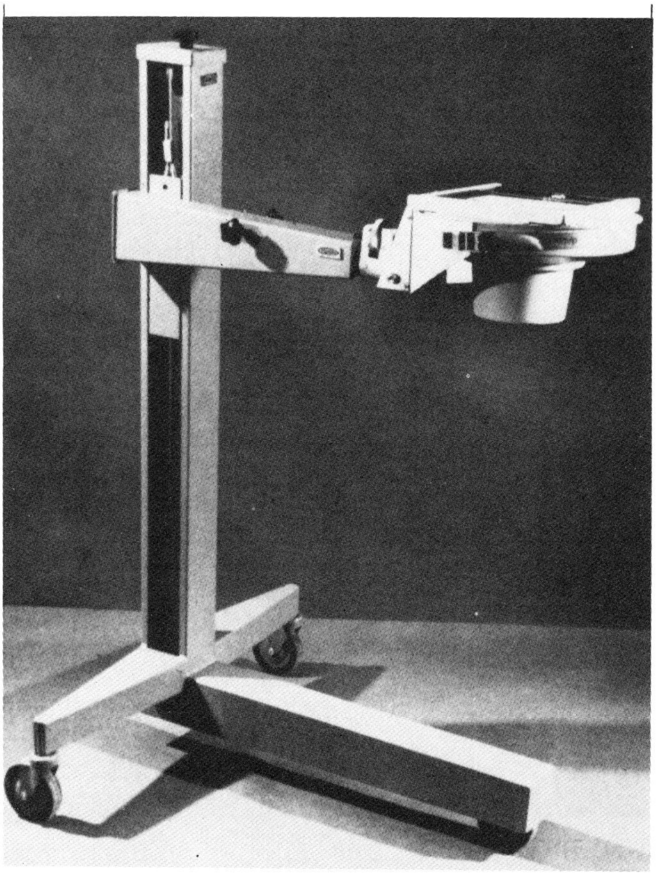

FIGURE 13. The Fresnel-zone tomographic camera. (From Holman, B. L., et al., *J. Nucl. Med.*, 16, 764, 1977. With permission.)

energy range of ^{99m}Tc. As suggested by the authors, a solution to this problem might be to image with a scintillation camera with the digital holograms decoded by computer. One problem, however, with the scintillation camera would be the high photon flux transmitted through the aperture under normal imaging conditions. Faster detectors such as a multiwire proportional chamber have been proposed as an alternative[44,45] to accommodate the higher detection rate needed. The use of small array processors to decode digital Fresnel zone-plate data[46] might also make this approach to limited-angle tomography very practical.

III. TIME MODULATED CODED APERTURES

Only limited clinical investigation of other coded apertures has been performed in nuclear medicine. Koral et al.[47] have imaged the thyroid with a time modulated coded aperture technique and have compared it to standard pinhole imaging. Their first clinical trial included a small group of 19 patients to determine the potential of the coded aperture imaging (CAI) approach in a clinical environment. A pseudo-random pinhole sequence (121 elements long) and time modulation were reported to give improved resolution and efficiency compared to the Fresnel zone-plate camera. Image reconstruction utilized a standard algebraic reconstruction technique (ART) and a simultaneous iterative reconstruction technique (SIRT). Multiple planar pinhole images were acquired (anterior 75° LAO and 35° RAO) and compared to CAI results. ^{99m}Tc-pertechnetate was injected intravenously and imaging was started ap-

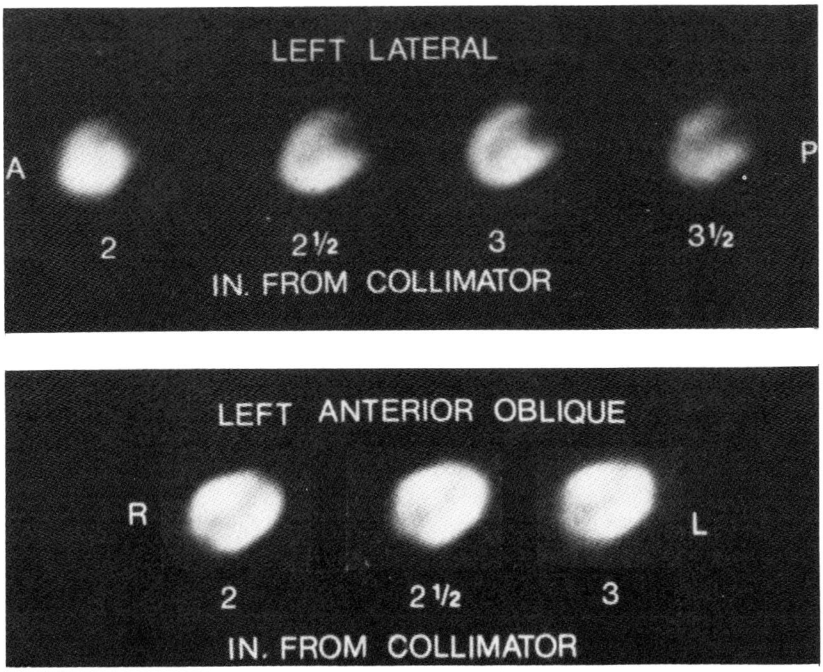

FIGURE 14. Myocardial perfusion images in normal dog made with the instrument of Figure 1. (Top) Left lateral; (bottom) left anterior oblique. (From Holman, B. L., et al., *J. Nucl. Med.*, 16, 764, 1977. With permission.)

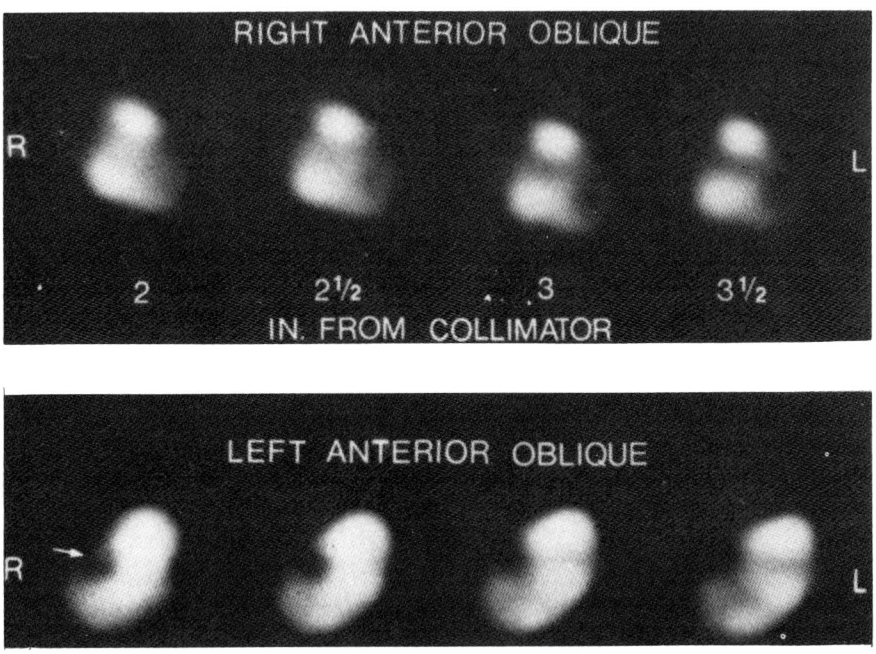

FIGURE 15. Myocardial perfusion images following occlusion of the left anterior descending artery. Perfusion defect involves anterior wall and apex: top is right anterior oblique; bottom is left anterior oblique. (From Holman, B. L., et al., *J. Nucl. Med.*, 16, 764, 1977. With permission.)

proximately $^1/_2$ h later. Planar pinhole images were acquired for 200 kcounts. Total data collection time with the coded aperture was arbitrarily set to the same duration as that used for the anterior single pinhole view. The aperture was positioned 1 cm from the anterior surface of the patient's neck, and 121 individual encoded images were collected into 64 × 64 matrices. Longitudinal planes were obtained at 1.2, 1.7, 2.3, and 3.3 cm and, in some cases, 4.3 cm depth from the skin surface. Planar pinhole images were acquired such that the thyroid image covered 75% of the field-of-view of the camera. The preliminary study of 19 cases was somewhat deceiving from a diagnostic point of view. CAI was visually judged better in 5 cases, equal in 13, and worse in 1 case.[46] In a second prospective study by Resinger et al.[48] encompassing a group of 136 patients, 109 pairs of studies comparing CAI to planar pinhole images using ROC analysis did not yield very encouraging results; both techniques had the same sensitivity and performed similarly. Nevertheless, CAI offered improved contrast, accurate sizing of the thyroid at different depths, no pinhole distortion, and faster data collection. The major limitation of CAI in routine clinical work was the very long computer processing time required for image decoding. Software improvements were able to reduce processing time by a factor of two from the initial trials.[47] If no special purpose hardware with parallel processing is used, however, the 2 h processing time remains impractical for clinical studies and provides no reasonable alternative to pinhole scintigraphy.

The clinical potential of time modulated coded aperture imaging for cardiac studies has also been investigated by Rogers et al.[49,50] Several advantages of CAI were reported; since images are multiplexed at the detector's face, the camera can be kept to a relatively small size, such as that of portable cameras for intensive care units. Furthermore, the use of time modulated coded apertures allows small organs to be placed within 1 to 2 cm of the aperture. The pseudo-random time coded aperture used for thyroid imaging was changed by the author to a dual-plate time coded aperture designed for cardiac imaging. Figure 16 depicts a multiple-pinhole geometry (73 elements long, pseudo-random, with a mean transmission of 12% used by Rogers et al.[50]). A code plate lies on top of an aperture plate, with both plates providing well-defined pinhole patterns. Multiple sequential steps consist of sliding the coded plate across the aperture plate and collecting a multiplexed image of an organ with a scintillation camera. The recorded pattern depends on the time modulated pinhole pattern as well as the distribution of activity in the object. The decoding step involves a digital correlation with the code sequence of each hole in the aperture plate. Longitudinal tomograms are then obtained by means of an ART algorithm. A photograph of the cardiac aperture is shown in Figure 17. A set of 12 tomographic planes obtained from one single-pass data set was reconstructed in 96 s in the University of Michigan's AMDAHL V470 computer. Postprocessing of tomograms with a median filter was performed to eliminate spurious noise, and a variable Chesler filter was applied to reduce noise without sacrificing resolution. A series of tests was done with phantoms, *in vitro* dog hearts, living dogs, and human myocardium to assess the validity of the method. Figure 18 shows ^{201}Tl tomograms of a living dog obtained after occlusion of the LAD artery. An anterior infarct is clearly visible in all four slices. Gated blood-pool tomograms at various depths are shown in diastole and systole in Figure 19. ^{210}Tl images of a patient with an apical aneurysm are shown in Figure 20. These preliminary myocardial perfusion studies with coded apertures looked promising, although the product of dose times data collection time was too long by a factor of 3 for the pinhole diameter (3 mm) used in the experiment. Comparison with the unmultiplexed seven-pinhole technique[18,20] was also performed. Simplicity of the seven-pinhole technique (no moving aperture, no decoding algorithms, and known sensitivity) makes it the easier approach to tomographic imaging of small organs. Because of signal multiplexing, it is very difficult to specify the sensitivity in the coded aperture technique. At a particular point the noise depends not only on the local source distribution, like unmultiplexed imaging, but also on distant sources. This contribution makes it difficult to specify the SNR for extended sources. At

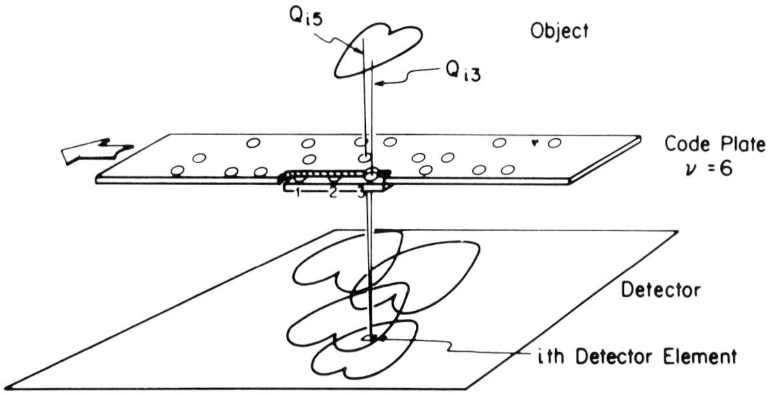

FIGURE 16. Illustration of cardiac-aperture geometry showing translating code plate and multihole aperture plate. Coded image, composed of overlapping pinhole images on camera face, is shown schematically. (From Rogers, W. L., et al., *J. Nucl. Med.*, 21, 371, 1980. With permission.)

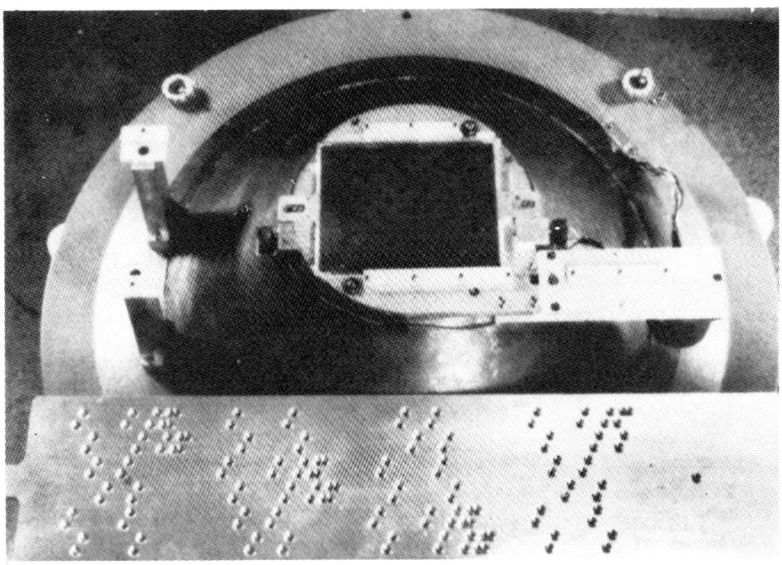

FIGURE 17. Photograph of cardiac aperture, with translating code plate removed, to show movable 72-pinhole aperture plate. Aperture assembly is shown attached to wide-field camera mount. (From Rogers, W. L., et al., *J. Nucl. Med.*, 21, 371, 1980. With permission.)

present, decoding would require hardware dedicated to make time modulated coded apertures clinically practical.

A second approach to time modulated coded apertures is the rotating-slit aperture introduced by Tanaka and Iinuma[14] and investigated more extensively by physicists at the University of Arizona.[15,16] Variations on the single-rotating slit, including rotating-slat collimators and hybrid slit-pinhole collimators, have also been investigated.[16]

Emission data accumulated with rotating-slit or rotating-slat collimators, illustrated in Figure 21, are similar to transmission data accumulated in computed tomography (CT). Decoding of the time modulated data to recover a single reconstructed image was done in a manner similar to the filtered backprojection methods of CT, since both systems yield data blurred by an l/r pointspread function. There is, however, a fundamental difference in

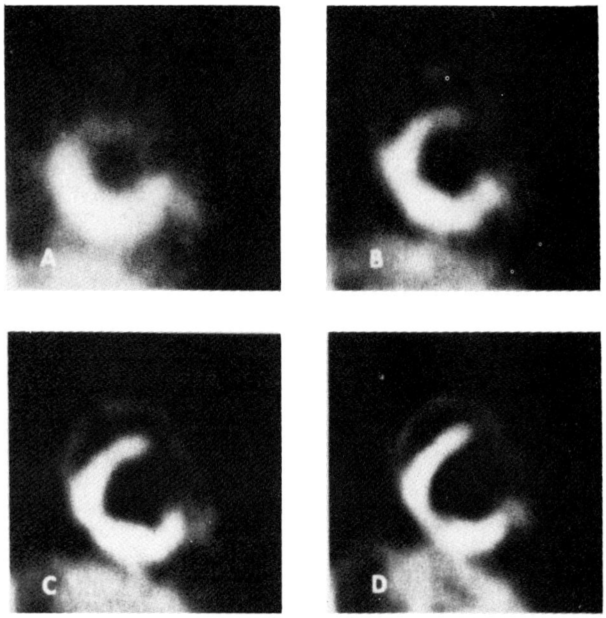

FIGURE 18. Thallium tomograms of living, intact dog, obtained with portable camera. Anterior infarct is clearly shown in four slices beginning near base (A) at 8 cm, and stepping in 1-cm increments toward apex. Dog is viewed from in front with 20° cephalad tilt, a projection that is equivalent to LAO in man. (From Rogers, W. L., et al., *J. Nucl. Med.*, 21, 371, 1980. With permission.)

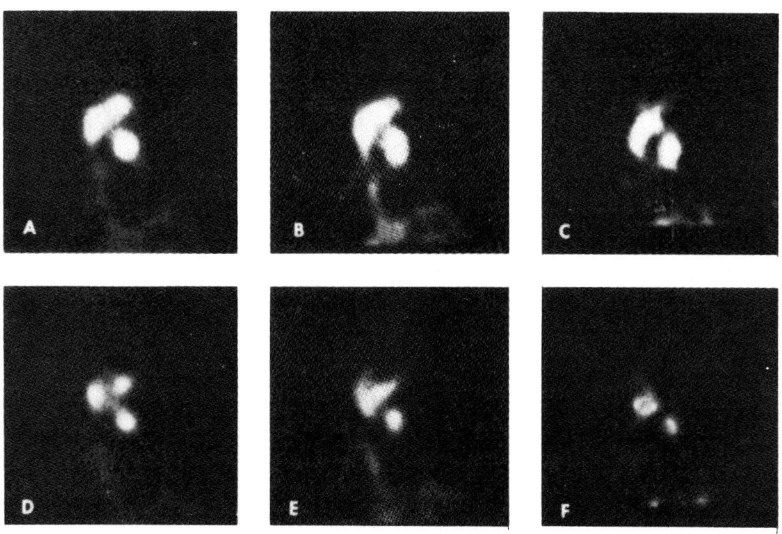

FIGURE 19. Gated blood-pool tomograms of normal dog obtained with portable camera. Diastolic images at 12, 11, and 10 cm are shown in top row, with corresponding systolic images in bottom row. Images were postprocessed with median and adaptive filters (10, 11). Corresponding diastolic and systolic images were photographed with same count-intensity scale. Dog was viewed from in front, with 20° cephalad angulation of camera. Note correspondence between thallium images in Figure 7 and blood-pool images. (From Rogers, W. L., et al., *J. Nucl. Med.*, 21, 371, 1980. With permission.)

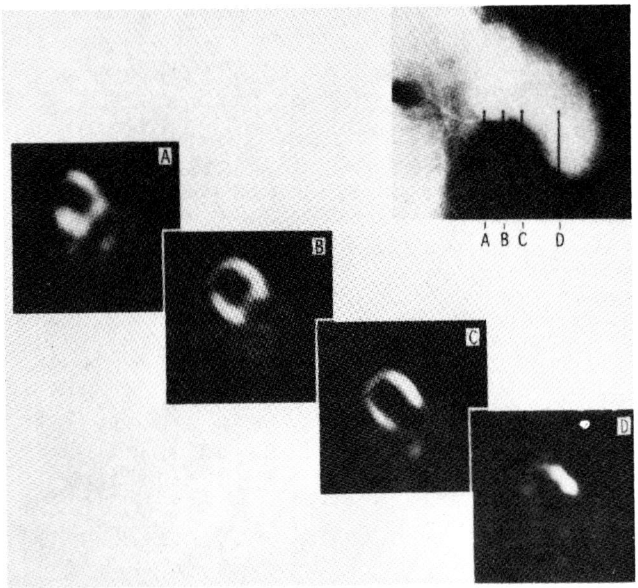

FIGURE 20. Coded-aperture resting thallium tomograms of patient with large apical aneurysm. View is from 30° LAO. Approximate slice depths are marked on 40° RAO ventriculogram, shown above for reference. Images were postprocessed with median filtering and adaptive filter using Chesler's algorithm. Approximately 20% background subtraction was used to discriminate against tissue background observed in resting thallium images. (From Rogers, W. L., et al., *J. Nucl. Med.*, 21, 371, 1980. With permission.)

rotating-slit emission imaging and CT transmission imaging. CT is inherently planar by the nature of data acquisition; the data collected are line integrals of linear attenuation coefficients through a preselected planar section. For the case of a slit passing through the axis of rotation, rotating-slit emission tomography, on the other hand, collects data nontomographically. Each plane through the object and parallel to the plane of the slit aperture emits photons collected by the system. Different planes parallel to the aperture are unresolved by the decoding process. All planes parallel to the aperture plane are collapsed into a single image, just as in transmission radiography or collimator-emission imaging.

Decoding of a planar section at a particular depth can be accomplished by using an off-axis rotating slit, as shown in Figure 22. Displacing the slit from the axis of rotation of the aperture provides a scale in relation to which depth may be measured. Planes out of the depth of interest are blurred by the off-axis slit, much like the blurring of out-of-focus planes in conventional transmission tomography.

Experimental investigations of rotating-slit apertures have been restricted to phantom studies. Rotating-slit images have been compared to single-pinhole images acquired over equal exposure times and equal magnifications. Figure 23 shows a comparison of these two methods of imaging using a 6-in. disk phantom with cold spots produced by round copper absorbers with varying transmittances and a square lead attenuator at the center. Image quality is similar with the two methods of data acquisition. In general, pinhole imaging appears to yield a slightly better SNR for cold spot imaging, while rotating-slit imaging gives a better SNR for hot spot imaging.[15]

IV. UNIFORMLY REDUNDANT ARRAY IMAGING

Uniformly redundant arrays (URAs) were developed by Fenimore and Cannon[5-7] at Los Alamos and have been used to record X-ray emission during laser-driven fusion experi-

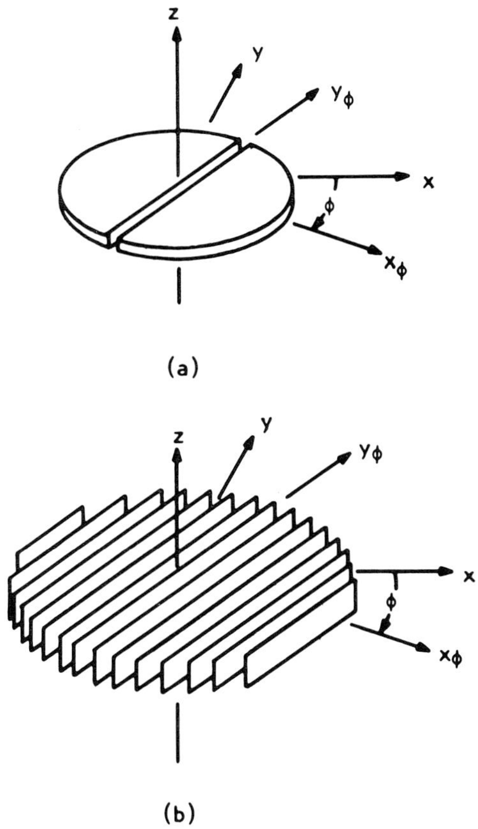

FIGURE 21. A rotating-slit aperture (a) and a rotating-slat collimator (b). (From Gindi, G. R., et al., *Med. Phys.*, 9, 324, 1982. With permission.)

ments.[51] Fenimore and Cannon have also done extensive theoretical studies on the expected performance of URAs.[5-7] Experimental work on the performance of URAs for nuclear medicine imaging is currently underway at the University of Colorado.[18]

URAs have several potentially promising advantages over other coded apertures used for medical imaging. One potential advantage is that with proper decoding methods,[5] finite-sized URAs can be constructed that have delta-function point-spread functions. As shown in Figure 24, this is an improvement over the point-spread function of Fresnel zone plates and random-pinhole arrays. Like Fresnel zone plates, URAs are approximately 50% transmitting and are thus superior in photon collection efficiency to nonredundant arrays and the time modulated coded apertures that have so far been applied to medical imaging. Like most other coded aperture, URAs can be used for tomographic reconstruction of planar images at a range of depths within the patient. Also, like most other coded apertures, fixed-geometry URAs suffer the limitations of a limited-angular view of the object and the reduction of SNR due to multiplexing when extended objects are imaged. The latter problem is illustrated in Figure 25 by a series of images of disk phantoms of increasing sizes acquired using a 61 × 59 URA at the University of Colorado. As the size of the disk increases from 1 to 4 cm, the SNR of the image degrades seriously. As pointed out by Barrett and co-workers,[25] this is a limitation of all filled (≃ 50% transmitting) arrays. Theoretical studies by Wagner et al.[21] find the URA to be superior to a "grand array" and a large open square when imaging point-like objects; however, the advantage of URAs disappears with increasing object size. Such a limitation makes the clinical task of imaging weak sources difficult in the presence

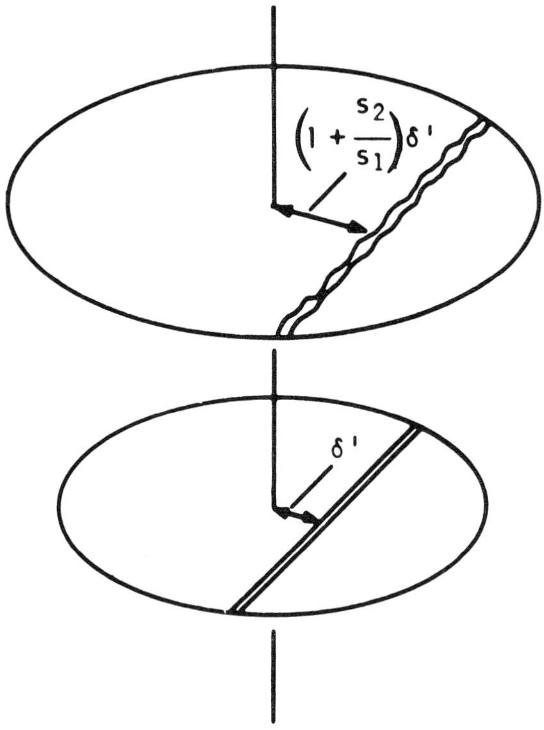

FIGURE 22. The off-axis slit. If the slit is translated as shown above, the stripe translates by a proportional amount. (From Gindi, G. R., et al., *Med. Phys.*, 9, 324, 1982. With permission.)

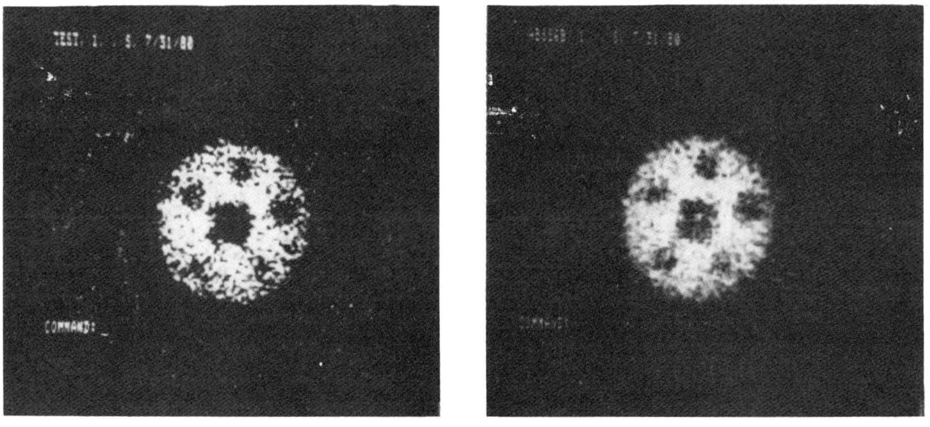

A B

FIGURE 23. (A) Pinhole image with 90,000 counts. (b) Rotating-slit image. For both images, the magnification is unity and the exposure time 40 s. The reconstructions are on a 128-×-128 grid. (From Gindi, G. R., et al., *Med. Phys.*, 9, 324, 1982. With permission.)

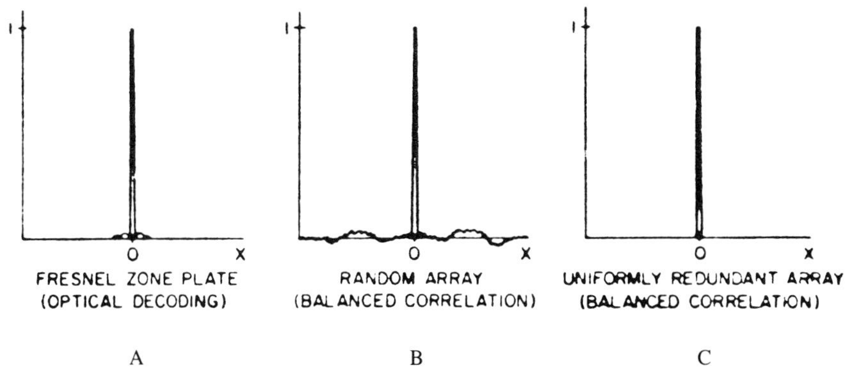

FIGURE 24. (A) The system point-spread function (SPSF) of an optically decoded 37-zone Fresnel zone-plate coded aperture. The size of the sidelobes diminishes as the number of rings in the aperture is increased. (B) The SPSF of a random array equal in size to the FZP of (A). Again, the sidelobe structure decreases as the random array is made larger. (C) The SPSF of a uniformly redundant array (URA). The sidelobes of the URA SPSF are always flat, regardless of array size. The central peak would be a delta function if infinitely small pinholes were used. (From Cannon, T. M. and Fenimore, E. E., *Opt. Eng.*, 19, 283, 1980. With permission.)

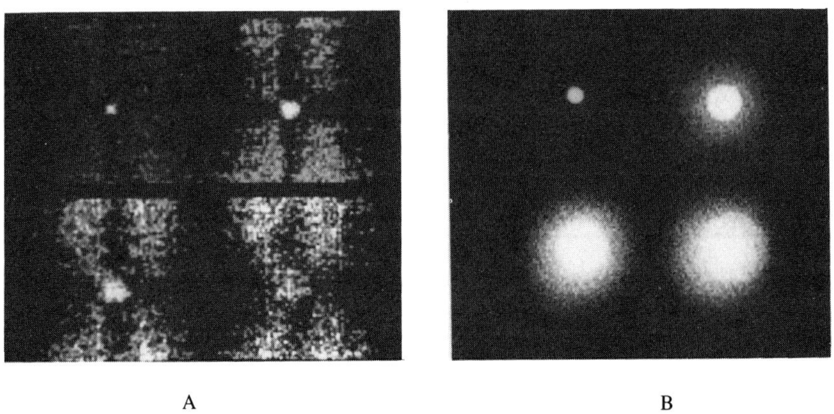

FIGURE 25. A comparison of performance of (A) uniformly redundant array, (B) single-pinhole, and (C) parallel-multihole collimator in imaging homogeneous disks of activity of 1-, 2-, 3-, and 4-cm diameters. The imaging time was 4 min for each acquisition. Note the decrease of the signal-to-noise ratio as object size increases for the URA image. (Preliminary results from R. E. Hendrick and U. Raff, University of Colorado Health Sciences Center, Denver.)

of distributed background activity. This problem is illustrated in studies of a simulated lesion of 1 cm diameter positioned in a planar background of activity.[18] Images acquired with a URA, single-pinhole aperture, and parallel-multihole collimator illustrate the failure of URAs to equal the performance of conventional apertures in this simple application.

V. PROBLEMS AND FUTURE OF CODED APERTURE TOMOGRAPHY

Two problems plague coded aperture imaging as developed to date: the limited-angle problem and the multiplexing problem. The limited-angle problem can be solved only by acquiring multiple views of the patient at widely different angles, either by moving a single-aperture-camera system or by employing several fixed-aperture camera systems simultaneously. Preliminary studies using several-aperture camera systems are underway at the University of Arizona.[17]

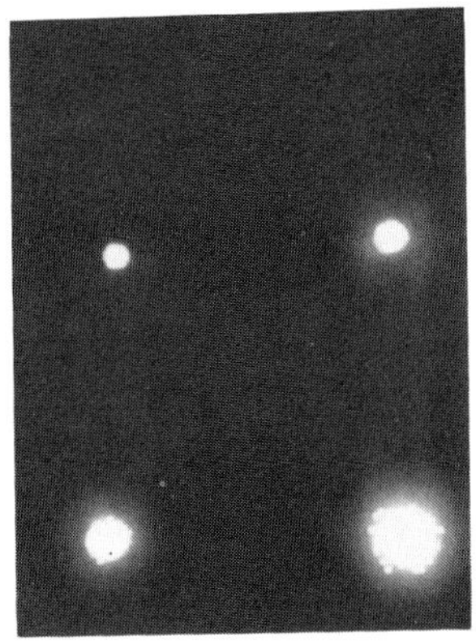

FIGURE 25C.

The multiplexing problem (i.e., the loss of SNR as the object increases in size when imaged with filled arrays) may be less serious than the limited-angle problem.[17,52] The multiplexing problem has been demonstrated to be a serious limitation of filled (50% transmitting) arrays such as Fresnel-zone plates and conventional URAs. An unanswered question in coded aperture imaging is, can coded apertures be designed with intermediate transmission factors (between a fraction of 1 and 50%) and with good point-spread functions? Because of reduced transmission compared to filled arrays, such apertures might not suffer from so serious a multiplexing problem as that experienced with filled arrays. They may also possess sufficiently high photon collection efficiencies to be superior to single-pinhole or parallel-multihole collimators in some clinical applications.

A related unanswered question is, what is the most efficient algorithm to perform SPECT imaging with coded apertures? That is, can an efficient algorithm be found to combine a number of coded aperture views, acquired at different angles, into a set of two-dimensional images or a single three-dimension image?

To date, an ideal coded aperture has not been found. The promise of coded apertures for tomography in clinical nuclear medicine remains to be no more than it has been in the past — a hope for the future.

REFERENCES

1. **Mertz, L. and Young, N. O.,** Fresnel transformation of images, *Proc. Int. Conf. Opt. Inst.*, 305, 1961.
2. **Dicke, R. H.,** Scatter-hole cameras for X-rays and gamma rays, *Astrophys. J.*, 153, L-101, 1968.
3. **Ables, J. G.,** Fourier transform photography: a new method for X-ray astronomy, *Proc. Astron. Soc. Aust.*, 1, 172, 1968.
4. **Golay, M. J. E.,** Point arrays having compact, nonredundant autocorrelations, *J. Opt. Soc. Am.*, 61, 272, 1971.
5. **Fenimore, E. E. and Cannon, T. M.,** Coded aperture imaging with uniformly redundant arrays, *Appl. Opt.*, 17, 337, 1978.
6. **Fenimore, E. E.,** Coded aperture imaging: predicted performance of uniformly redundant arrays, *Appl. Opt.*, 17, 3562, 1978.
7. **Cannon, T. M. and Fenimore, E. E.,** Tomographical imaging using uniformly redundant arrays, *Appl. Opt.*, 18, 1052, 1979.
8. **Barrett, H. H.,** Fresnel zone plate imaging in nuclear medicine, *J. Nucl. Med.*, 13, 382, 1972.
9. **Barrett, H. H. and Horrigan, F. A.,** Fresnel zone imaging of gamma rays; theory, *Appl. Opt.*, 12, 2686, 1973.

10. **Barrett, H. H. and DeMeester, G. D.,** Quantum noise in Fresnel zone plate imaging, *Appl. Opt.*, 13, 1100, 1974.
11. **Koral, K. F., Rogers, W. L., and Knoll, G. F.,** Digital tomographic imaging with time-modulated pseudorandom coded aperture and Anger camera, *J. Nucl. Med.*, 16, 402, 1975.
12. **Simpson, R. G., Barrett, H. H., and Fisher, H. D.,** Decoding techniques for use with annular coded apertures, in *Applications of Holography and Optical Data Processing,* Marom, E., Friesem, A. A., and Weiner-Avnear, E., Eds., Plenum Press, New York, 1977, 87.
13. **Simpson, R. G. and Barrett, H. H.,** Coded-aperture imaging, in *Imaging in Diagnostic Medicine,* Nudelman, S., Ed., Plenum Press, New York, 1980, 217.
14. **Tanaka, E. and Iinuma, T. A.,** Image processing for coded aperture imaging and an attempt at rotating slit imaging, *Proc. 4th Int. Conf. Inform. Process. Scintigr.*, 43, 1975.
15. **Gindi, G. R., Arendt, J., Barrett, H. H., et al.,** Imaging with rotating slit apertures and rotating collimators, *Med. Phys.*, 9, 324, 1982.
16. **Smith, W. E., Barrett, H. H., and Paxman, R. G.,** Reconstruction of objects from coded images by simulated annealing, *Opt. Lett.*, 8, 199, 1983.
17. **Paxman, R. G., Schmith, W. E., and Barrett, H. H.,** Two algorithms for use with an orthogonal-view coded-aperture system, *J. Nucl. Med.*, 25, 700, 1984.
18. **Hendrick, R. E., Raff, U., and Hendee, W. R.,** Comparison of Uniformly Redundant Arrays, Multihole Collimators, and Single Pinhole Collimators in Gamma Camera Imaging, paper presented at the 1984 meeting of the Radiological Society of North America, Washington, D.C., November 1984.
19. **Vogel, R. A., Kirch, D., LeFree, M., and Steele, P.,** A new method of multiplanar emission tomography using a seven-pinhole collimator and an Anger scintillation camera, *J. Nucl. Med.*, 16, 6, 1978.
20. **Kirch, D. L., Vogel, R. A., LeFree, M. T., Sklar, J., Hasegawa, B. H., and Johnson, P. C.,** A gamma-camera for medical applications using a multiwire proportional counter, *J. Nucl. Med.*, 25, 1003, 1984.
21. **Wagner, R. F., Brown, D. G., and Metz, C. E.,** On the multiplex advantage of coded source/aperture photon imaging, *SPIE,* 314, 72, 1981.
22. **Chiu, M. Y., Barrett, H. H., Simpson, R. G., Chou, C., Arendt, J. W., and Gindi, G. R.,** Three-dimensional radiographic imaging with a restricted view angle, *J. Opt. Soc. Am.*, 69, 1323, 1979.
23. **Tam, K. C. and Perez-Mendez, V.,** Tomographical imaging with limited-angle input, *J. Opt. Soc. Am.*, 71, 1981.
24. **Davison, M. E.,** The ill-conditioned nature of the limited angle tomography problem, *J. Appl. Math.*, 43, 428, 1983.
25. **Barrett, H. H. and Swindell, W.,** *Radiological Imaging, The Theory of Image Formation, Detection and Processing,* Vol. 2, Academic Press, New York, 1981, 490.
26. **Shulman, A. R.,** *Optical Data Processing,* John Wiley & Sons, New York, 1970, 387.
27. **Goodman, J. W.,** *Introduction to Fourier Optics,* McGraw-Hill, New York, 1968.
28. **Rogers, W. L., Han, K. S., Jones, L. W., and Beierwaltes, W. H.,** Application of a Fresnel zone plate to gamma-ray imaging, *J. Nucl. Med.*, 13, 612, 1972.
29. **Barrett, H. H., DeMeester, G. D., Wilson, D. T., et al.,** Recent advances in Fresnel zone plate imaging, in *Medical Radioisotope Scintigraphy,* Vol. 1, International Atomic Energy Association, Vienna, 1973.
30. **Tipton, M. D. and Dowdey, J. E.,** Coded aperture imaging of large extended gamma-ray objects with an on-axis Fresnel zone plate, *J. Nucl. Med.*, 15, 538, 1974.
31. **Farmelant, M. H.,** Improved anatomical definition by a Fresnel zone plate imager, *J. Nucl. Med.*, 14, 393, 1973.
32. **DeMeester, G. D., Barrett, H. H., and Wilson, D. T.,** Imaging of large organs with a Fresnel zone plate, *J. Nucl. Med.*, 14, 391, 1973.
33. **Farmelant, M. H., DeMeester, G. D., Wilson, D., and Garrett, H. H.,** Initial clinical experiences with a Fresnel zone-plate imager, *J. Nucl. Med.*, 16, 183, 1975.
34. **Leith, E. N. and Upatnieks, J.,** Recent advances in holography, in *Progress in Optics 6,* Wolf, E., Ed., North Holland, Amsterdam, 1967, 46.
35. **Macdonald, B., Chang, L. T., Perez-Mendez, V., and Shiraishi, L.,** Gamma-ray imaging using a Fresnel zone plate aperture, multiwire proportional chamber detector, and computer reconstruction, *IEEE Trans. Nucl. Sci.*, NS-21, 678, 1974.
36. **Budinger, T. F. and Macdonald, B.,** Reconstruction of the Fresnel-coded gamma camera images by digital computer, *J. Nucl. Med.*, 16, 309, 1975.
37. **Blake, R. L., Burek, A. J., Fenimore, E. E., et al.,** Solar X-ray photography with multiplex pinhole camera, *Rev. Sci. Inst.*, 45, 513, 1974.
38. **Dance, D. R., Wilson, B. C., and Parker, R. P.,** Digital reconstruction of point sources imaged by a zone plate camera, *Phys. Med. Biol.*, 20, 747, 1975.
39. **Wilson, B. C., Parker, R. P., and Dance, D. R.,** Digital processing of images from a zone plate camera, *Phys. Med. Biol.*, 20, 757, 1975.

40. **Singleton, R. J., Ransom, P. L., and Mittra, R.,** Digital imaging of gamma-ray sources with depth information, *IEEE Trans. Bio. Eng.*, 23, 239, 1976.
41. **Budinger, T. F.,** Physical attributes of single-photon tomography, *J. Nucl. Med.*, 21, 579, 1980.
42. **Farmelant, M. A., DeMeester, G., Wilson, D., and Barrett, H.,** Initial clinical experiences with a Fresnel zone-plate imager, *J. Nucl. Med.*, 16, 183, 1975.
43. **Holman, B. L., Idoine, J. D., Sos, T. A., Tancrell, R., and DeMeester, G.,** Tomographic scintigraphy of regional myocardial perfusion, *J. Nucl. Med.*, 18, 764, 1977.
44. **Perez-Mendez, V., Kaufman, L., Lim, C. B., et al.,** Multiwire proportional chambers in nuclear medicine: present status and perspectives, *Int. J. Nucl. Med. Biol.*, 3, 29, 1976.
45. **Lacy, J. L., LeBlanc, A. D., Babich, J. W., et al.,** A gamma camera for medical applications using a multiwire proportional counter, *J. Nucl. Med.*, 25, 1003, 1984.
46. **Polak, J. F. and Holman, L.,** Limited angle tomography using rapid digital processing of Fresnel zone plate data, in *Emission Computed Tomography: Current Trends*, Esser, P. D., Ed., Society of Nuclear Medicine, New York, 1983, 227.
47. **Koral, K. F., Freitas, J. E., Rogers, W. L., and Keyes, J. W., Jr.,** Thyroid scintigraphy with time-coded aperture, *J. Nucl. Med.*, 20, 345, 1979.
48. **Resinger, W. W., Rose, E. A., Keyes, J. W., Jr., Koral, K. F., Rogers, W. L., Brady, T. J., Kline, R. C., Sisson, J. C., and Thrall, J. H.,** Tomographic thyroid scintigraphy: comparison with standard pinhole imaging, *J. Nucl. Med.*, 22, 638, 1981.
49. **Rogers, W. L., Koral, K. F., Nayans, R., Leonard, P. F., and Keyes, J.,** Coded aperture imaging of the heart, *J. Nucl. Med.*, 19, 730, 1978.
50. **Rogers, W. L., Koral, K. F., Nayans, R., Leonard, P. F., Thrall, J. H., Brady, T. J., and Keyes, J. W., Jr.,** Coded-aperture imaging of the heart, *J. Nucl. Med.*, 21, 371, 1980.
51. **Fenimore, E. E., Cannon, T. M., Van Hulstryn, D. B., and Lee, P.,** Uniformly redundant array imaging of laser driven compressions: preliminary results, *Appl. Opt.*, 18, 945, 1979.
52. **Barrett, H. H., Barber, H. B., Ervin, P. A., Myers, J. H., Paxman, R. G., Smith, W. E., Wild, W. J., and Woolfenden, J. M.,** New directions in coded-aperture imaging, private communication, 1984.

ADDITIONAL READING

Akcasu, A. Z., May, R. S., Knoll, F. G., Rogers, W. L., Koral, K. F., and Jones, L. W., Coded aperture gamma-ray imaging with stochastic apertures, *Opt. Eng.*, 13, 117, 1974.

Barrett, H. H., Fresnel zone plate imaging in nuclear medicine, Letter to the editor, *J. Nucl. Med.*, 15(3), 1974.

Barrett, H. H., Barber, H. B., Ervin, P. A., Myers, J. H., Paxman, R. G., Smith, W. E., Wild, W. J., and Woolfenden, J. M., New directions in coded-aperture imaging, a private communication, 1984.

Barrett, H. H., Garewalk, K., and Wilson, D. T., A spatially-coded X-ray source, *Radiology*, 104, 429, 1972.

Barrett, H. H., Wilson, D. T., DeMeester, G. D., The use of half-tone screens in Fresnel zone plate imaging of incoherent sources, *Optics. Commun.*, 5, 398, 1972.

Bottema, M., Fresnel zone-plate diffraction patterns, *J. Opt. Soc. Am.*, 59, 1632, 1969.

Brown, C. M., Mutiplex imaging with multiple-pinhole cameras, *J. Appl. Phys.*, 45, 4, 1974.

Brown, C. M., Multiplex Imaging and Random Arrays, Ph.D. thesis, University of Chicago, Chicago, IL, 1972.

Chou, C. and Barrett, H. H., Gamma ray imaging in Fourier space, *Opt. Lett.*, 3, 5, 1978.

Chou, C. and Barrett, H. H., Gamma ray imaging in Fourier space, *Opt. Lett.*, 3, 5, 1978.

DeMeester, G. D., Wilson, D. T., and Farmelant, N. H., Tomographic imaging with a Fresnel zone plate system, in *Tomographic Imaging in Nuclear Medicine*, Freeman, G. S., Ed., Society of Nuclear Medicine, New York, 1973, 106.

Gaskill, J. D., *Linear Systems, Fourier Transforms, and Optics*, John Wiley & Sons, New York, 1978.

Gindi, G. R., Reconstruction of a two-dimensional slice from its one-dimensional coded image, in Tech. Rep. TR83/03, Yale University, New Haven, CT, 1983.

Gindi, G. R., Use of *A Priori* Information For Improved Tomographic Imaging in Coded-Aperture Systems, Ph.D. thesis, University of Arizona, Tucson, 1982.

Groh, G., Hayat, G. S., and Stroke, G. W., X-ray and gamma-ray imaging with multiple pinhole cameras using a posterior image synthesis, *Appl. Opt.*, 11, 191, 1972.

Koral, K. F., Knoll, G. F., and Rogers, W. L., Emission tomography with timecoded apertures, in *A Review of Information Processing in Medical Imaging*, Brill, A. B., Price, R. R., McLain, W. J., and Lindsay, M. W., Eds., 1977, 252.

Koral, K. F. and Rogers, W. L., Application of ART to time coded emission tomography, *Phys. Med. Biol.*, 24, 879, 1979.

Lang, L., Kaplan, S. H., Macdonald, H. H., Burns, F., Perez-Mendez, V., and Shiraishi, L., A method of tomographic imaging using a multiple pinhole-coded aperture, *J. Nucl. Med.*, 15, 1063, 1974.

Leith, E. N. and Upatnieks, J., Reconstructed wavepoints and communication theory, *J. Opt. Soc. Am.*, 52, 1123, 1962.

Levy, G., Fresnel zone plate imaging in nuclear medicine, letter to the editor, *J. Nucl. Med.,* 15(3), 1974.

Macdonald, B. and Perez-Mendez, V., Axial tomography and three-dimensional image reconstruction, *IEEE Trans. Nucl. Sci.,* NS-23, 568, 1976.

Macovski, A., Gamma-ray imaging system using modulated apertures, *Phys. Med. Biol.,* 19, 523, 1974.

May, R. S., Akcasu, Z., and Knoll, G. F., Gamma ray imaging with stochastic apertures, *Appl. Opt.,* 13, 2589, 1974.

Mertz, L., Applicability of the rotation collimator to nuclear medicine, *Opt. Commun.,* 12, 216, 1974.

Miller, E., Radially Symmetrical Coded Apertures, M.S. thesis, University of Arizona, Tucson, 1978.

Milster, T. D., Selberg, L. A., Easton, R. L., Barrett, H. H., and Rossi, G. R., A modular imaging system for use in nuclear medicine, unpublished.

Renaud, L. J., Michael, L. G., and Gilday, D. L., Fourier multiaperture emission tomography (FMET), *J. Nucl. Med.,* 20, 986, 1979.

Rogers, W., Jones, W., and Beierwaltes, W. H., Fresnel zone plate imaging in nuclear medicine, letter to the editor, *J. Nucl. Med.,* 15, 1974.

Rogers, W. L., Han, K. S., Jones, L. W., and Beierwaltes, W. H., Use of incoherent holography for gamma-ray imaging, *J. Nucl. Med.,* 13, 464, 1972.

Rogers, W. L., Adler, R., and Koral, K. F., A rational for optimal coded aperture design, *Proc. Int. Opt. Comp. Conf.,* Book 1., Vol. 231, Bollingham, SPIE, Washington, D.C., 120, 1980.

Simpson, R. G., and Barrett, H. H., Coded aperture imaging, in *Imaging in Diagnostic Medicine,* Nudelman, S., Ed., Plenum Press, New York, 1980.

Simpson, R. G. and Barrett, H. H., Noise Analysis of Annular Aperture Imagery, unpublished.

Steinbach, A., An Analysis of the Depth Resolution Problem in One-Dimensional Coded Aperture Imaging, Ph.D. thesis, Stanford University, Stanford, CA, 1977.

Stigliana, D. J., Jr., Mittra, R., and Semonin, R. G., Resolving power of a zone plate, *J. Opt. Soc. Am.,* 57, 610, 1967.

Tipton, M. D., The ODCAT: one dimensional coded aperture tomography, *Proc. SPIE,* 152, 113, 1978.

Tipton, M. D., Dowdy, J., and Stokely, E. M., Background suppression of multiple pinhole-coded aperture scintigrams, *Proc. 4th Int. Conf. Med. Phys. AAPM,* Ottawa, July 1976.

Walton, P. W., An aperture imaging system with instant decoding and tomographic capabilities, *J. Nucl. Med.,* 14, 861, 1973.

Webb, S., Longitudinal emission tomographic imaging using a three-pinhole aperture and an Anger camera, *Br. J. Radiol.,* 54, 673, 1981.

Wild, W. J., Dilute uniformity redundant sequences for use in coded aperture imaging, *Opt. Lett.,* 8, 247, 1983.

Wouters, A., Simon, K. M., and Hirschberg, J. G., Direct method of decoding multiple images, *Appl. Opt.,* 12, 1871, 1973.

Young, N. O., Photography without lenses or mirrors, *Sky Telescope,* 25, 8, 1963.

INDEX

A

B

C

D

M

N

P

Q

R

S

T

U

W

X